SUBSTANCES, WELFARE, AND SOCIAL RELATIONS

Breaking Stigma, Pursuing Hope

I0135790

Substances, Welfare, and Social Relations uses intimate, complex portraits to tell the stories of people who have lived some part of their life course while using or recovering from using substances (such as alcohol or illicit or prescription drugs) while being part of a family and experiencing poverty.

Through these multifaceted stories, layered with a critical analysis of welfare policy, the book probes the deeply entrenched stigma of living with addiction and with low income. Amber Gazso argues that (1) addiction is part of everyday life; (2) if we believe that people are not their addictions, then stigmatizing addiction has no place in society; and (3) destigmatizing addiction and providing better, more imaginative programs and services invites and supports actionable hope. Reflecting on qualitative data, both narrative interviews and policy discourse, *Substances, Welfare, and Social Relations* illuminates how stigmas can be overturned through a collective praxis of hope.

AMBER GAZSO is an associate professor of sociology at York University.

Substances, Welfare, and Social Relations

Breaking Stigma, Pursuing Hope

AMBER GAZSO

UNIVERSITY OF TORONTO PRESS
Toronto Buffalo London

© University of Toronto Press 2023
Toronto Buffalo London
utorontopress.com

ISBN 978-1-4875-4677-9 (cloth)   ISBN 978-1-4875-5096-7 (EPUB)
ISBN 978-1-4875-4753-0 (paper)   ISBN 978-1-4875-4941-1 (PDF)

Library and Archives Canada Cataloguing in Publication

Title: Substances, welfare, and social relations : breaking stigma,
    pursuing hope / Amber Gazso.
Names: Gazso, Amber, author.
Description: Includes bibliographical references and index.
Identifiers: Canadiana (print) 20230164609 | Canadiana (ebook)
    20230164684 | ISBN 9781487546779 (cloth) | ISBN 9781487547530
    (paper) | ISBN 9781487550967 (EPUB) | ISBN 9781487549411 (PDF)
Subjects: LCSH: Substance abuse – Ontario. | LCSH: Addicts – Services
    for – Ontario. | LCSH: Addicts – Rehabilitation – Ontario. |
    LCSH: Welfare recipients – Ontario. | LCSH: Public welfare –
    Ontario. | LCSH: Stigma (Social psychology) – Ontario.
Classification: LCC HV5000.C32 O6 2023 | DDC 362.2909713 – dc23

Cover design: Liz Harasymczuk
Cover illustration: Franzi/Shutterstock.com

We wish to acknowledge the land on which the University of Toronto Press
operates. This land is the traditional territory of the Wendat, the Anishnaabeg,
the Haudenosaunee, the Métis, and the Mississaugas of the Credit First Nation.

University of Toronto Press acknowledges the financial support of the
Government of Canada, the Canada Council for the Arts, and the Ontario Arts
Council, an agency of the Government of Ontario, for its publishing activities.

Canada Council   Conseil des Arts
for the Arts   du Canada

ONTARIO ARTS COUNCIL
CONSEIL DES ARTS DE L'ONTARIO
an Ontario government agency
un organisme du gouvernement de l'Ontario

Funded by the   Financé par le
Government   gouvernement   Canada
of Canada   du Canada

Contents

vi   Contents

Acknowledgments

Many people were involved in or supported me in writing this book, and I wish to thank them all. I will do my best to do so and ask forgiveness if I overlook anyone. The study that is this book has taken a long time to come together (2015+), and the book itself has taken some time to write (2019–22). Any oversight on my part will be because of how my memory has blurred with the passing of time.

I begin by acknowledging with gratitude the people featured in this book. I am ever thankful to the twenty-eight people who agreed to meet and be interviewed by me, and to share their stories about working through their alcohol or drug use and while accessing welfare or social assistance, what is known as Ontario Works in Ontario. Among other things, they told me stories about their experiences of policy rules and regulations when known as a substance user; their raising of children and how they are part of families when receiving benefit incomes below the poverty line; their recommendations for changes to how Ontario Works supports substance users who are often facing other barriers to employment; and their hopes and dreams for their futures. I am most thankful for the benefit recipient participants' time and energy, notably their emotion and identity work to capture their experiences for me; an outsider and someone who listened to, further probed, and tried to understand their stories. I am acutely aware that the honourarium I provided each participant only compensated a small portion of the wealth of knowledge they shared and that was produced in our interview talk. I am equally grateful to the Ontario Works caseworkers I interviewed. Through their perspectives I learned about policy discourse on addiction and their enactment of policy rules and regulations for people who defined as, or were seen as, struggling with managing their alcohol or drug use. But I also learned about their discretionary kindnesses and ongoing support of benefit recipients, without which some people would certainly be worse off.

I now turn to the people who supported me in writing this book. I start with a focus on people representing institutions who made the research I undertook possible. I am grateful to people I met at the Toronto Employment and Social Services (TESS) department, which administers and manages Ontario Works for people living in the City of Toronto. My TESS contacts agreed with the importance of my research and through our adoption of ethical procedures of informed consent, supported my recruitment of benefit recipients and caseworkers. While I completed my data collection and analysis independently, I am also thankful for how TESS welcomed us learning together about my findings (shared in anonymous and in aggregate form) at various meetings and to inform current and future casework practice and other potential policy change. I also thank anonymous reviewers at my home institution, York University, for their support of my research by awarding me internal research grants. Through this monetary support, I was able to hire research assistants to help me with a review of relevant literature as well as assist with analysis of public-use policy discourse; provide honourariums to participants; and hire a transcriber. As well, I am grateful to the sociology graduate program committee who assigned me research assistance support as part of the Graduate Assistance program. And I am thankful for the way that the small support fund that faculty members receive each year can be put towards hiring research assistants. To conference audience members who heard findings from my study that were later published as journal articles, thank you for thoughtful and constructive feedback. To all the graduate and undergraduate students who I kept inundating with stories from my research as they completed introduction to sociology, sociology of the family, gender and social policy, and qualitative methods courses with me: thank you for listening and for your interest.

I wish to thank some very specific people. I thank Anna Lippman for transcribing my interviews with caseworkers and for sharing her wealth of experience accrued as a social services youth worker. Through conversations with Anna I learned to see the boundaries and discretionary opportunities of case management differently. I thank Daniel Blais and Keith Joe for being MA students in sociology and working as graduate assistants with me to understand what has been studied in the United States and Canada about people who use drugs or alcohol and are on welfare. I thank undergraduate student Kalisha Mohamed for working hard to help me unravel how addiction is conceptualized in the American and Canadian policy context and policy specific to social assistance and health care. Sue Hamilton, an independent contractor, provided me with invaluable assistance, transcribing at least half of my interviews with Ontario Works benefit recipients. Finally, I bestow my most heartfelt thanks on Sabina Mirza. Sabina began working with me as a research assistant when I had concluded my research and began writing this book and while she was still a PhD candidate. Now Dr. Mirza (Education, York University), Sabina has been a consistent presence in my life as my friend and colleague even up until the moment I wrote these acknowledgments, steadily assisting me with the ongoing nature of literature reviews when writing a book over a few years and assisting me to work through the sheer number of public-use policy documents I sampled. Sabina read drafts of chapters several times, and I am so thankful for her academic, reflexive, and critical engagement with my work. To others who have generously and freely given their time to read early chapters and comment on them out of genuine care, thank you: PhD candidate Amber-Lee Varadi (Sociology, York University) and friend and colleague Dr. Dean Herd.

It would be remiss to conclude without three more thank yous. First, I am so thankful that my editor, Jodi Lewchuk, was as keen as me to see this book come to fruition – even when it existed on paper as a draft outline and mostly in my mind. I am grateful for all the editorial support I have received from the University of Toronto Press, including their facilitation of the very thoughtful comments and suggestions that three anonymous reviewers provided on an earlier version of this book. I thank members of the University of Toronto Press production team, for example, artists who created this book's cover, and others who crucially supported me through the final phases of making this book into what it is. Second, I am thankful to the friends in my life who just happen to be academics and who listened as I talked about the book I was working on – for several years: my mentor and friend Susan McDaniel (and my PhD supervisor!); my friend and colleague Katherine Bischoping, who always teaches me a great deal about qualitative methods; and my friend Jason Webb. Jason had to keep hearing about this book as he finished his PhD in Sociology under my supervision; now Dr. Webb, Jason always had thoughtful comments to inspire me. Finally, I thank those who are "nearest and dearest" to me. Michael and Mac's unwavering love and support mean so much to me every day, then, now, and into tomorrow. My partner and child made my work on this book possible, most memorably by supporting my taking a few "writing retreats" in the form of short three- to four-day getaways to some other place where I could just sit and write for unlimited hours. I thank my parents, whose curiosity about what I am working on continues to fuel me. I am thankful to my extended family for the support and understanding provided to me every time I squirreled myself away to work in their homes (when I should have been visiting). I thank the fur- and scale-covered family members I live with for taking my attention elsewhere. And I thank Bosley, my horse. He might not talk to me, but he is a steady character with a spirit open to all my emotions and always receptive to us escaping it all, through riding, riding, riding.

SUBSTANCES, WELFARE, AND SOCIAL RELATIONS

1 Introduction

A person is not their addiction.

Unknown

Stigma is fueled by ignorance and fear.

Randy Davis, Coordinator of Gay/
MSM Sexual Health, The Gilbert Centre

If we ever stopped hoping, we would no longer be human.

Zygmunt Bauman, sociologist and philosopher

If you're an addict, then you're an addict. You're just as bad as the addict over there and the addict over there and the addict over there. Even though it's a complex issue, that everybody is different. Everybody has their own reasons for having become an addict. Everybody has their own demons that they're fighting. It's just ridiculous the way I feel that a lot of people just lump – like "a junkie is a junkie." No.

Jules, lone mother, Ontario Works benefit
recipient and research participant

No. No, indeed.

These are quotes that have stayed with me as I thought about and wrote this book. Simply stated, this is a book about what it is like and how it feels to live with addiction to alcohol or drugs while simultaneously on welfare and engaged in multiple social relations. And this is an understatement in so many ways. More accurately and quite complexly, this book tells the stories of people's lives *as lived* at one point in their life course when using substances (i.e., alcohol or illicit or prescription drugs) or recovering from substance use, as part of families, and in the midst of pover*ties* – receiving below poverty level social assistance incomes and experiencing a lack of other services and supports.

Approximately 21 per cent of Canadians will experience addiction in their lifetime (Pearson et al., 2013). In 2012, roughly 6 per cent of the population relied on social assistance (Kneebone & White, 2015), also known colloquially as welfare (Béland & Daigneault, 2015). What we know about living with addiction while experiencing low income in Canada, however, is limited. Existing sociological research that focuses on individuals' welfare use when they are also working through addiction is largely American. Other disciplines (e.g., health, criminology, social work) may take up the focus on the relationship between addiction and social assistance use in Canada but often in a less concentrated fashion, such as when a health study on addiction operationalizes individuals' low income as social assistance receipt but does not focus on experience of this receipt. Exceptions exist, such as Boyd's (1999) *Mothers and Illicit Drugs: Transcending the Myths*, in which she carefully analyses the experiences of women drug users on welfare and how the welfare system, and by extension social services, regulate their mothering. On balance, however, there is not yet a book offering a qualitative in-depth exploration of the experiences of women and men who are impoverished, receive social assistance in Ontario – Ontario Works – and *are constructed and perceived* to be "addicts," whether by policy and caseworkers or the lay public.

Indeed, in the way that this book centres people's complex, unfolding, and simultaneous experiences of navigating the rules and regulations of social assistance policy discourse (in order to survive) and the management of substance use, this is a book not yet written by others. In the contents of its chapters, I honour and capture the experiences of people through their own poignant and moving stories about hardship and resilience and new beginnings. In so doing, I wrestle with the very construction of addiction and its stigmatization, working to dismantle especially the latter. My goal in writing this book is to inspire others to adopt my central argument: we can change how we see, understand, support, and live with addiction in our own lives and the lives of others – through a collective praxis of hope.

In total, this book will appeal to critical scholars who themselves seek to unpack the risks of reducing addiction and poverty to only individual problems or pathologies, instead of as seeing these problems as relationally, situationally, structurally, and discursively constituted. This book will intrigue scholars who wish to eschew the seeming impartial and objective quantification of lives (or statistics), and convince them to embrace the meanings, perceptions, and experiences of the self in relation to other individuals and institutions invited by qualitative research. Finally, this book will appeal to others who seek social change, specifically social justice, and social inclusion.

My desire to learn, listen to, understand, and share these stories stems from a decade of qualitative research with low-income individuals, many of whom were parents of young children. In past research, I have comparatively explored how parents experienced social assistance receipt, and specifically welfare-to-work programming, in British Columbia, Alberta, and Saskatchewan and to what extent gender expectations shaped their participation in employment or employment programming and the resulting consequences (Gazso, 2007a, 2007b, 2009). With colleagues, I have focused on how low-income parents manage to make ends meet by creating networks of social support that consist of formal supports (government or community programs) and informal supports (family and friends) and involve exchanges of instrumental and expressive support (Gazso et al., 2016). In both these projects, I kept meeting people who were experiencing a life of low income and caring for children *and* sometimes working on managing their use of substances. People living with addiction on social assistance, also known as welfare in Canada (Béland & Daigneault, 2015), caught my attention. Specifically, what would it be like to follow the rules and regulations of social assistance or welfare in Ontario – known as Ontario Works (OW) – and meet the conditions set upon oneself while also using or attempting not to use substances? What would it feel like to conform to the construction of addiction that is inherent in OW policy? And what is this construction anyway? And, even more than that, what if children were also being raised amid all this? Indeed, I was curious about individuals' experiences of and feelings about simply living their lives as engaged in social and family relations, especially the raising or co-parenting of children, while ensuring their continued receipt of OW and somehow managing their substance use. This is what I set out to discover with the research study that is presented in this book.

The Study

I collected and analysed two forms of qualitative data, personal narratives and policy discourse, to explore the everyday experience of living with substance use, as part of families, and in the midst of poverties. Between fall 2016 and fall 2017, I completed in-depth interviews with seven OW caseworkers and twenty-eight OW benefit recipients. I undertook narrative analysis of benefit recipients' stories about their simultaneous experiences of managing substance use and receiving welfare. I focused on the choices and chances and external factors that shaped individuals' coming to use substances and receive social assistance by incorporating insights from a life course perspective. I was attentive to how benefit recipients' stories highlighted performances of emotional labour and changing senses of self, these differentiated by gender and family relations. Invoking principles of discourse analysis too, I was especially curious how benefit recipients' stories of emotional labour suggested conformity to OW policy discourses or discourses about family, addictions, and poverty in the broader social milieux. In total, I understood benefit recipients to be sharing stories of their agentic pursuit of their personal biographies over their life course at the same time I saw their access to OW as constraining, regulatory, and prolonging their low income in the ways their lives were enmeshed within OW policy and broader discourses.

I collected and analysed public-use policy documents concerning social assistance in Ontario over the period 2009–17 (see Appendix A for my sources). My discourse analysis of these policy documents sought to unravel the construction of people living with addiction as an object of focus in OW policy discourse and then targeted in policy design and administration. I also worked to uncover the subjectivity constituted in OW policy discourse for persons living with addiction and whether and how it changes if policy discourse has shifted over time. I undertook interviews with seven OW caseworkers to yield their stories of case management and supporting people living with addiction, but these stories also represent the policy discourse(s) in which their caseworker practices were situated (see Appendix B for my interview guides). The bulk of this book is my sharing of people's narratives about living with addiction while on OW and the discourses that interact with and shape them (see Appendix C for a comprehensive review of my methods, including sampling).

A Note on Theory

At the broadest level, I began this study with the understanding that individual ways of being and becoming in this contemporary moment are shaped by individualization, a process of social change (Dawson, 2012). Individualization captures how life courses and mechanisms of regulation and resource allocation, including the welfare state, are transformed in contemporary, post-industrial, Western societies and individuality is enhanced in the process (Howard, 2007). Individualization runs parallel to the dis-embedding and re-embedding of the industrial social order into the present modernity, or what is called reflexive modernization (Beck et al., 1994). That is, previously "normative" structures like class, gender, and the nuclear family do not disappear but are de-traditionalized, weakened, and so less deterministic of identities and social interactions. Within this milieu, the ways individuals have more opportunity to create their own biographies (Beck et al., 1994, p. 13) or pursue what Giddens (1991) calls "a reflexive project of the self," creating and choosing trajectories, are part of individualization.

In *The Normal Chaos of Love*, for example, Beck and Beck-Gernsheim (1995, p. 5) write that individualization means that conceptualizations of family, marriage, parenthood, sexuality, or love are no longer definitive and "vary in substance, exceptions, norms and morality from individual to individual and from relationship to relationship." Individualization is suggested by how heteronormative nuclear families are less the norm, common law and lone parent families are increasing in numbers, and people increasingly live alone in Canada (Statistics Canada, 2017). In turn, relations of instrumental support (the giving and receiving of physical or material aid) and expressive support (the giving and receiving of love, guidance, and affection) are increasingly with kin <u>and</u> "fictive kin" and seen as defining families rather than simply relations of blood and marriage (Gazso & McDaniel, 2015; Morgan, 2011). A discourse of "the family" is no longer monolithic, if it ever was (see also Eichler, 1997). The family and household composition of benefit recipients I interviewed, ranging from being on welfare as a single individual, a lone parent, or part of a common-law union, reflect these broader trends.

And yet, Bauman (2007) argues that individualization produces inequalities too, precisely because individuals do not all share equal resources in their pursuit of their own biographies. Individuals may seemingly pursue their biographies with more freedom, but they experience this agentic project of the self differently dependent upon their social positioning. Not just their class and citizenship or relationships with the state, but their race, ethnicity, gender, sexual orientation, age, generation, and ability intersect and interact with related social, structural hierarchies (e.g., "the gender order" as per Connell, 1987; or capitalism, ongoing colonization, etc.). Amartya Sen, though not an individualization scholar, persuasively argues that if social position inhibits an individual's capability "to live a decent life," they ultimately experience poverty and may experience other, related deprivations, such as stigma and loss of freedom (Sen, 2000). As this book makes clear, deep economic inequality and stigma indeed texture the experience of people accessing welfare and managing substance use challenges.

Scholars Beck, Giddens, and Lash (1994) generally concur that individualization promises agentic choice in a life lived and to be lived but does not mean existing structures and ideologies disappear (recall reflexive modernization). We are, for example, still witnessing and/or personally experiencing pay inequity among women and men in the labour market (see also Beck & Beck-Gernsheim, 2001). Lash (2001) provides another example of these tensions in observing that people may pursue intimate relations that reflect their own self projects but, in some cultures, these very choices (exclusive of religious values) would invite stigmatization and criminalization. Reith (2004, p. 285) further points out that with individualization there are still cultural norms and institutions to which individuals' "subjective states" and "inner desires" must accord. Considering the experiences of people receiving welfare and living with addiction, I am therefore attuned to assuming their agentic decision-making but seeing it as still connected and shaped by the rules and regulations they must follow in order to receive OW benefits each month.

Indeed, that people face new demands, controls, and constraints that include those of welfare state institutions is also part of the process of individualization (Beck & Beck-Gernsheim, 2001; Beck, 2007; Howard, 2007; Klett-Davies, 2007). Zinn (2002) observes that with individualization, welfare states create new choices through new institutional arrangements. Brodie (2007, p. 159) persuasively argues that the transition towards an "active" welfare state in Canada is reflective of individualization and voices broader concerns about how individualization actually "serves to embed neo-liberalism in social policy thinking and practice." The ways in which the emphasis on reflexivity and choice in individualization can fit too comfortably with neoliberal principles of self-sufficiency and individual responsibility with implications for governance of the self (Dawson, 2012) is a focus I take up further in chapter 3 of this book. More so echoing Brodie's (2007) concerns, Van der

Veen (2012) maintains that welfare states create new social risks, such as welfare loss, for example, the loss of social security coverage. As I will show in the case of Ontario, these new risks include the perpetuation of poverty through exercises of neoliberal welfare reform. Tonkens et al. (2013) make a different and compelling argument that there is an emotional subtext of the individual experience of welfare reforms shaped by individualization, illuminating this by applying Hochschild's (2003) theorizing of emotional labour. Later in this book I too argue that OW policy discourse and other discourses impose feeling rules on people in receipt of welfare benefits such that they engage in emotional labour to comply with them (see also Kampen et al. 2013).

The process of individualization and even its meaning is rife with tensions, contradictions, and contestations (Dawson, 2012; Howard, 2007; Lash, 2001). For Howard (2007), then, individualization can be more appropriately thought of as a discursive field; many discourses make up individualization and shape individual experience and social relations, including the discourse of neoliberalism. I find utility in Howard's (2007) perspective and consider individualization to be the broad lens through which I can situate and tap into people's stories of choices and chances of living with addiction on welfare and the discourses which infiltrate their storied lives. Throughout the chapters of this book, I further draw in theorizing on, for example, neoliberalism and social exclusion, the life course, identity and the self, emotional labour, stigma, and narrative and discourse, and privilege an understanding of human experience as diversified by social positions and identities and corresponding systems of social stratification (see also Choo & Ferree, 2010). Overall, I develop a robust theoretical and methodological bricolage, meaning a pragmatic and eclectic approach that I saw to best fit my research questions about the experiences of living with addiction and on welfare when seeing them as situated within the process of individualization (see also Appendix C for how I account for drawing in multiple paradigms).

The Argument(s) and Scholarly Contribution

In my final analysis of people's lives as lived at one point in their life course when using substances (i.e., alcohol or illicit or prescription drugs) or recovering from substance use, as part of families, and in the midst of poverties, I arrive at three points of argumentation. I present them in summative form here, noting that the weightiness of their worth is unravelled chapter by chapter in the very organization of this book. In this book I argue:

- First, living with addiction is part of everyday life. Of all our lives no less: whether we ourselves have a problem with alcohol or drugs or a person close to us or people we share our communities with. While living with addiction can be seen (even sociologically and criminologically) as "deviant," morally wrong, or abnormal and may be constituted as such in social-assistance policy, it is but one part of individuals' exceedingly complex lives. People are not their addiction.
- Second, if we believe people are not their addiction – they are not simply "an addict on welfare" – the stigmatization of addiction is incomprehensible. If we stigmatize addiction and reduce an individual's identity to that of addict alone, we limit human potential in our moral imaginings and we exclude in our social relations. All based on identifying human worth through a binary: one is an addict or not.
- Third, de-stigmatizing persons living with addiction while accessing OW, the de-stigmatization of addiction in general, is possible through a collective praxis of hope. I conclude this book by outlining this praxis to invite others, given my study findings, to not just assuage but dismantle the stigmatization of addiction. I want individuals who are working through substance use challenges to have hope. I want others to share my view. But it is not enough for us to try to instil this hope in others – we need to want to have hope for others. Or, more bluntly, we have to have hope for others.

Let me be clear, there are near tipping points suggestive of how something has "got to give" in how we live with addiction, whether we experience it directly or indirectly. Canada is experiencing an opioid crisis made stark by climbing opioid-related deaths during the COVID-19 pandemic. The pandemic, though originating long after the study featured in this book was completed, has profoundly changed the management and experience of supportive services for people living with addiction in our communities, including safe injection sites. As well, the historical stigmatization of addiction carries forward into the present, making it difficult for workplaces and social programs to even entertain how to make paid work *work* for people living with addiction, or implicating custody and child welfare decisions such that parents may feel less able to parent their children and pursue recovery. At the utmost extreme of living with addiction while being impoverished – people are dying. In homes, hotels, parks, and on our streets.

If we have collective hope, we, as a society, will facilitate human potential. We will see in others capacity and possibility. We will create better opportunities for persons living with addiction to begin, again, and if and when they want (not us wanting) to try something different with regard to using substances. We will have better community resources and services for people living with addiction, more accessible and imaginatively organized treatment programs, and adequate employment programs, such as for persons on methadone who can work for pay if work was organized to accommodate them, to name just a few. Through collective hope for our fellow humans, we support and create potential and can open space for actionable hope.

My Place in This Book

Reflexivity is a quality of feminist qualitative research. It is the practice of asking oneself how they are part of the research process: how the standpoint or social location of them as a researcher, assuming their subjectivity matters too, shapes the research in its design, from questions to method to interpretation. The practice of reflexivity requires researchers to make their place in the production of any knowledge transparent. In a book like this one, that infiltrates the intimacies of people's lives for knowledge gain, I practise ethical responsibility and accountability, to my interview participants, readers, and knowledge communities, by writing my place with and into it (see also Doucet & Mauthner, 2002).

I begin with my standpoint and social location at the time of this writing. If asked to define myself as simply as possible, to acknowledge the identities that matter to me and from which I approach the social world, I would reply: I am a feminist, tenured academic. I am a cisgendered and heterosexual white woman, and nearing the middle of my life (e.g., 45+). I am a mother and a partner in a committed relationship. I am a daughter and a sister. If I were probed about my family history, including my class, I would answer: I grew up in, and am the product of, a working-class nuclear family made up of me, my brother, and my parents. My father and mother worked for pay, my father full time and my mother part time. They were married (and still are) when I left home. I have reproduced the nuclear family in my own life, though I am now ensconced more in the "middle class" than my family of origin.

Perhaps there will therefore seem few identities and social locations I share with some of the people I interviewed for this book. Specifically, I have not yet experienced an addiction to alcohol or drugs. As I observed in my field notes while doing this research, the embodiment of addiction to alcohol or drugs seems completely foreign to one who has never suffered from it. As well, I have never had to rely on accessing the larger system that is social assistance. The closest I have experienced to low income is when I was a graduate student and made very low wages as a teaching assistant, but my family members could provide a financial safety net when needed.

Some may not see me as the right person to do this research and therefore see the findings I share as less valid. I can understand this point of view, how it is linked to broader insider-outsider debates on experiential knowledge researcher positioning, and respect it. However, while my backstory and the self I cultivate diverges from those of the OW benefit recipients I interviewed in so many respects, I do not think this is reason alone to see the findings and interpretations I highlight as purely circumspect. When I thought about what can possibly be common in human experience between myself as a researcher and the people I interviewed, especially benefit recipients – and from a sociological perspective – I first became stuck. Undoubtedly, each person I interviewed had their own standpoint, family histories, and sense of self in the present. With some sociological musing, however, I concluded that what I also shared with people living with addiction was our very being and existence, of living a life of change, of seeking a sense of self, and of *feeling* our experience. In each interview I undertook, it therefore became natural for me to share about myself and my life in ways that furthered conversation and in an effort to embrace how myself as a researcher and people as participants share how we are immersed in the social relations of existence. Our lives, no matter how (importantly they are) different, were and are lived through relationships with other people, including kin and non-kin, and institutions and textured by and situated in an ever-changing social-historical context. In my efforts at sharing too, I sought to show what I assumed – that while I, caseworkers, and benefit recipient participants have multiple, unfixed identities that unfold in tandem with interactions, events, and transitions in our lives, each of us are irreducible to one identity, to one category. It is from these assumptions that I write this book about the lives of others who have lived differently than me. What I will continue to pursue in this book is a sketching out of deeper and often moral similarities in lives lived with an emancipatory and hopeful outcome.

While I focus on individuals living with addiction and in low income and so seem to reproduce categories that potentially reify stereotypes, this is an analytical move. First, this language narrows the scope of my research. Though sociology opens up the imagination and invites deconstruction of social "reality," we remain limited by our language in doing so. I can recall as if it were yesterday the discussions I had about the problematic use of "addict" and "addiction" with a colleague who facilitated my meeting OW caseworkers and benefit recipients. While we agreed we could make many arguments for using new terms, from her experience on the front line, she learned that these are still the terms used by the majority of people who use substances or have a problem using substances. In my past research, I had also learned that people identify with "addict" and having an "addiction." Addiction is the language used in OW policy and by caseworkers, as I will show in this book, and it is exactly how it feels to experience the labelling of "addict" and regulation associated with it that inspired it. I therefore adopt these categories, this grouping of people, at the same time that I maintain a healthy suspicion of categorical thinking and appreciation for the philosophical tensions therein. I try to demonstrate this throughout the book by using interchangeably alcohol and/or drug "addiction" with "dependency" and (perhaps) the less charged terms of "user," or "substance use," or "people who use drugs." For the most part, I refer to study participants on OW as "living with addiction." I recruited benefit recipients who self-identified as having an addiction to drugs or alcohol, whether they were sober, in recovery, or still randomly using and were constructed, labelled, and targeted as such by OW policy. I use this "living with addiction" classification to further capture individuals' ongoing management of their use, which can include their use patterns, practices of harm reduction (as simple as their use of strategies to reduce negative effects of their use), or engagement in other treatment. I also see "living with addiction" to capture the energy and emotion needed to work through a process of recovery, however long, as well as to refer to the experience of a person years sober. I do distinguish at times between sobriety and recovery, defining sobriety as a person not engaged in use and not intoxicated by a substance, and recovery as involving an ongoing process of addressing problematic use behaviour and involving abstinence from the substance or reduction of harm associated with its consumption.

Moreover, I create still greater analytical tension as I pursue the overarching arguments of this book, which I further outline below: the need to overturn the stigmatization of addiction and pursue hope. I seek to make clear that individuals living with addiction to substances and on OW are simply individuals living complex – burdensome and rewarding – lives, much richer than miserabilist interpretations and stigmatization of addiction would suggest. And though each person I interviewed had unique life experiences, their lives were also similarly shaped and challenged by OW rules and regulations; their experience of poverties; their relationships of support with others, including family or lack thereof; and systemic, structural barriers inhibiting their efforts at recovery should they pursue it. If I succeed in revealing how benefit recipients live with addiction (even if just a beginning, of touching on the infinite ways), I create room for pause; for all of us to critically disrupt and break apart stigma associated with addiction. I create opportunity to resist seeing people as defined by their addiction and of lives as limited to addiction, and rather addiction as an experience of all our social relations. And if I can achieve this critical break for others, I can create momentum for hope, and specifically hope that produces change.

Doing and sharing research such as this, of course, connects to questions of voice. I want to make another point about voice here. While I am centred by my academic training in sociology, I draw in relevant research from other fields, such as medicine, psychiatry, psychology, political science, social work, and gender and sexuality studies in this book. My use of other scholarship (of which I am not expert) is primarily for contextualization purposes rather than explanatory ones. Where possible, I do acknowledge if what I have found seems to be discussed similarly in disciplines outside of sociology.

Second, and what I feel to be a more important point about voice, I completed interviews with women and men, both OW caseworkers and benefit recipients, to hear their stories, from their social location, through their voices. Through narrative research, we are taught that we can especially listen to empower voices that have not been heard or that we rarely hear and may be deliberately silenced. I align myself with this perspective. Yet, I am the one writing this book. I have made the choice to share these voices in a book written in *my* voice. I tell a "big story" of living with addiction while on OW and seemingly displace those originally doing the storytelling in doing so. I hold a keen awareness of the potential ethical pitfalls of this. My analytical – and ethical and moral – choice was therefore twofold: (1) to feature lengthy excerpts of participants' transcripts so the story remains told as it was; (2) to be present throughout this book. In terms of the latter, readers will find I move between third person and first person and from participants' experiences and thoughts to my own and try to do so as seamlessly as possible. My presence signals that while the voices of participants are being shared, they have been organized and interpreted through decisions of my own.

My voice comes most to the fore of this book in its last chapter, when I turn to the arguments I extrapolate from my findings. These I write with less trepidation than I would have ten or more years ago. I do follow academic convention concerning research on problems of a policy nature, for example, I note the policy implications of my research. I then present arguments for change that are, to me, most broadly about creating social inclusion. At varying times, my arguments may be read by others as left-leaning, polemical, idealistic, romantic, and/or perhaps even radical or moralistic. I embrace this reading. I think it important to explain why. Once while at a work and family policy conference, I presented a paper about lone mothers' experiences on social assistance. An audience member commented (and I roughly paraphrase): "Why are we always hearing yet another paper about single mothers? Hasn't enough been done?" At another conference, I shared qualitative research that identified the social support networks that low-income lone mothers create to simply survive to argue for improved welfare incomes and accessible community supports. An audience member misconstrued my intent and commented to the effect of: "Shouldn't we avoid making these networks known, so that mothers don't face greater scrutiny from caseworkers?" In sharing these experiences, what I am trying to make clear is that I have felt the deeper social justice implications of my research findings curtailed by others' apparent discomfort, frustration, and I dare say stigma. Throughout my career I have subsequently felt a certain tiredness set in from trying to change and resist the trotted out cultural tropes that can be a response to research about people experiencing low income. With the big story I present in this book, I felt a shift, an opening, an excitement, a determination – I felt hopefulness – about what I learned. So, I set aside my apprehension, I overcame my tiredness, and now I stand firm: my desire for a shift in *understanding* and *attitude* about, and *support* of, a life lived differently than perhaps one's own, a life of so much more than addiction and economic marginalization, fuelled much of each sentence I wrote.

Organization of Book

This book is organized into three parts. In Part 1, *Contextualizing and Embedding Experience*, I "set the stage." Chapter 2 offers a review of the relevant broader literature that connects to and contextualizes the specific study of substances, welfare, and social relations that I undertook. I focus more narrowly on the meaning and definition of addiction as researched in chapter 3. At the end of this chapter, I shift to how addiction is subjectively understood by the benefit recipients I interviewed, their definitions assumed in the remaining two parts.

Part 2, *Lives as Lived*, shares the findings of my research. The way in which I sought stories from benefit recipients living with addiction while accessing OW, and then ruminated over their stories alongside those of caseworkers *and* the findings of my discourse analysis inspired me to see the "big story" that I wanted to tell as that of a collective narrative arc or trajectory of the life course. This arc moves from *becoming* to *being* to *beginning anew* and is covered over five chapters. I explore the *becoming* of a substance user in chapter 4 and turn to *being* a substance user on OW in chapters 5, 6, and 7. I juxtapose how one is constructed to be living with addiction and an object of OW policy discourse and practice (chapter 5) with the many ways of being that make up living a life everyday while accessing OW (chapter 6). I narrow my focus to benefit recipients' being part of families and social support relationships (while living with addiction and accessing OW) in chapter 7. *Beginning anew*, or starting a different chapter in one's life through the work of recovery, is the focus of chapter 8. In the final section of each of these five chapters, I interpret my findings and extrapolate their broader significance; beyond just descriptive accounts of what is, I offer what is, in my view, their meaning and significance. These extrapolations offered serve another and larger purpose: each chapter conclusion unravels a piece of the foundation that buttresses my final points of argumentation taken up in Part 3.

Indeed, Part 3 is the capstone of this study. In this part, *Destigmatization, Hope, and Potential for Change*, I dwell on how I arrive at the argument for a collective praxis of hope from this study. Only one chapter and largely offering a framework for praxis, I see my discussion here as a beginning. I invite others to join me in imagining how we may move forward, valuing the whole person working through substance use challenges and meet them with hope when they themselves begin to formulate a different way of being to pursue.

PART ONE

Contextualizing and Embedding Experience

2 Situating the Study of Substances, Welfare, and Social Relations

Into the 2000s, great gaps have grown between those who have a lot and those without enough (Aldridge, 2017; Younglai & Yukselir, 2017) in Canada. Living without enough remains a problem for some Canadians regardless of which relative measure of low income is used. In 2019, 10.1 per cent of Canadians lived in poverty (Employment and Social Development Canada, 2021) or had incomes that did not permit them to afford a basket of goods and services to meet their own or their family's needs and so achieve a modest standard of living; they were poor according to Canada's official definition of poverty (Government of Canada, 2018, the Market Basket Measure [MBM]). Using the After-Tax Low Income Cut Off (LICO), Grant et al. (2017) found that while the low-income rate remained fairly stable for Canada in total, it increased in the province of Ontario between 2006 and 2016. In 2018, the city of Toronto's poverty rate was 20 per cent and higher than the national average of 16.8 per cent when it was calculated with the Census Family Low Income measure (Citizens for Public Justice, 2018). Across Canada, single working-age adults, children, unattached seniors (particularly women), and lone mother households are the groups most likely to experience low income (however measured) (Aldridge, 2017; Grant et al., 2017), with lowest incomes experienced unequally by new immigrant, racialized, and Indigenous persons, especially women, within these same groups (Smith-Carrier & Mitchell, 2015).

The low income experienced by some Canadians is linked to the changing, global labour market. Zizys (2011) defines the economy as an "hourglass" or "two-tier," characterized by the disappearance of mid-level jobs and the corresponding polarized expansion of higher-skilled, well-paying knowledge jobs and lower skilled, lower-paid entry-level positions (or, precarious forms of employment). Only two thirds of those employed in 2012 held full-time and permanent jobs, and among them, there were fewer women and racialized workers (Broadbent Institute, 2012). Unemployment or under-employment can, in turn, create the experience of low income.

Low-income individuals and families can access provincially administered social assistance or "welfare" across Canada. Ontario's social assistance program of "last resort" for unemployed adults with or without children staves off absolute poverty but does not raise individuals in receipt of it above low-income thresholds. Monthly Ontario Works (OW) benefit rates for singles (basic needs and shelter), for example, total just over $700 (City of Toronto, 2020, 2023). This is also the case for all family types (e.g., lone parent or two parent) in Ontario; this information is jarring given census data that reveals that lone parent households are growing in numbers, and for the first time in census history, since 2016, more people are living alone than in a household with children (Statistics Canada, 2017; Statistics Canada 2022; Tang et al., 2019). Narrowing the focus to the 2016–17 time period in which interviews were completed for the study presented in this book, singles on social assistance in 2017 received the lowest amount of "welfare income," which included social assistance and other government transfers in each province; for singles in Toronto, their welfare incomes reached just 45 per cent of the MBM threshold (Statistics Canada, 2019; Tweddle & Aldridge, 2018). Among individuals aged twenty to thirty-four who lived alone in 2015, close to one half (48 per cent) had shelter (housing) costs that were 30 per cent or more of their average monthly household income (Tang et al., 2019). Recent research revealed that single individuals on OW accessed fewer and less generous benefits outside social assistance compared to other family types in Toronto (Herd et al., 2018; Kim et al., 2018). And even though lone parent families across Ontario saw their welfare incomes increase in 2017 with the new child benefit, they were still well below low-income thresholds; in Toronto, at 71 per cent of the MBM (Tweddle & Aldridge, 2018).

My purpose in the remainder of this chapter is rather precise. I seek to ground the importance of this sociological study and its theoretical framing through a review of what is already known about the relationship between poverty, addiction, and welfare. Note that I place a deeper exploration of literature on addiction itself in the subsequent chapter as a point of entry and conceptualization for this study. This chapter also establishes the broader political, economic, and policy context in which OW does not meet individual or family needs and challenges therein. It is not just problematic that low income is not relieved by the receipt of OW but how OW regulates the experience of benefit receipt too. The need to considering this experience for persons also living with addiction is made especially clear.

Poverty, Substance Use, Addiction

The Canadian Mental Health Association estimates that about 21 per cent of the total Canadian population (six million), will experience addiction in their lifetime. In Ontario, about 10 per cent of the population uses substances problematically (Canadian Mental Health Association, 2021). Addiction can be experienced by individuals of any socio-economic status. The North American literature, however, suggests that people who are experiencing poverty are at significantly higher risk for using and abusing substances (Bungay et al., 2010; Long et al., 2014; Roy et al., 2012; Virokannas, 2011; Wincup, 2011) than those who are not.

Luck et al. (2004) observed that there is some debate about whether substance use creates welfare use or vice versa, though I find that the former seems less likely. For example, Long et al. (2014) found that the majority of injection drug users in Vancouver, British Columbia (BC), who participated in their study did not tend to experience decreased income status associated with their use. Higher income injection drug users, however, would turn to high-risk income-generating activities, for example, sex work and drug dealing, to make ends meet even while still maintaining their employment.

American scholarship recognizes that there is a proportion of the welfare caseload that are substance users (Montoya & Atkinson, 2002; Schoppelrey et al., 2005) and who often repeat welfare use on and off over time (Schmidt et al. 2007). Scholars have been especially interested in how persons using substances experience welfare-to-work requirements (e.g., employment and education training) and in view of how time limits on welfare receipt were legislated with the *Personal Responsibility and Work Opportunity Act* (PROWA) and its introduction of Temporary Assistance for Needy Families (TANF) in the mid-1990s. For the most part, substance dependence is understood as a barrier to employment and therefore an exit from welfare (Danziger et al., 2000; Gutman et al., 2003; Reuter, 2006).

Women substance users are understood to face greater challenges in exiting welfare than men (Hogan et al., 2011; Metsch et al., 1999; Schmidt et al., 2007). When additional obstacles intersect with substance dependence, such as domestic violence, accessing childcare, or their own or their children's serious mental and physical health conditions, researchers find that mothers often have trouble leaving welfare rolls for paid work (Gutman et al., 2003; Hogan et al., 2011; Luck et al., 2004; Schmidt et al., 2007). Based on their quantitative analysis of mothers who were part of the Welfare Client Longitudinal Study in California, Schmidt et al. (2007) found that it was not substance use problems that shaped mothers' exits from welfare into paid work or subsequent return to welfare, but rather their entrance into poorly paid and short-lived employment. For both women and men on welfare who used substances, the most consistently documented challenges to employment included limited education, poor job-search skills, lack of prior work history (also associated with having a criminal record or language problems), lack of childcare and transportation, and lack of effective drug abuse treatment (Montoya & Atkinson, 2002; Schmidt et al., 2007).

Other structural barriers to employment for woman substance users include welfare services' negative views of them (Bush & Kraft, 2001). Following the introduction of welfare-to-work initiatives under PROWA, Dohan et al. (2005) found that California caseworkers perceived the reforms to have ended the enabling of substance abuse, encouraged clients to "bootstrap" their way into jobs, and allowed clients to claim personal responsibility for their substance abuse problems. In other work, they show how caseworkers' day-to-day work conditions and unstated stigma surrounding substance abuse can create an environment in which welfare recipients with substance dependence are not identified and therefore not supported through referrals to social services and treatment (Henderson et al., 2006). Focusing on the experience of substance users on welfare in the United Kingdom, Bauld et al. (2012) observed employers' reluctance to hire anyone with a substance use problem as another structural barrier to paid employment.

Canadian research does not share the same degree of concentration on the simultaneous experience of living with addiction and receiving welfare. Social science research (including my own past research) may note that people experiencing substance use dependency face more challenges when on social assistance yet not reveal the specificity of these (see Lightman et al., 2005), or may recognize substance use as a barrier to employment but not offer much in-depth discussion (McMullin et al., 2002). There is some scholarship on welfare receipt and changes in use patterns. Krebs et al. (2016) found that drug intensification followed receipt of benefits in Vancouver, BC. The risk of overdose at a supervised injection site in this same city was also higher following "cheque day" than other days of the week (Zlotorzynska et al., 2014). Long et al. (2014), however, found no indication that individuals' social assistance receipt increased their overall injection drug use.

Other Canadian research considers the connections among substance use, poverty, and social assistance receipt but specifically for street-involved individuals (e.g., homeless, temporarily homeless, living and working on the street). Researchers observe that the amount of social assistance street-involved women receive each month is not enough to meet their basic needs (Bungay et al., 2010; Roy et al., 2012). Others find that many crack cocaine users develop income-generating strategies dependent on the informal street economy, such as petty theft, panhandling, sex work, and drug dealing, and may use their welfare payment to support some of them (Roy et al., 2012). Bungay et al. (2010) observed that the poverty of a racially and ethnically diverse sample of street-involved women who used illegal drugs, that is, crack cocaine, in an inner-city neighbourhood in Western Canada, was compounded by their experiences of racism, sexism, violence, challenges in accessing health services (e.g., harm reduction), personal health problems (e.g., dental care), and social isolation.

Although the experience of living with addiction and a life shaped by social assistance receipt is not the focus, still other Canadian research carefully documents how Indigenous peoples have much longer histories of experiencing gendered and colonial violence, including the intergenerational trauma of residential schools, that disproportionately shapes their poverty (and employment trajectories) and drug use (Boyd & MacPherson, 2018/9; Jacobs & Gill 2002). Culhane (2003) powerfully reveals the injustice associated with how Indigenous street-involved women who use drugs in Downtown Eastside Vancouver experience stigma, violence, and murder because of their survival strategies (e.g., sex work, drug dealing). Meanwhile, Culhane (2003) argues, the poverty-level welfare cheques they receive drive them into these very strategies. In their study of this same location, Benoit et al. (2003) found that care provided by services like Sheway that support women's traditional and spiritual practices were crucial to Indigenous women's survival since social assistance only kept them in poverty.

Overall, existing scholarship reveals that the experience of living with addiction while impoverished is replete with challenges. Lone mothers seem to weather these experiences at the risk of further harm. Black, Indigenous, and people of colour, especially women, more acutely experience harms to their self and health and well-being when impoverished, using substances, and relying on social assistance to survive on Canada's streets. Other research, to which I will now turn, narrows the focus still further to the intersections of addiction, poverty, and family lives.

Family Lives

There is considerable room for improvement in the sociological focus on Canadian family relations, and addiction too, especially how the two intersect with poverty. An inter-disciplinary review yields research findings that emphasize the health and well-being of children of parents living with addiction and, perhaps less so, of parents themselves. Social workers Lander et al. (2013) argue that an individual's substance use disorder affects their families and family members. Others show that children of parents who experience addiction are at greater risk for developmental issues, impaired attachment, mental health issues, behavioural problems, violence from the user, or developing a substance use problem; all which may impact their own parenting abilities later in their own lives (Benoit & Magnus, 2017; Lander et al., 2013;Lussier et al., 2010; Rutherford & Mayes, 2019). Families may also experience economic hardship, legal problems, and an overall unpredictable environment (Lander et al., 2013).

When the focus turns to prospective parents or substance-using parents, research attention can be placed on the actual and perceived quality of their parenting (Benoit & Magnus, 2017; Grant et al., 2011a). Pregnant women and mothers who engage in substance use are often viewed by others as engaging in morally wrong behaviour (Benoit et al., 2015; Grant et al., 2011; Parolin & Simonelli, 2016; Sderstrm, 2012), which has implications for their parenting practices. Indeed, women, and especially racialized and Indigenous women, who use criminalized drugs have long been more vilified than men who engage in the same behaviour (Boyd, 2007; Boyd & MacPherson, 2019). Other research, however, reveals that mothers' drug abuse is often associated with other factors (e.g., higher rates of serious psychopathology, depression, disorders of attachment, some of these stemming from childhood histories of trauma) that compromise their ability to parent and place their children at risk of neglect and/or being removed into foster care (Grant et al., 2011b; Strathearn & Mayes, 2010). Sometimes mothers feel ambivalence, tempered by strong feelings of guilt, anxiety, anguish, and blame, about their mothering and treatment. Silva et al.'s (2013) qualitative study shows how when mothers feel this ambivalence, they can adopt merely functional roles for their children. They may control their dosage of methadone to meet the child's basic needs but show little willingness to emotionally engage or talk and play with them (Silva et al., 2013).

Since people who use especially illegal drugs are still viewed as "deviant," this "deviance" is further compounded if they are on social assistance and parents too (see also Boyd, 1999). As Virokannas (2011) puts it, they are "triply deviant." Existing interdisciplinary literature does tend to convey (and perhaps wholly unintentionally) that parents living with addiction are likely to inadequately parent and negatively shape a child's development. While I acknowledge that these findings cement the need for establishing the safety and security of children in households – and see this as paramount in importance – I am drawn to other research that is quite novel in revealing the practices of parenting actually performed and the importance of it to parents' identity and everyday life. In more recent qualitative research, Benoit and Magnus (2017) focused on how parenting and substance use (drugs or alcohol) was problematized by low-income parents themselves. They found that fathers saw themselves to perform responsible fathering when they provided material provisions and were positive role models for their children. Mothers defined the substance use of fathers as problematic when it specifically exceeded moderation, invoked risks for children, compromised fathers' own capabilities, or seemed to precipitate their partner's acts of domestic violence towards them.

Mothers and fathers may do much to work against others' stigmatizing perceptions of their parenting capabilities and practices. Boyd's (1999) interviews with low-income mothers on welfare who used illicit drugs revealed the efforts they made to resist welfare policy and therefore caseworkers' allegiance with dominant constructions of mothering – and seeing their mothering as outside these ideological bounds. In research with Israeli fathers on methadone, Peled et al. (2012) found that they valued their paternal status and created evolving, multifaceted identities as fathers amid pejorative constructions of their fathering as "less than" or deficient. The work of performing as a mother or father for social or child welfare workers and its implications is also powerfully taken up by Virokanna's (2011) study of nineteen mothers in Finland. Virokanna found that mothers who had been using illegal drugs but were now in recovery had to (re-)produce their mothering identities in relation to their case workers' perceptions – which were often distorted, mistrusting, and overbearing. Mothers' own activism is most obviously an example of resistance to others' perceptions of them as "triply deviant." In downtown eastside Vancouver, Indigenous mothers and allies, including other mothers, annually march in the Women's Memorial March to honour women from their community who have disappeared or been murdered and to reclaim and demand others' awareness of their identities as mothers, daughters, and sisters (Culhane, 2003).

There is a growing awareness of the importance of understanding how parents who use substances parent and see themselves as parents when accessible and non-judgmental supports are in place instead of exclusionary and stigmatizing ones (Benoit & Magnus, 2017; Peled et al., 2012; Virokanna, 2011). Chapter 7 in the second part of this book is inspired by this research that attempts to move beyond, set aside, or deeply and critically engage with the moral evaluation of parents who use substances or are in recovery. My interest now is to consider and discuss the wider post-war social policy context in which this study is situated.

Neoliberalism and Social Policy Restructuring

Stemming from the income instability of the early twentieth-century economy (e.g., the Great Depression of the 1930s), a growing consensus emerged among politicians and other social actors that risks of poverty and unemployment were collectively experienced. Following the Second World War, a social contract began to emerge in Canada, largely infused with a notion that other risks, too, such as old age and poor health, required government intervention and/or support (Rice & Prince, 2013; Yalnizyan, 1994). The initial design of the post-war welfare state was further informed by the work of economist John Maynard Keynes, who argued that governments had the specific economic responsibility of spending to boost the economy and facilitate full employment (e.g., through investment) and to cushion any negative effects through corresponding changes in levels of taxation (Rice & Prince, 2013; Simeon, 1994). Over several years, specific social programs were rolled out to support and consolidate Canada's Keynesian welfare state partially framed by universalism (e.g., Old Age Pensions, Medicare) (Brodie, 2002). This is not to say that all social and economic inequalities were curbed; this was far from the case. Some racialized groups faced considerable hardship because of exclusionary immigration policies (e.g., Chinese men subject to the Chinese Head Tax and corresponding deterrence from establishing families in Canada). Particularly, Indigenous peoples continued to experience ongoing colonization of their land simultaneous to the emergence of the apparently "benevolent" welfare state. Accounting for this history of racism and social exclusion, I am nonetheless simply (and rudimentarily) establishing the general political economic and policy context before neoliberalism as an economic doctrine and ideology (Hartman, 2005) began driving post-1980s welfare state reform and restructuring in Canada.

With its prioritization of free trade and market competition, neoliberalism has signalled a paradigmatic shift away from Keynesianism

(Garrett, 2018; Harvey, 2007). Alongside this economic doctrine, its political ideology assumes that the role of the state should be limited, smaller; variable governance patterns are normative; and individuals are responsible for their social and economic welfare (Hartman, 2005). The tone of neoliberalism and its implications are widely recognized as sedimenting with Thatcher and Reagan's governance in the late 1980s, in the United Kingdom (UK) and in the United States (US), respectively.

Room for neoliberal restructuring was partially made possible by a growing crisis mentality surrounding the architecture of the Canadian welfare state, one that flourished among critics with different social and economic viewpoints and political party allegiances (Rice & Prince, 2013). As Pollack and Caragata (2010) put it, neoliberalism is effective in responding to a crisis in social spending because the state becomes a mechanism through which markets can be expanded, instead of a mechanism through which social policy constrains market risks. Rice and Prince (2013) pinpoint the advance of obvious neoliberal programmatic retrenchment to the election of a federal Conservative government in the early 1980s. Beginning then and even throughout the 1990s under the Liberals, this retrenchment, including the cutting of the size and expense of social programs, implementing more restrictions into program design, and further shifting policies into a residual direction – sometimes without taxpayers' knowledge – is why Battle and Torjman (1989) define this period of welfare state change as "social policy by stealth."

Canada's current neoliberal policy framework (Larner, 2000) is not without inherent contradictions. For some scholars, the welfare state has undergone such additional change that post-2000 it takes the form of a social investment state. Jenson and Saint-Martin (2003), for example, make the case that the post-war welfare state "social rights" citizenship regime has slowly been replaced by a newer, pro-market "social investment" citizenship regime. Where the former was concerned with providing access to a safety net and protection, the latter is concerned with state supplementation of individuals' low wages through activation initiatives (e.g., employment and skills training) that will integrate people into the labour market; a "trampoline" welfare state as opposed to a "safety net" (Jenson & Saint-Martin, 2003, p. 89). Simon-Kumar (2011) further argues that the social investment state is characterized by investing in policy, modernizing the public sector, and interlinking community partnerships and citizen participation (e.g., through volunteering) in the delivery of policy, services, and supports. Concerning social assistance, reforms that aim to improve the employability potential of citizens (what I will refer to as welfare-to-work or workfare below) are seen to be placing an investment in individuals and to signal a positive shift in policymaking and delivery. The 2000s onward introduction of benefits in support of women's reproduction, childcare, and work–life balance are often cited as other examples of investment (Béland & Daigneault, 2015; Dobrowlsky & Jenson, 2004).

The notion that governments have a role to play by investing in human resources and infrastructure, and to even develop an entrepreneurial culture, is not limited to Canada. The logic can be linked to Anthony Giddens's conceptualization of social investment as part and parcel of the Third Way, a middling approach between old-style social democracy and neoliberalism, neither of which he sees as functioning in a manner that entirely benefits citizens in capitalist nation-states (Giddens, 1998; Simon-Kumar, 2011). The social investment state is also understood to be characteristic of European and Latin American countries post-1990 (Jenson, 2010). And yet some scholars are sceptical of the extent to which social investment is a new policy paradigm with considerable sway, especially in Canada. White (2012), for example, finds that even in apparent social investment states there is also evidence of continuity with past policy practices. White (2012) further notes that the argument that social investment as a paradigm has replaced neoliberalism is belied by continued, strong adherence to traditional market norms in policy.

Peck and Tickell (2002) recommend scholars see neoliberalism as not universally defined or applied and instead characterized by "vagaries" specific to social-cultural context. They define this by the apparent "roll out" and "roll back" of neoliberal reforms within a welfare state. Applying their perspective to social policy change in Canada, there has been political embracement of the "roll back" of government support and prioritization of individual choice and responsibility for self-sufficiency; reduced state support, in turn, translates into governments' greater competitive edge in the market. At the same time, there is a continued "roll out" of new social programs, such as those "investments" I discussed earlier. Coupling the perceived trend towards social investment with Peck and Tickell's (2002) insights, I contend that the tightening of eligibility for some social programs as well as the greater surveillance of benefit recipients continuing into the 2000s means that while we may perceive investment through activation initiatives, investment is nonetheless underscored by the questionable and negative implications of the neoliberal responsibilization of the individual subject, a point I will return to below.

Social Assistance (or Welfare) Reform

Social assistance policy has always been differently designed and administered by provincial governments (Boychuk, 1998), with variable funding support from the federal government. However, there have been several common trends concerning policy rules and outcomes, if not outright convergence, that demonstrate how all provinces engaged in social assistance reform (or "welfare reform") in the 1990s (Béland & Daigneault, 2015), a project that I see as shaped by neoliberalism.

One key reform of the federal welfare state that drove provincial social assistance reform was the replacement of the Canada Assistance Plan with the Canada Health and Social Transfer. Under the 1966 CAP, the funding of social assistance was to be 50/50 cost-shared by the provincial and federal governments (Baker & Tippin, 1999). CAP's "entitlement model" obligated provinces to base receipt on a needs-test and to recognize five rights of citizens: the right to an adequate income; the right to assistance when in need; the right to appeal decisions made about their assistance; the right to claim assistance whatever one's province of origin; and the right to assistance without forced participation in work and training rogramms (Klein & Montgomery, 2001, p. 7; Morrison, 1998; Pulkingham & Ternowetsky, 1999; Rice & Prince, 2013). Through negotiation, a 1985 agreement enabled provinces to add work incentives into their social assistance programs to shape citizens' improvements to their labour market potential (Lightman & Riches, 2000); the federal government committed money to skills training through the Canada Job Strategy program. Between 1990 and 1995, a 5 per cent ceiling on CAP was introduced in the wealthiest provinces of Ontario, BC, and Alberta. Boychuk (1998) explains that if CAP had not been "capped," for example, Ontario's social assistance program would have become even more costly. The right to assistance without forced participation in work and training programs, however, ended in 1995 when the Liberal government budget replaced CAP and the Established Programs Financing (EPF) (the agency responsible for shared provincial and federal costs for health and education) with the Canada Health and Social Transfer (CHST). Notably, the CHST ended all rights but one: the requirement that provinces could not impose minimum residency requirements for access to social assistance (Battle & Torjman, 1995). The CHST has since been divided into the Canada Health and Canada Social Transfer. The CHST essentially created greater opportunities for provincial experimentation with social assistance design and delivery.

Boychuk (2015) cautions against crediting the restructuring of social assistance across Canada solely to the end of CAP because to do so would be to ignore the diverse social, economic, and political context of each province that further shaped their reform trajectories. I concur and note that as my own research has shown, social assistance policies in the Western provinces of BC, Alberta, and Saskatchewan were subject to reforms for two other reasons: provincial economic deficits experienced by all provinces and spikes in social assistance caseloads (Gazso, 2006). Similar cost conditions were a concern for many provinces in the 1990s. Post-CAP reforms that seemed generally shared across the provinces included restrictions of eligibility, a steady dose of cost cutting, and increased mechanisms of surveillance (Béland & Daigneault, 2015). Some provinces' reforms nonetheless stand out by comparison. Two different waves of welfare reform in BC, 1995 and 2002, involved cutting benefit amounts and requiring lone mothers to seek employment when their children were increasingly younger ages (three years in 2002). BC was the only province to introduce time limits to benefit receipt in 2002, a punitive eligibility requirement borrowed from American reforms under PROWA (Gazso, 2006); exemption criteria were introduced before they were to officially take effect in 2004 and they were removed in 2012 (Pulkingham, 2015). Most obviously, and like massive welfare reforms in the United States in the 1990s more generally, employment activity became increasingly mandatory across all provinces; a condition of benefit receipt solidified in the use of "employment plans" completed between caseworkers and benefit recipients in BC and Ontario. Moreover, neoliberal hallmarks of individual responsibility and an invalidation of social rights of citizenship became increasingly embedded in social assistance reform via the discourses of social investment and activation.

Responsibilization and Curtailment of Social Rights. If an individual is deemed responsible for their social and economic welfare, states need not at all, or barely, intervene in people's lives, surely evidenced in the below poverty-level incomes one receives on social assistance. The discourse of welfare dependency, which rests on several ideas, including the notion that the individual suffers from moral deficiencies or failings that precipitate their unemployment and idleness (Gazso et al., 2019), can fuel this orientation and, as we will see, was powerfully used to shape reforms in Ontario. In turn, if economic insecurity and dependency is the fault of the individual, then they alone are logically responsible for correcting it. Thus, responsibilization is inherent in the making of social assistance receipt contingent upon an individuals' investment – operationalized as an able-bodied person participating in employment activity programming. As Ilcan (2009) explains, neoliberalism invokes this "responsibilizing ethos." Elsewhere, I have also noted that Giddens's Third Way view that the contemporary welfare state is to produce "responsible risk takers" has relevance for Canadian neoliberal social assistance reform (Gazso, 2006a; Giddens, 1998).

Almost two decades ago, Brodie (2002) observed that once individuals are perceived as responsible for their own welfare, social responsibility is undermined. Some facets of the social rights of citizenship (some, given the historical exclusions that made this regime imperfect and unequal, as I observed earlier) were lost in the neoliberal turn and have been repeatedly curtailed in the 2000s. As conceptualized by Marshall (1963, p. 74), social rights emerged in the twentieth century and ranged from the right to a modicum of economic welfare and security to the right to share in the collective culture of society, especially in terms of living according to the standards of society; education and social services were institutions that provided this social element of citizenship. Social rights were not without responsibilities for Marshall, these including the responsibility of engaging in the labour market and obeying and upholding the law in capitalist society. And they had and have a particular gendered quality (Gazso, 2007a,b; Gazso & McDaniel, 2010). A heteronormative nuclear family was assumed and gender and citizenship encoded so that men's wage earning was equated with "independence" and a basis to claim support and women's lack thereof, and participation in caregiving responsibilities was equated with "dependence" and a lesser claim to support (Ilcan, 2009; O'Connor et al. 1999; Orloff, 1993). It bears repeating that social rights did not correct market-generated, class-based inequalities or even gender- and race-based inequalities. However, they could dampen inequalities, particularly if they represented a relationship between individuals and the state that was not conditional, contractual, or tied to the market (Dwyer, 2002).

With responsibilization and the conditioning of social assistance benefit receipt, there has been an overturning of the recognition of an individual's social right to support when in need. The slow evolution of this shift in welfare design and administration in the UK over the 1990s and early 2000s is referred to as "creeping conditionality" by Dwyer (2002). This conditionality no longer creeps in Canada but is entirely entrenched. The continued neoliberal design and administration of Canadian social assistance policy largely aims to construct identities and eligibility based on labour market citizenship (Gazso & McDaniel, 2010). Considerable research documents how women and men are differently affected when market citizenship eclipses social citizenship (Bezanson, 2006; Brodie, 1997; McDaniel, 2002; O'Connor et al., 1999), with my own past research emphasizing how the apparent gender-neutral conditioning of income support on parents' employability efforts (e.g., attendance in welfare-to-work programs) produces deeply gendered consequences, such as lone mothers' differential experiences of work–family conflict (Gazso, 2006b, 2007b).

Post-1990s Social Assistance in Ontario

I have good reason for narrowing this study's focus to being about how people living with addiction experience social assistance only in Ontario. While social assistance reform shares trends associated with the paradigm of neoliberalism that are observable across the provinces, Ontario's 1990s reforms were infamous for their severity of cuts to benefit amounts and the dramatic way in which eligibility was over-hauled through the introduction of an obvious "work first" approach. Into present day, OW is still a primary case in point across Canada of social assistance reforms that have and do produce the questionable and regulatory treatment of especially lone mothers, strict eligibility expectations, punitive techniques of surveillance, and a bleakness of survival for benefit recipients.

By the early 1990s and associated with the broader economic reces-sion of the time, social assistance caseloads in Ontario and their cost were increasing. The province's spending reached $6 billion annually in 1995. In that year's provincial government election, the winning party, Mike Harris's Progressive Conservatives, made strategic use of the wel-fare dependency discourse in their party platform. *The Common Sense Revolution* campaign, outlined in a 1994 document of the same name, "played on rumours of lazy deadbeats cheating the welfare system" (Bradburn, 2015, np).

Through the coupling of a social spending crisis with the plight of welfare dependency, Harris's government justified its reforms. The Social Assistance Reform Act (SARA) replaced the Family Benefits Act and the General Welfare Assistance Act in 1997, the first major change in social assistance administration and delivery in Ontario in just over three decades (Morrison, 1998). SARA introduced Ontario Works (OW) and the Ontario Disability and Support Program (ODSP). The *Ontario Works Act* (OWA), in turn, marshalled in a new "work first" orienta-tion to social assistance receipt directed at able-bodied persons, while ODPS targeted those deemed as disabled under new eligibility criteria. Although OW and not ODSP is the policy of focus in the remainder of this book, it is noteworthy that under ODSP, addiction no longer quali-fied as a disability.

The OWA transformed what was perceived to be a "passive" financial assistance program into an "active" one "that emphasized self-reliance and return to work through employment assistance" (Bill 142, Schedule A, OWA, s. 39, 1). Employable recipients were to participate in some form of welfare-to-work programming, or specifically "workfare," in order to remain eligible for benefits (Gorlick & Brethour, 1998). While welfare-to-work programming can include a range of employment-oriented activities (e.g., education, skills training, job search or job readiness programs), workfare is the term used to refer to when programming is compulsory and mandated; workfare has the objective of "enforcing work while residualizing welfare" (Peck, 2001, p. 10). Indeed, Harris's government made explicit the seeking of employment or participation in the first available job as a condition of OW receipt, what Graefe (2015) also sees as evidence of its "work first" discourse. In placing the onus of responsibility for self-sufficiency squarely on the shoulders of individuals, the province absolved itself of recognizing the structural conditions that create poverty (Community Development Halton, 1998).

Two decades ago, Morrison (1998) maintained that SARA was a perfect example of the dismantling of the social rights of citizenship as a shared vision in Canada. I concur, and in my own archival research I found that specific language was changed to make clear that OW would no longer be perceived as a guaranteed entitlement as under the old legislation. The word "shall" (as in shall receive income support) was replaced with "may" (as in *may* receive income support) in all new legislation (Ministry of Community and Social Services, 1997). The OWA also was written in such a way that entitlements and program standards can be limited, restricted, or abrogated by regulation. New regulations and policies may even be promulgated; that is, changes proposed or made need not be scrutinized by the legislature or through political process (Morrison, 1998).

Harris's reforms in the most populous province were soon infamous because of their perceived punitiveness and problematic outcomes. Notably, the introduction of OW was accompanied by a 21.6 per cent reduction in benefit rates. Benefit amounts were later subject to freezing (Coulter, 2009). The effect over time has been that of pushing benefit recipients' social assistance incomes even further below measures of low income. Fast forward into the 2000s: people are even worse off now than under the Harris government (Smith-Carrier et al., 2020; Tiessen, 2016). Graefe (2015) calculates that a single employable person received less in benefit income in 2013 than even in 1993.

Compared to the *Family Benefits Act*, lone parents were seen as employable once their children were school-age ready (e.g., previously children age six; now children beginning all-day kindergarten at age four) under the *Ontario Works Act*. As I have written about elsewhere, the 1990s assumption that women and mothers specifically are earners is not unusual given women's increased entrance into the labour market post-1970 and agentic choice to be autonomous and self-sufficient. However, the requirement that lone mothers especially demonstrate their employability efforts when their children are quite young and have inadequate or inconsistent supports for childcare is problematic (Gazso, 2012). Several scholars have also documented these and other injustices, especially lone mothers' experience with these reforms (Bezanson, 2006; Gazso & McDaniel, 2010; Little & Marks, 2006; McMullin et al., 2002; Smith-Carrier, 2017). Moreover, in the way that scrutiny coincides with the imposition of new expectations of employability, these changes confirm that the discourse of "deserving/undeserving" continues to be a part of the moral regulation of mothers through welfare policy in Ontario (Little, 1994, 1998) and productive of differences in eligibility experiences (Boychuk, 1998, 2015).

People deemed deserving of OW continue to be required to engage in mandatory practices, including meeting their caseworker every three months to review their eligibility conditions and providing monthly reports of their participation in welfare-to-work activities. They may be subject to random audits of their assets, income, and expenses to prevent fraudulent behaviour (or welfare fraud) (Ministry of Community and Social Services, 2011a). Should any benefit recipient be perceived to not meet the conditions of their benefit receipt (as documented in employment plans), they may face sanctions for "non-compliance" and then a complex process should they want to appeal these. The death of Kimberly Rogers remains the most disturbing example of the extreme harms associated with the regulation of eligibility. Rogers had plead guilty to welfare fraud and was sentenced to house arrest. While she managed to re-instate her OW benefits with legal help, the amount she received each month was insufficient to live upon; she had only $18 for food after paying her rent. In August 2001, she overdosed from ingesting an anti-depressant, while pregnant and amid a heat wave (Gilhula, 2006).

The most obvious example of workfare in the OWA is the expectation that benefit recipients work without pay for non-profit organizations or other municipal projects in order to receive benefits (Morrison, 1998). The Community Placement program continues to exist today and can obligate employable lone mothers to perform up to seventy hours of unpaid work per month to receive their monthly benefit (Little & Marks, 2006; Ministry of Community and Social Services, 2011a). Overall, the OWA facilitates contentious relationships among caseworkers, benefit recipients, and the general lay public. The "snitch line" was a provincial telephone line introduced and designed to allow citizens to anonymously report suspected fraud by social assistance recipients as part of their civic duty (Little & Marks, 2006). Still in use, the telephone line directly involves the public in regulating social assistance recipients' behaviour. Citizens may report "bad" people on OW, including those who they perceive to receive benefits and other sources of income (e.g., from paid work) each month (see also Gazso, 2012; Ministry of Children Community and Social Services, 2019). Though now defunct, the "spouse in the house rule" assessed the deservedness of lone mothers' receipt of benefits. Under this rule, any man who appeared to live with a lone mother was understood to be her spouse unless proven otherwise. Even male roommates or boarders were assumed to have a sexually intimate relationship with mothers or to share social and financial responsibility for their children (Little & Morrison, 1999).

Another change with the launch of OW has bearing for the findings reported later in this book: technology became a greater part of the caseworker–client relationship. For example, the province contracted an outside consulting firm to launch a computerized service delivery of programming in 1996 (Morrison, 1998). By 2001, the Service Delivery Model Technology (SDMT) was introduced for case management, an electronic duplicate of a benefit recipients' file. Maki (2011) explains that the collection and management of information and evaluative potential of SDMT – e.g., to confirm if a recipient was receiving payments erroneously – was perceived as a primary defence against welfare fraud. It was replaced in 2014 with SAMS, the Social Assistance Management System. In 2016, SAMS made news headlines for overpayment of recipients, a technological and social mistake that cost millions to correct (Jones, 2016). Technologies of surveillance require human involvement and so are not without the absence of caseworker discretion (Morrisson, 1998), a point that will be returned to later in this book. Beyond SDMT, Maki (2011) reviewed other forms of computerized technology that were used to surveil and regulate benefit recipients' lives in the early 2000s and, ultimately, contribute to the construction of any person who failed to be a "good market citizen" (e.g., conform to employability expectations) as "deviant."

By 2016, the year in which I began the research featured in this book, there had been no major changes in OW since those brought about under Mike Harris's Progressive Conservative government. The OWA continues to be largely delivered municipally with funding support from the provincial and federal governments. Though each municipality must follow the rules set out in the Act, there is room for considerable regional variation in delivery standards (Morrisson, 1998), including the contracting out of services, for example, employment programming. Only in 2010 did the province begin a process of review of OW as part of its Poverty Reduction Strategy under the Liberal government. Prior to this, there were some revisions to OW Directives made, and new initiatives introduced, such as the Addiction Services Initiative. As well there is evidence to suggest that a new discourse other than "work first" is driving administration and delivery of OW in Toronto.[1] The significance of these latter two changes for persons living with addiction will be discussed at length in the second part of this book.

Stigma

Goffman (1996, p. 3) defined stigma as any "attribute that is deeply discrediting" and prompting of others to see a person with this attribute as "tainted" and to be "discounted."

Observing that stigma is varyingly researched and defined across disciplines, Link and Phelan (2001) put forth their own sociological re-conceptualization of it. They argue stigma is tied to processes of labelling, stereotyping, separation, status loss, and discrimination. Differences that are thought to matter socially are created and labelled as such by individuals; what is different therefore becomes a culturally created category and hegemonic over time. "Addicts" and "welfare users" are such categories. Stigma further occurs when a label is applied to an individual to denote for others that they possess the negative attribute(s); a stereotype of said label becomes entrenched in

---

1 Canada's history is that of a capitalist nation constructed and therefore characterized by ongoing income (and social) inequality, a trajectory most obviously initialized through settler colonialism. It is beyond the scope of this book to write more deeply of this, but this much longer historical context must be reminded. Offering this footnote largely as a postscriptum to my study, I note here that in Fall 2018, Premier Ford's Progressive Conservative government announced the intention to reform social assistance (Crawley, 2018; Ontario 360, 2019). By 2021, the government was pursuing changes in technology-based provision, centralization of services, and expectations of municipal and provincial roles in service delivery (Government of Ontario, 2021). As of 2022, the government announced that employment supports associated with social assistance would be integrated with Employment Ontario (a provincial system) and that a new model where Employment Ontario caseworkers support and work with OW clients and caseworkers would be tested (Government of Ontario, 2022). Piloting of some of these newer arrangements began to take place in 2020 and specifically in the Peel, Hamilton-Niagara, and Muskoka-Kawarthas regions (Taekema, 2020). These reforms seem increasingly driven by a "life stabilization" framework (Government of Ontario, 2022), which is further suggestive of shifting discourses in policy design and delivery; noteworthy is how "life stabilization" was discussed by some OW caseworkers in my interviews with them in 2016 and 2017, as will be shown in the second part of this book.

discourse. In this, Link and Phelan follow Goffman in seeing stigma as a relationship between an attribute and stereotype. They make the additional and crucial point that labelling and stereotyping creates separation, and in turn, people are thought to be the thing they are labelled. Thus, people are "addicts" rather than a person who lives with addiction, a point that resonates with my discussion throughout this book. Status loss and discrimination are an outcome of stigmatization, including individuals' deepening perceptions of their own social exclusion, or their experiences of discrimination by others or structured within institutions (e.g., systemic racism). These processes of stigmatization, as argued by Link and Phelan (2001), are produced by and operate within relations of power.

Like Link and Phelan (2001), Fraser et al. (2017) are interested in processes of labelling and separation on the basis of constructions of difference and the power relations therein, but where they differ is in their stronger argumentation that stigma is politically productive and achieves something. For them, stigma is a biopolitical technology of power that constitutes conditions under which subjects emerge. Stigma operates in the service of normative social relations; stigma excludes to uphold that which is to be included, that which is "normal." The moral quality and experience of stigma is also considered by Link and Phelan with colleagues Yang, Kleinman, Lee, and Good. They argue that the act of stigmatizing others can be an individual and institutional response to "perceived threats, real dangers, and fear of the unknown." Stigmatizing others occurs when the stigmatizer is faced with considering what is at stake for them in their social world (Yang et al., 2007, p. 1528). For the stigmatized, stigma can compound their suffering given their sense that what is at stake for them is discredited or devalued by stigmatizing others.

Wincup and Monaghan (2016) focused on the stigmatization of low-income persons who also use substances and offered one example of the attitudes that give shape to it: people who "choose" to pursue their habit while on welfare are seen as doing so at the expense of "the hard-working taxpayer." Welfare dependency is condemned, while simultaneously drug users are made underserving. As we saw above, the welfare dependency discourse and notions of deservedness have shaped social assistance reform in Canada and Ontario. So, too, has the stigmatization of persons on social assistance been a constant in Canadian society.

Calnitsky's (2016) study of the 1970s Manitoba Basic Annual Income Experiment gives historical context in that it reveals how some participants thought their receipt of "Mincome," a basic income program separate from social assistance, to be less stigmatizing than receipt of social assistance itself. In qualitative research I undertook with colleagues to explore the intergenerational dynamics of OW receipt (i.e., participants' and their own parent and/or adult child's receipt), our participants recognized that they were stigmatized and specifically identified stigma as the weight of shame to be carried and an element of humiliation to be endured in order to receive benefits (Baker Collins et al., 2019). Garrett (2018, p. 33) convincingly argues that the degradation and humiliation endured by those on social assistance is a form of what Bourdieu calls "symbolic violence," that which stigmatizes and devalues a group of individuals.

There are other tangible implications of the double stigma of being on social assistance and living with addiction. As noted earlier, clearly women who are Black, Indigenous, or a person of colour, on welfare and using substances and perhaps mothering children are among the most stigmatized, facing greater difficulty in accessing services and at higher risk than men of losing custody of their children and/or risk of violence at the hands of others (see also Jones et al., 2015; Pinedo et al., 2020). Building on existing research that has established that health care providers may be prejudiced against people who use drugs (see also Madden, 2019), Dassieu et al. (2020) found that the stigma attached to drug use shaped the meaning that health care providers gave to the actions of Montreal drug users who also suffered from chronic pain. This was the case for Randy, whose pain made it difficult for him to walk. Others interpreted his inability as simply his "laziness." If labelled foremost as "addicts," people who suffered from chronic pain could therefore be denied pain management (Dassieu et al., 2020).

Pivot: From a Context for Stigmatizing Addiction to Breaking Stigma

People living with addiction are undoubtedly a heavily researched population. Attention has been given to the experience of addiction and welfare receipt, most notably in American research, and broadened to include how the two experiences intersect with family lives. What is missing in Canadian research, however, is an awareness of what it is like to be known as an "addict" on welfare, regulated as such by policy and caseworkers, perhaps parenting children too, and what this feels like. The study presented in this book is one step forward to narrowing this gap in knowledge. Moreover, I situate this study in Ontario because, quite bluntly, neoliberal reforms in Ontario are widely understood to have produced a punitive, regulatory, and stigmatizing social assistance system. As noted, one disturbing impetus for these reforms was the discourse of welfare dependency. Stigma was and is its corollary.

Low-income persons on welfare experience stigma when others perceive them as failing to participate in the labour market, be self-sufficient, and be responsible for their own economic wherewithal, and consequently, as "dependent" on the state. As Hogue et al. (2010) observe, under neoliberal welfare regimes, worklessness is viewed as inherently problematic or even a sin. Substance users experience stigma too when they are perceived to violate norms of behaviour associated with a rational, self-sufficient, and productive neoliberal subject and engage in a "deviant" use of drugs or alcohol. The normative neoliberal subject may occasionally imbibe in the use of substances for pleasure but certainly does not lose control and not at the cost of their participation in normal activities of daily life, for example, employment or relationships with children, family, and friends.

While existing research importantly understands and establishes the lived experience of stigma, one of my difficulties is that the end point of some published research, my own included, may be just a naming, and a knowing of stigma. Returning to much earlier discussions in this chapter, I note how existing research on people living with addiction and/or people on welfare can even contribute to stigmatization with the way findings have the potential to be read as offering hopeless and even miserabilist interpretations of people's lives. I intend for something different with the big story in this book. I resist or upend the processes of labelling, stereotyping, separation, status loss, and discrimination that seem to bound the experience of living with addiction. I contend that resisting stigmatization requires overturning and re-constructing what has been conventionally known as deviant, different, or "other" – living with addiction and in poverty – into different meanings. It requires dismissing the idea that people can be reduced to a label and stereotype, for example, "the addict," and constituting different conditions under which subjects emerge. I aim to do all the above with the findings I present and the big story I tell in this book – with hope.

3 Knowing Addiction

One of the difficulties in taking on a project like this one as a sociologist is entering into an area of research inquiry about which much has been researched and written *elsewhere*. If we divide up scholarly inquiry in academia through the simple division between the hard sciences and social sciences, it is clear that even within an area, experts and scholars are not fully in agreement about what constitutes addiction, or its causes. In essence, addiction is socially defined, and its definition varies across culture and time (Fraser et al., 2017; West, 2001). In this chapter, I reveal how addiction is understood at least in North American and some European scholarship. Doing so establishes a backdrop to then shift to how living with addiction is understood by the people accessing Ontario Works (OW) that I interviewed and throughout the remainder of this book.

A Disorder, a Disease, a Body Pathologized

Based on an analysis of scholarship in Medline and the Science and Social Science Citation Index, West (2001), a health psychologist, maintained that there are five main theories of addiction. These include theories that: (1) conceptualize addiction and outline its biological, psychological, and social processes broadly speaking and those that focus on (2) effects of additive stimuli, for example, pleasure, relief; (3) individual susceptibility, for example, genetic predisposition to addiction; (4) environmental factors, for example, stressors, social roles, and opportunities that shape addictive behaviour; and (5) recovery and relapse, for example, psychological conditioning of substances and/or the effects of withdrawals. West (2001) argues that existing scholarship that can be grouped to correspond with these five main theories can be further split into either behavioural and social approaches or biological ones.

West's distinction seems to hold well still today. Many of us experience daily life as replete with social interactions and exposure to, and consumption of, media (e.g., the Internet; Netflix streaming or television; newspapers) whether face to face or mediated through Facebook or Instagram. It seems fair to say that each of us has most likely learned of at least one or more of these theories.

The theory of addiction as a mental health condition or disorder is rooted in the "psy" sciences (i.e., clinical psychology, psychiatry). Individuals can have "substance abuse disorders" where patterns of use interfere with their motivation and therefore everyday life (Cheetham et al., 2010;

In psychiatry, substance-related disorders are operationalized in a specific way in the *DSM-5*, the *Diagnostic and Statistical Manual of Mental Disorders, Fifth Edition*. It outlines the classes of drugs associated with substance-related disorders, including but not limited to alcohol, cannabis, hallucinogens, opioids, and stimulants (e.g., cocaine). The symptoms and diagnostic features of illnesses and pathological behaviours that constitute substance-related disorders are also described. Psychiatry draws on medical research that has established that using these substances activates the brain's reward system (see also below), leading to reinforcement of behaviours and facilitating the construction of memory; the activation produced by using substances produces the corresponding feeling of a "high" (*DSM-5*, 2013). However, whereas some disorders in the *DSM-5* fit the definition of "disease" – a problem that impairs functioning and is primarily biologically caused – notably, addiction does not.

In clinical psychology, it is understood that while addiction is understood as an illness that is also linked to dysregulation, Cheetham et al. (2010) observe that addiction is bound up with individuals' experiences and emotions. They also note that individuals who are diagnosed with affective psychopathology (e.g., mood and anxiety disorders) demonstrate high rates of comorbid substance abuse disorders. Said differently, emotional distress further prompts substance abuse. The emphasis on comorbidity of substance use disorders and other physical and mental health problems is widely recognized (see, for example, WHO, 2004). Adults with comorbid substance abuse disorders may suffer a myriad of mental health problems and problems with psychosocial functioning that can be complex to treat (Kelly et al., 2012).

In psychology, other psychological and social-cultural factors are understood as constitutive of and related to addiction, placing more emphasis on individuals' wrestling with these multiple factors productive of their substance use problems and often through talk therapy.

Psychologists Hill and Leeming (2014), for example, focused their research on "the self" and personal habits of those who defined as "addicts" (i.e., loss of control over substance use) and in recovery. They found that all participants struggled with overcoming a stigmatizing "addict" identity despite their years of sobriety. Participants felt they were perceived by others as having little education, a lack of will power, loss of morals, and being "unstable."

Health Canada (2023) outlines an approach and understanding of substance use as a spectrum, moving from non-use on one end of the spectrum and addiction or substance use disorder on the other. Substance use disorder is defined as a pattern of use that persists despite an individual's awareness of the negative consequences that follow with their use, such as failure to fulfil major roles at work, school, or home and continued use despite social or interpersonal problems caused or intensified by alcohol or drugs (see also Pearson et al., 2013). Noteworthy is how Health Canada (2023) observes substance use disoder as a treatable condition that impacts the brain. Other negative consequences for the individual using include substance dependence, increased tolerance, and risk of withdrawl. Reith (2004) reminds us that the WHO re-defined addiction in 1964 as "dependency" to shift attention to individuals' needs and subjective evaluation of their "loss of control" as key to their being diagnosed. The Centre for Addiction and Mental Health (CAMH) defines addiction by the four Cs: Craving; loss of Control of amount or frequency of use; Compulsion to use; and use despite Consequences (CAMH, 2020). It recognizes that substance use can create physical dependence, but dependence itself does not imply addiction (CAMH, 2023). Statistics Canada's 2012 Community Health Survey on mental health endeavoured to uncover the degree to which Canadians experience substance use disorders. Employing the WHO Composite International Diagnostic Interview (a standardized instrument used to assess substance use disorders as per the *DSM-4*) led to the estimate that substance use disorders affect six million Canadians, with males understood as more likely affected than females (Statistics Canada, 2013).

Neuroscientific research firmly establishes addiction as a brain disease. Drug seeking, consumption, withdrawal, and relapse are understood in the broader neurobiological context of the dopamine reward system, which then affects perceptual, emotional, and motivational process of the brain (Buchman et al., 2010). This brain disease is seen as chronic, often relapsing, and characterized by compulsive drug seeking and use with impairments in social and occupational functioning (Schwabe et al., 2011).

Scholarship that advances this neurobiological understanding has been recognized to give rise to the possibility of reducing societal stigma towards addiction (Buchman et al., 2011; Fraser et al., 2017). An understanding of addiction as a brain disease, for example, allows for people struggling with substance use to receive the same level of compassion and access to health care services as those living with other diseases, and possible changes in policy and legal responses (Buchman et al., 2011). However, while a brain disease model legitimizes addiction as a medical condition and reduces the responsibilization of people for their "bad" choices, it can promote neuro-essentialist thinking. It can remove an awareness of the psychological factors, agency, and social context involved in substance use outlined earlier, and therefore undermine an understanding of the complexity of developing an addiction (Buchman et al., 2010, 2011). While loss of control over the amount of substances used, their duration of use, or compulsion to use are symptoms of addiction (or dependency) for many (CAMH, 2020; WHO, 2020), Buchman et al. (2010) caution over how neurobiological understandings of addiction can ensure loss of control is no longer any part of an individual's responsibility.

The distinction between the psychiatric disorder and disease model of addiction are complex. Not all scholars (or service providers) share the opinion that addiction is a brain disease alone or is created by a disorder of the mind. While the cause of addiction is highly debatable across disciplines, consensus does seem to have emerged in terms of the individual behaviours and patterns that are seen to constitute addiction, especially the aforementioned loss of control and/or dependence.

Our exposure to these biomedical explanations may conflict with our own individualistic, social and even moral explanations of addiction (e.g., drug use is a personal choice; people chose to socialize with the wrong crowd). Besides the medical model of addiction, Erickson and Callaghan (2005) maintain that the moral view of addiction continues to be pervasive and places the onus of blame for substance dependence squarely onto the shoulders of individuals who voluntarily chose to use. Campbell (2010) adds that there continues to seem an incommensurability between claims that addiction is a matter of individual choice and claims that it is a neurochemical disorder disruptive of volition. She contends that while figuring out "what's going on in the brain" is foundational work, neuroscience should place more attention on the social-situational contexts and relationships within which addictions are experienced. In many ways, the sociological study featured in this book is exactly that: a focus on the social relations that persons who define as living with addiction experience.

The social as it connects to addiction does seem to be of some focus, too, across disciplines other than sociology; if certain behaviours and actions are defined as addiction, or if suggestions are made to improve the disease model of understanding, such as those above. I can remember one specific example of how the social relations of addiction are present in broader discourse while I was undertaking the research for this book. On 24 October 2018, I was listening to Metro Morning (the CBC Radio morning show in Toronto) while hurriedly driving to the train station to then get to the university campus. Dr. Diane Rothen was being interviewed by (then) host Matt Golloway about a new addictions program, ALAViDA, that administered medication to those with an alcohol addiction in order to inhibit their pleasure responses from alcohol and aid in their recovery. Once parked, I spent a few precious minutes quickly jotting down information about the interview so I could return to the recording/transcript because of Dr. Rothen's statement: "drinking is a learned behaviour, it is learned … people lose control over time." I was intrigued by the scientific, medicalized response of ALAViDA being partially informed by an understanding of the socialization of drinking.

Sociologically Speaking

As I first indicated in this book's Introduction, I am not interested in assigning the cause of addiction to the brain, individual choice, or the social environment alone. I review the literature above to establish the breadth of interdisciplinary scholarship on addiction and as a point of departure for the sociologizing of addiction I endeavour to undertake in this book. Here, I shift away from the scientific and medicalized attention to addiction towards showing that addiction as researched and theorized in sociology has an interesting past and a still-growing future. The sociology of addiction or substance use is not, I dare say, a full and historically defined area of inquiry and remains rather ambiguous at the time of my writing this book. According to Weinberg (2011, p. 298), not all sociologists study addiction as the "putative enslavement to a substance" as Lindesmith (1938) did, whom he calls "the father of addiction." Instead, there is constant slippage towards studying addiction as deviant or a disapproved activity. I admit, I am more interested in the latter because it resonates with my study's focus on social relations.

My first exposure to studying drug or alcohol addiction was in sociology and criminology undergraduate courses I completed in the 1990s, where substance use was introduced as deviant behaviour. This was before Bendle's (1999) article "The Death of the Sociology of Deviance" but years after Becker's (1953) "Becoming a Marihuana User" article. The idea of drug use especially and alcohol use potentially as deviant has strong roots in sociology. For example, if deviance is understood as Becker (1963) defines it, as a violation of social norms, then any behaviour that strays from the norm can be potentially deviant. Since the requirement of sobriety, alongside rationality and autonomy, invades many aspects of daily life (Fraser et al., 2017; Room, 2011), using substances to alter this sobriety can therefore be thought of as deviant. The "addict"engages in behaviour and a lifestyle in stark contrast to the social norms of mainstream society (Järvinen & Miller, 2010). The addicted person transgresses the management of alcohol or drug use in ways that are socially approved and may ingest substances that are illicit or illegal (regarding criminal law), both of which inhibit rule-abiding behaviour. Becker (1963) was clear that social groups and relations construct what is normative and what is therefore deviant by contrast; so, for Becker, actions like using alcohol or drugs in and of themselves were not deviant. Long before West (2001) maintained addiction is socially defined, Becker (1963) argued that even what is deviant is socially defined.

Sumner (1994), in his text *The Sociology of Deviance: An Obituary*, argued that the sociology of deviance died in 1975. For Sumner and others, established theories of deviance, including those applied to problematic substance use, were too relativist or rooted in behaviourism. These theories seemed to fall apart in view of post-modern and post-structural thought that deconstructed the very notion of "the social" and "society" and so the mainstream, or idea of universal social norms to which persons were to abide. As Bendle (1999) writes, confidence in the theorizing the sociology of deviance was also lost, for example, by disagreement as to whether the focus should be on the behaviour as deviant or what socially constitutes deviant behaviour (the latter being Becker's interest) and the inability to pinpoint causality of deviant behaviour. As to whether "deviance is dead" or has the resonance it once did in sociology, this is still a matter of debate. The continued relevance of perceiving some substance use as deviant behaviour, drug use in particular persists and may in part be because the buying and selling of illicit drugs has not been decriminalized in Canada. Notwithstanding the legalization of cannabis consumption, procuring or creating illicit drugs as a business and profiting from it is still in contravention of social norms and criminal law. As well, some research on the prison industrial complex continues in the vein of the sociology of deviance (see, for example, Bendle, 1999).

While somewhat of a digression, this brief foray into the sociology of deviance provides some context for then understanding how, if addiction is not seen as deviance, is there a sociology of addiction, as Weinberg (2011) maintains there is? Or a sociology of substance use? Part of the difficulty in pinpointing how addiction is understood in sociology is that scholars, like in other sciences and social sciences, use addiction interchangeably with other terms like substance use, overuse, problem use, (drug) misuse and (drug) abuse, and deviant drug use (Järvinen & Miller, 2010; Weinberg, 2011). It seems that, in general, the sociology of addiction emphasizes social relations as shaping drug or alcohol addiction and/or as interspersed in patterns of individual use. Weinberg's (2011) review of sociological literature led him to conclude that many theories of addiction (e.g., symbolic interactionist, social constructionist, and even in a way functionalism) see it as a condition that is influenced by social forces and the wider society. Peralta and Jauk (2011), for example, theorize how the social construction of excessive alcohol consumption involves its association with masculinity and violence. They argue that this construction confirms how substance-related problems materialize through societal power structures and gendered sources. And yet, since sociology has such far-reaching scope, what is being made to be the sociology of addiction or substance use seems limitless in scope. I outline only a few directions here. Some sociologists intentionally make a deliberate move away from the language of addiction. I note, for example, the edited volume *The Sociology of American Drug Use*, now in its third edition, in which Faupel et al. (2013) are careful to unpack how use itself has been problematized over time. Other scholars are concerned with the social construction of substance use as that of addiction.

Reith (2004) traces the "birth of the addict" as a distinct and deviant identity to late nineteenth-century discourse construed by the medical profession in relation to the industrial nation-state. In this medical-moral discourse, addiction was a disease of the will and the "addict" one "whose consumption was characterized by frenzied craving, repetition, and loss of control" (p. 289). Today, addiction is an uncomfortable part of the paradox of Western society; it sits awkwardly amid the values of freedom and autonomy and choice associated with consumerism and oppositional discourses that curtail these very principles. That is, while addiction and "addict" identities have been historically constructed through some discourses (on par with Foucault's analytic of the discursive constitution of subjects), other broader contours of the market economy continue to encourage individuals' consumption with abandon (Reith, 2004, p. 284). Reith asks us to see addiction as a product (or object) of discursive social relations: addiction is "a discursive device that transmits the notion of disordered consumption, and that articulates a sense of loss of control; a subordination of personal agency to some external or unwilled mechanism" (p. 286). The importance of Reith's geneaological analysis of the making up of addiction cannot be understated. Related argumentation is taken up by others. Bourgois (2000, p. 167), for example, maintains that addiction disciplines bodies. Methadone maintenance as treatment and in place of heroin use is Foucaultian biopower at work. The state has defined methadone use and heroin use as different – one is medicine, the other a drug – to socially control and govern the pleasure and productivity of bodies (Bourgois, 2000).

While conceptualizations of addiction today may diverge in so many ways, biomedical and sociological ones still seem to converge around one historicized marker of "addict" behaviour: loss of control. Piennar et al. (2010) note that discussions of addiction in general often contain narratives of social and individual harm, loss of control, autonomy and free will, and these narratives all relate to the modern neoliberal subject. Reith (2004, p. 286) further analyzes contradictions in freedom for the neoliberal subject who is an "addict" in noting that the individual is no longer "realizing the self through consumption but is consumed by consumption; the 'addict' is forced to consume." Järvinen and Miller's (2010) study of persons addicted to methadone illustrates how when addiction is constructed as a condition where the individual is not free or autonomous in decision-making, the individual then becomes viewed as irrational and unable to manage risks to themselves or others. People can then find themselves in circumstances that are self-fulfilling: they come to see their addictive behaviours to resemble life through the neoliberal lens of potential risk and harm, which in turn, leaves them to feel socially excluded and isolated (Järvinen & Miller, 2010).

In the risk and governmentality literature more popular in critical criminology, neoliberalism has also been theorized to produce a particular conceptualization of the "criminal addict" and their subjectivity. Moore (2007) argues that whereas the "addict" was a pathological substance abuser under what they term welfarism, neoliberal restructuring of the criminal justice system (e.g., privatization, funding cuts) has produced a rational choice subject that errs in judgment. When substance use is constructed as individual choice, responses are directed at teaching and reforming the individual through treatment specifying non-use. Said differently, neoliberalism creates opportunities for the governance of the drug user as a normal subject of government (O'Malley, 2004). Whenever drug and alcohol consumption become a social problem, it is no longer about simple pleasure seeking but is associated with irrational and compulsive behaviour, with individual physical and mental pathology, that conflicts with (neo) liberal governance and assumptions of responsibility, rationality, and independence (O'Malley & Valverde, 2004).

Drawing in other sociological concepts, some scholars theorize substance use behaviour as socialized, mirroring views held by many of us, including Dr. Rothen, mentioned above. Just as we learn to "fit in" and conform to the broader social norms and mores of society over time, we can learn to use alcohol or drugs. In 1953, Becker theorized that in becoming a marijuana user, one had to learn the behaviour from others: the technique, the effects, and the enjoyment of the effects. Becker (1955) also wrote that deviant behaviour comes into being through the breakdown of social controls, which often happens in subcultures. Linking drug use to subcultural norms continues today, though some call for the retirement of this connation since drug users and practices have diversified to such an extent (Moore, 2004). Still, research continues to emphasize the learning of use through social interaction. For example, Oetting and Donnermeyer (1998, p. 998) argue that adolescent drug use stems from peoples' weak social bonds with primary agents of socialization (e.g., family, schools, peers) that teach conformity to social norms.

In a quite popular and debatable conceptualization of substance use, Parker et al. (1998, 2002) and others argue that use has been normalized among youth in particular. Normalization here refers to the incorporation of elements of "deviant" behaviour previously marginalized into the mainstream or everyday "normal" life. Based on their study of British youth culture in the 1990s, Parker et al. (1998) argue that youths' recreational use of illicit drugs – cannabis use at the time of their study – has been accepted as a normal part of youth interaction. Others have explored how the use of club drugs has become normalized within club culture (e.g., the EDM or rave scene) (Kelly, 2006; Sanders, 2005). In some ways, the normalization thesis fits in well with the death of deviance arguments outlined earlier. Parker et al.'s work has also done much to push the shift towards the language of "user" rather than "addict" and even connects to harm-reduction arguments, as we will see much later in this book.

Before I continue, a quick exercise of foreshadowing is important here. I can see how as they are revealed the findings of this study may be read as implying a variation of the "make drug use normal" argument. And, if not just recreational use but substance use dependency is normalized, this may even feed into an argument for improved harm-reduction services and de-stigmatization of use too. However, the argument I will develop throughout this book is different. The people I interviewed were adults, many of whom had experienced distinct and negative events in their life courses that confirmed that in wider

Canadian society their substance use was not normalized. For example, they had been incarcerated for drug dealing or their children were involuntarily relinquished from their care by child welfare officials because of their patterns of use. Instead of normalizing use, I argue that my findings permit the development of the understanding that living with addiction is but one facet of a complex self with limitless potential. It may impact any one of us over a life course writ large. My findings are the impetus for me to invite others to re-imagine how our societal responses to living with addiction may be transformed and through the sharing of hope.

Thus far, it is clear that social relations are constitutive of addiction, whether the emphasis is on the problem being constructed or the social relations as partially shaping addictive behaviour. I want to now turn to a review of literature that establishes these social relations as interspersed in patterns of individual use. Research in sociology does emphasize the experience of or feelings associated with alcohol and drug use. Addiction may be best and ultimately located within subjective criteria and subjective evaluation of loss of control (Reith, 2004). In sociology, there is growth in scholarship that situates this subjective sense of addiction socially, by attending to how individuals identify with or resist the "addict" identity or addicted body constructed by others and discourse.

For Järvinen and Miller (2010), addiction is not simply agentically chosen but also something that is suffered as a disjuncture between a person and their social environment. Participants in their study felt that those who have never used substances keep drug and alcohol users at a distance and that their difficulty in making friends with non-users was related to how people view users as to be avoided and not trustworthy. This suffering can then be part of a "process of loss, hopelessness and non-becoming" (p. 817). Weinberg's (2011) years of research with drug and alcohol users led him to conclude that they did not uniformly depict their use as a self-governed activity and often characterized it as deeply troubling and associated with their mysterious loss of self-control. Individuals can further associate using substances with feelings of guilt, shame, disgust, and self-loathing when they consider the harm to self and others that coincides with their substance use. Hughes's (2007) qualitative interviews with current or past heroin users revealed how grafting (i.e., doing crime to purchase drugs) could produce their feelings of shame, particularly because their grafting was of friends or family. Besides engaging in criminal activity, individuals who use substances uncontrollably may neglect personal hygiene or neglect family members (Nettleton et al., 2011). Living with addiction transforms social networks too. Hughes (2007) also found that when heroin users become caught up in "chaotic use," a six- to twelve-hour cycle around their obtaining and using the drug, their engagement with non-users dissipated. They had little or no contact with family members or friends and could experience joblessness and homelessness (Hughes, 2007). Family members' or a friend's lack of understanding about the experience of using can also contribute to users' feelings of isolation (Dassieu et al., 2020; Hughes, 2007).

Meanwhile, alongside research that highlights suffering, the concept of pleasure has been reclaimed in the study of the subjective and embodied experience of drug use and largely from a post-modern/post-structural perspective. Duff (2008), for example, takes umbrage with how medical discourses can assume that pleasure is produced only in "recreational" drug use and that "problematic" use is devoid of pleasure. They argue for the need to focus on drugs as experience, of being and doing and becoming, accompanied with an understanding of pleasure as emergent and developed within specific contexts. Emphasis can be on "the kinds of practices and experiences drugs facilitate, as well as the ways these drugs make one feel" (Duff, 2008, p. 391). Researchers nonetheless observe the tensions brought forth by focusing on pleasure. The larger fear is that to recognize pleasure in problematic use would mean that suffering is invalidated (Dennis, 2019) or to encourage the use of drugs (Malins, 2017).

Other research that can be generally thought of as part of the PWUD movement also embraces the subjectivity and experience of "people who use drugs" and, if not focusing on pleasure, critically disrupts the limitations of perspective that have been created in the construction and study of addiction. As someone who has not shared in the substance-using experiences of those I sought to interview and my knowledge often clouded by academic discourse, the politics of this shift in meaning of substance use resonates with me. Rudzinski et al. (2017) argue against the tendency in the broader academic literature to portray drug use as synonymous with lack of skills or potential. They establish the importance of acknowledging the strengths and accomplishments of people who use drugs and recommend a strength-based resilience lens in research with PWUD. Research with crack cocaine users, for example, shows that they may face the greatest adversity and victimization as drug users but are active participants in their surroundings and skilled at navigating life on the street. They can report joy in daily successes and hope for their futures (see, for example, Ribeiro et al., 2010; Windsor et al., 2011), a finding I echo in the big story I share and the argumentation I pursue in this book.

By embracing individuals' understandings of their use, opportunities for learning and unlearning are created. For example, the history of colonization, including the ongoing intergenerational harms of residential schools, becomes understood as connected with the present inequalities experienced by Indigenous PWUD (Barker et al., 2019). The gendered context experienced by PWUD is revealed in the ways women who inject drugs (WWID) are stereotyped as passive victims with harmful negative interactional and societal consequences then created (Gibson & Hutton, 2021). Ti et al. (2012) are clear in stating that the only way to create stronger and informed health policy and programs for PWUD is to involve them in the very design of policies and programs for them. Collins et al. (2017) further argue for a shift in research practice itself. Instead of researcher–participant, if researchers view their studies as transactional, this creates space for PWUD to assert some power over the research process. They find that PWUD enact agency and power and manage others' stigmatization of them when they assume the role of expert for which compensation is seen as equitable.

I think it useful to end this section with a further refinement of my choice to use the language of "living with addiction" in my study and this book, especially given the inclusive scholarship I have reviewed above and how I conclude on the promise of hope associated with the de-stigmatization of addiction. In other research, I have met people on OW who self-define as having an addiction to substances, whether drugs or alcohol. Thus, when I set out to do this study, I took on this language too. I also began my study knowing that social assistance policy constructs categories of claimants in the determination of eligibility and administration of benefits, including rules and regulations coinciding with these. Moreover, one of my main contributions in this book is to show how people living with multiple barriers, and therefore living with addiction, are one of these such categories in Ontario social assistance policy or, as I reveal, became and are an object of OW discourse. As time passed in doing the actual research and writing this book, I became more critically aware of the limits of my choice. I think Lofland (1973, p. 15) best elucidated why I chose to retain the language of "living with addiction," know and accept its limits, and endeavoured to critically engage with them too. Over five decades ago, he wrote: "Analytic distinctions and definitions are intended to create clarity out of the confusion of reality. To the extent they are successful, to that extent 'reality' has been distorted. Nonetheless, they are indispensable intellectual tools, the sine qua non of human thought." To be clear, I wanted to establish conceptual boundaries on my work. Simultaneously, I deliberately sought to understand how OW policy used the language of addiction and how caseworkers applied it, including in their relationships with benefit recipients. Moreover, while I approached my study as one about "living with addiction," I did so while still questioning this "reality" and caring exactly about trying to create space in conversations for participants to identify with or resist or subvert policy, caseworkers, and still others' constructions of addiction and the limiting of their lives to the "addict" identity alone.

Knowing Addiction Intimately

As Reith (2004, p. 292) writes, "despite its status as a discursive object, the whole idea of 'addiction' nevertheless becomes something 'real' for those who subscribe to its deterministic influence." To conclude this chapter, I deliberately switch the analytical gaze from what is made known in existing research, to how living with addiction is known and perceived by those who identify with it and are accessing OW. In interviews when I raised the question "How do you define addiction?" I learned:

Painful. Time consuming. The devil period. *Charise*

Oh, if it's crack, the devil. *Bianca*

It just ruins everything in its path. It's all consuming. It will own you. *Trevor*

Using something and not having the choice whether you want to use it or not. Because it's something that's in your body I guess, and your body cries out for it. So, to me it's not something you just quit. Your body is dictating. *Shawn*

Physically, mentally, emotionally, everything. Every fucking one of them. Just everything. When you're an addict, your whole world is consumed by it, right? *Dante*

It just consumes everything – and anything about your life ... you'll sacrifice or sabotage anything, just for the addiction. Regardless of what the addiction is. *Adrienne*

It means that you will spend your time fighting. Without trying to fight to get up and keep the little bit that you have, like you lose everything. You lose your family. You lose good friends. You lose your place to live. Like, you just lose. *Tara*

For the people I interviewed who were randomly using or identified as in recovery, addiction was not universally knowable. Any definition given was purely experientially constructed and emotionally embodied but, collectively, seemed to coalesce around three themes. Addiction is:

(1)   an internal or external force to be reckoned
(2)   the consumption of the self
(3)   a loss of social relations

Given that Bianca overcame a crack cocaine addiction and Charise still randomly used crack when I met her, it is possible both women were referring to crack with its synonym slang name of devil. And yet, even adopting this image of the devil made it seem that, for them, addiction is a force external (perhaps also supernatural, see Szott, 2017) to the individual; it is threatening to the self. Desiring to consume a substance and feeling consumed by this desire suggest a battle of mind and body (see also Reith, 2004). Shawn invoked a tension-filled mind–body dualism in conveying that, in his view, in the internal war with a substance of choice, the mind of the individual seems to lose to the body. Of all participants, Shawn was the most closely aligned with a biomedical explanation. Shawn's view also seems to lend credence to Weinberg's (2011) caution that sociologists must not forget the involuntary enactment of embodied use. For Dante and Adrienne, however, it seemed that the self in its entirety is consumed by addiction such that the mind–body binary dissolves. Meanwhile, Trevor and Tara equate addiction with loss: the person using loses their sense of self and especially the self in relationship with others. Tara especially hints at how the self is made up of multiple identities (e.g., mother, friend). Identities can be fractured, hollowed out, or even destroyed when using substances.

In the remaining parts of this book, I adopt these definitions of addiction that OW benefit recipients shared. I assumed their understandings of how they lived their addiction, how they gave meaning to addiction individually and socially, or how they "made up" what is addiction for themselves based on their personal experiences with substances, others, and policy discourse. And I hold these assumptions in most of my writing about persons "living with addiction." There is one exception in Part 2. I leave more room for other and different interpretation when I explore how living with addiction was and is constructed as an object of OW policy discourse and practice in chapter 5. Finally, I acknowledge that sometimes I also use the language of "substance use dependency" in the remaining parts of this book when it seemingly captured the experiences of the people I interviewed.

PART TWO

Lives as Lived

4 Becoming a Substance User

It was in asking people questions about their childhood and adolescence that I heard stories that called into focus significant behaviours, interactions, and events that were tied to their first use of substances. In this chapter, I thematically trace out the becoming of a person who uses drugs or alcohol and eventually develops a sense of their self as having a problem with or being addicted to substances. Through participants' narratives, I highlight their social relationships with others, including family and friends, as well as their emergent relationships with the substances they used. I present a tentative typology based on these themes, which suggests that there is more than one process involved in the becoming of a substance user. While different and unique to each of them, participants' stories of becoming coalesced into one major finding of my research: no one wills their experience of addiction.

I ask readers to acknowledge three interrelated caveats here. First, I spend time providing some backstory and a brief demographic profile for each participant who is a benefit recipient when I first introduce them and their experiences in this chapter or in others; Appendix D is meant as a "cheat sheet" recapping this information and for further reference. Second, while I group stories by themes in this chapter, I caution that I do not see these themes as single causes of problematic substance use. Noteworthy is how Ontario Works (OW) benefit recipients could draw on two storylines or more in telling the story of their becoming a user, a phenomenon reflected by quotes from their interview categorized into more than one theme. Third, in my discussion of becoming a substance user, I do not adopt the convention of "pathways" of becoming, as seen in scholarship on pathways of drug use (see, for example, Richardson et al., 2016). I instead offer a typology and intend for it to clearly and sociologically illustrate why any individual's problems with substance use cannot be limited to pathology and must be historically, structurally, and socially contextualized.

Behaviours, Interactions, Events

Trauma[1]

The World Encyclopedia (2014, np) defines trauma as: "Any injury or physical damage caused by some external event such as an accident or assault. In psychiatry, the term is applied to an emotional shock or harrowing experience." In *Trauma and Its Wake*, Figley (1985) observes that the term stems from the original Greek meaning of the word "wound" and defines trauma as "an emotional state of discomfort and stress resulting from memories of an extraordinary, catastrophic experience which shattered the survivor's sense of invulnerability to harm" (p. xviii).

Definitions of trauma, however, are notably absent in sociological dictionaries. When taken up, scholars seem to draw from its conceptualization and treatment in psychiatry, developed through the work of "trauma pioneers" who completed research on survivors of child abuse, the Holocaust, rape, and combat zones and war (Figley, 2006). Dena T. Smith's (2011) more recent sociological conceptualization of trauma is useful here. She describes trauma as felt and exhibited as individuals' suffering, including mental illness, after their experiencing and surviving events (e.g., personal injury or threat of injury; witnessing others' death or injury, or perceiving threat of either to others) external to them. These events or traumatic stressors may yield symptoms that can be diagnosed as posttraumatic stress disorder, or PTSD (Smith, 2011). I further heed Comas-Diaz et al.'s (2019) articulation of racial trauma as related to but different from PTSD, inclusive of perceived threats of, or actual harm caused by, injury, humiliation, and shame, or witnessing of any of the above, and as experienced specifically by people of colour and Indigenous persons.

I heard participants tell stories of past events and experiences that seemed traumatic and productive of their suffering in some way. However, I do not argue trauma as the only cause of substance use dependency experienced by participants, nor can I categorize any participant as suffering PTSD. My interest lies in how some participants shared trauma narratives that were meaningful to them in their reflections about their emerging substance use or their perception of their

---

1 Readers are asked to take care in reading, feeling, and understanding the stories of trauma some participants shared in reflecting upon how they came to use substances.

development of an addiction. In my interpretation of these stories, I observe Smith's (2011) suggestion that a sociologically nuanced understanding of suffering and trauma is necessary to move away from the medical model of psychiatry and its tendency to dominate understandings of suffering with biological explanations. Thus, I endeavour to further understand participants' trauma and therefore suffering as linked to social structures (as likely to be produced through certain social conditions) (see also Smith, 2011), or vis-à-vis the sociological imagination, the connection between personal troubles and public issues.

Death. When I first connected with Alexei on the phone, he seemed ambivalent about my request to meet: "We can meet if you want to. Or not. It's okay." We agreed to meet at a coffee shop in north Toronto. A white man with startling blue eyes and short greying hair, Alexei wore a jogging (or athleisure) suit and gold chain around his neck. He was forty-seven years old, fit, and single. He had been divorced from the mother of his son, who had full custody, for over ten years. I learned that Alexei had immigrated to Canada from the Soviet Union (now Russia) in the early 1990s while he was in his early twenties. Alexei was open and honest about his patterns of heroin use and being in and out of treatment or pursuing sobriety at different moments in his life; he was still using heroin when we met. As we neared the end of our interview, we were discussing how his father continues to offer him support emotionally and financially. I had already kept Alexei talking for an hour and before wrapping up, I quickly thought to ask about his relationship with his mother. The first two lines of the quoted excerpt should be read as us talking over each other:

ALEXEI: Yeah, it was a long time ago, but yeah, it was good relationship.
AMBER: We're at the end [of the interview].
ALEXEI: When I was in treatment, they told me that maybe I have this thing, why I'm using and stuff, we were sharing past experience and stuff – when I was sixteen, we got into the car accident. My father let me drive the car. At that time, I didn't have driver's license, so we had accident and my mother died.
AMBER: Oh, I'm so sorry. And you were driving.
ALEXEI: Yeah, so I kind of felt guilt.

I remember feeling dumbstruck by Alexei's sudden disclosure and did not know what to do but offer sympathy. I could not help but immediately wonder in that moment: how does a life unfold after such an event and at such a young age? Alexei claimed he was in the process of coming to see the accident as somehow linked to his use. In their qualitative study, Chapple et al. (2015) found that when a person loses someone to a violent death, such as that created by a road crash like what Alexei experienced, they may question the acceptability of their grief, especially when they perceive an element of responsibility for the death. Chapple et al. (2015) further note that, for the person left behind, deaths associated with guilt, shame, or responsibility are especially burdensome. Alexei's brief story of how a complete shattering of family relations might link to substance use was but one of many that I had trouble letting go and why I rarely interviewed more than one person a week.

Trevor, age twenty-six, also seemed to experience trauma associated with the death of several people in his life over a short period of time. Trevor identified as single, using methadone and in recovery, and had been on and off OW for about six years prior. Trevor recalled: "A bunch of my family members, they all passed away. Like within the same year. And that's when I started using." Before this time, Trevor had been going to college, had a girlfriend, and had an entrepreneurial spirit. He was taking courses in business and had been developing a business opportunity with a friend. Though his own parents were not wealthy, as a young, white man with business acumen and direction, the future seemed bright. Trevor explained how his life unfolded quite differently. I present quite lengthy excerpts from my interview with Trevor to highlight his own suffering over and processing of these deaths and their connections to his use for him.

> TREVOR: And during the time I was in college, my mom and dad, they, we had to move out of the place we were living in because they hadn't been paying rent because my dad was an addict. So, we were living in this really small bachelor apartment with my grandma. Like, so I couldn't go to school, right? Because I had to make money because I was living like at the foot of my grandma's bed, right? So, my dad ended up dying. We ended up finding him dead in his bed.
> AMBER: Oh my god. I am so sorry.
> TREVOR: Naw, naw, it's okay. So, and then, after he passed away, then my mom started using a lot of drugs.... And I was taking the odd Percocet [combination pill of acetaminophen and oxycodone] or what have you, hey.
> AMBER: Yeah, like prescription?
> TREVOR: Because my grandma, who I was staying with, she was really sick. And she had lots of the prescriptions. So, and then a few months after that, my cousin who I grew up with.... She ended up dying in a car accident like five months after that.... And that's when my addiction for me really spiraled out of control.... And then my grandma died like six months after that. So, all of them, boom! Dead.

Our exchange confirms Trevor's perception of his emergent addiction as *that* dramatic. Considering his social and financial situation, he saw these deaths and the pressure to earn money as not only directly contributing to his use, but his escalation of use, from OxyContin to heroin, as well. That is, drugs cost money. Experiencing suffering and then not having money to purchase a drug of choice to mitigate this suffering can lead to changes in use patterns and unintended consequences, including the ingestion of an illicit and higher-risk drug. Trevor explained: "So one OxyContin, one like 80, is $80. For one pill. You know. Whereas ah, a bag of heroin, like a gram of heroin, is like $80."

Gendered Trauma. I heard stories of gendered trauma that could evoke strong emotions among some women I interviewed – and correspondingly within me – even years after the events happened. This gendered trauma specifically stemmed from their experiences of, sometimes not mutually exclusive, reproductive challenges, rape, and other forms of gender-based violence. My findings echo research that has observed that women's substance use can be linked to past experiences of victimization, notably sexual assault, pregnancy loss, and intimate partner violence (Gueta & Addad, 2013; Martin, 2010; Testa et al., 2003). Though the women I interviewed did not make a definitive causal connection between their experience of gendered trauma and substance dependency, they saw their trauma as somehow linked to their escalating use over time.

I met Smitri as she was finishing up her participation in Drug Treatment Court, a program that alleged offenders can complete in lieu of jail time for drug-related offences. Introducing herself as a forty-three-year-old Jamaican and Caucasian woman and mother of three children in the care of her own mother, Smitri was beautifully "put together" in her presentation of self (e.g., her hairstyle, clothing, carefully applied make-up). Her warm and self-assured presence drew me in and did wonders to ease my concern that she might find our meeting at an OW office uncomfortable. My interview with Smitri was one that I let take shape organically. While I approached all interviews in a semi-structured way, I found I could not ask as many questions of Smitri as I would have liked. We instead spent most of our hour and a half following the stories she wanted to tell, regardless of the question asked. After I shared that we would speak about her history of use, beginning with her childhood and growing up, it was clear that she had a way of approaching our conversation through sharing, in her own words, "little flashbacks." Smitri recalled that at age thirteen, she was raped by several men.

> Full grown-assed men.... And this one particular day I remember lying to my mom ... "I'll tell my mom that I'm sleeping over," but I knew we were

going to this adult dance kind of thing.... And I thought I'd be sleeping over with my friend, but the older sister dropped her little sister home and said, "you can come with me." They bring me back to this after-hours place where all these guys resided that I knew.... And they started feeding me vodka with rum with wine.... And I was so embarrassed to even tell them I felt sick.... The one guy said, "you can lie in the basement" and brought me to the basement. [I] fall asleep and I woke up, pitch dark and there's somebody on top of me, helping themselves to me … and I never told anybody I was so embarrassed.... [W]hen I was sixteen, one of my boyfriend's brother-in-law, older guy, heard about it … And that's when he told me it was five guys who had actually just taken their turns with me and I caught the last one.... All these years I did not know that. So, I remember going home that particular day when I was informed of this. My mom was drinking wine and I was late. "Really sorry I'm late mom but I have something to tell you...." "I was raped by 5 men...." I don't think she cried or cared or anything.

I struggle with Smitri's story every time I revisit it and even read it on the page. I am taken back to our interview and remember how we both sat quietly with this story immediately after Smitri shared it. I am still overcome with emotion when I recall our moment of silently honoring Smitri's suffering and her resilience and fortitude of spirit.

At the time of our interview, Smitri seemed to be puzzling a loose connection between this trauma and how easy it seemed for her to later turn to crack cocaine. She shared another "flashback" about one day after school when she was fourteen: "Some guy came on the school yard and introduced me to crack. Lured me with it. I went with him. I was supposed to go on the school bus, and I went with this random stranger." Indeed, Smitri seemed to be coming to terms with how her experience of trauma at such a young age somehow connected to her subsequent life choices and chances. I wonder too, but cannot know, if her mother's reaction to her sharing about her experience of gendered and racialized sexual violence is somehow layered into how her life course unfolded thereafter.

Adrienne lived as a single mother with her seventeen-year-old son when I met her at her spacious apartment. A white woman, thirty-three years old, she self-defined as nine months sober. Adrienne had an open and relaxed presentation of self, a languidness to her movements that sometimes jarred with how quickly she spoke in conversation with me. As we sank into her comfortable couch, she told me that she was actively pursuing recovery from an opioid addiction with a suboxone treatment program and one-on-one counselling. Adrienne recalled an earlier experience of miscarriage during her adolescence as a profoundly frightening time and connected this event with her opioid use over several years.

> I had a miscarriage at fifteen and didn't even know I was pregnant. My parents don't even know.... I told my dad, obviously "call the ambulance" thing.... I just had really, really, really bad cramps and just like, really bad bleeding and – but I'm pretty sure the doctor knew when I had the exam. Like, clearly the doctor's gonna tell.... I felt bad about it, but then I was like, I didn't know what to do, so I kinda just, obviously, ya know, self-medicated with that issue there.

Adrienne had a way of telling her story so evocatively that I felt like we had both stepped back in time through her recollection. Of course, I could not perfectly feel what she felt or see what she saw. I was an outsider, someone looking in on her memories. However, I could appreciate her fear and the worry she had about telling someone about her miscarriage. Having had a miscarriage, and remembering how I felt at the time, I can perceive the emotional burden it would have been for Adrienne to carry the experience with her without receiving emotional support from others; I felt I could understand her use of substances as a coping strategy.

On a very rainy fall day, I drove to midtown Toronto to meet Tynesha at a McDonald's near to where she was living, to sit and chat over food and coffees. By this date, I was getting quite good at having participants complete necessary paperwork, like the consent form, and recording interviews without drawing too much attention in each setting. Tynesha was in her mid-twenties, described herself as mixed race (Caucasian and Trinidadian), and had mothered three children who were in the custody of and living with their biological father. Tynesha experienced gendered trauma at the hands of the father of her children.

> TYNESHA: He [her ex-partner] uses alcohol, but in the beginning, he was like my knight in shining armour, almost.... But as soon as he found out I was pregnant that's when I saw the change in him.
> AMBER: So, when you got pregnant with your first, how did he change towards you?
> TYNESHA: More controlling, more not wanting me to do anything, not wanting me to go out with my friends and stuff like that.... I didn't really pay too much attention to it because I'm like "Oh I'm pregnant, he's just looking out for me, blah-blah-blah." And by the second one, that's when I knew ... he assaulted me the first time when I was pregnant with her.

Tynesha left the father of her three children in 2014, when her third and youngest child was an infant. She was honest and forthcoming that she engaged in alcohol use during their relationship but did not define herself as addicted to alcohol. Tynesha made it clear that she used alcohol to manage her emotional pain, particularly when she became pregnant with their fourth child and she chose to have an abortion instead of subjecting another child to witnessing their father's abuse of her. She explained: "It's not like I don't have the control to not drink. I chose to [drink] because I just didn't want to feel at that time." Tynesha was also blunt in saying that others' perception of her problematic use of alcohol was why her children were placed in the care of their father by the Children's Aid Society (CAS) of Toronto. In many ways, I heard Tynesha to be contextualizing her children's experience by the racialized trauma she had also experienced in her relationship with this system, a finding echoed in the wider literature on child welfare (Adjei et al. 2017; Maynard, 2017). While Tynesha defined her alcohol use as a coping strategy in the face of trauma in her life, she was then re-traumatized by the loss of her children through others' judgments of her patterns of use.

Household Environment. Tynesha was also one of a few participants who linked their early use to the living environments they grew up in. She first used alcohol at age fourteen, and not just part of hanging out with her friends: "That's what I used to do because growing up was so destructive when I look back at it.... I probably drank every single day until I was nineteen. But ... after going through counselling, I seriously chalked it up to that's my way of coping." When I asked about her early childhood, Tynesha recalled that her biological father sexually abused her from age four until age eight and even after he moved out of her home.

> He lived with us until I was five ... he was a drug addict. I can even remember walking into the bathroom and he's smoking out of a pop can.... My mom – I remember being shipped around to so many different homes as a kid because she was always gone or doing something. Later on, she got turned into a full-blown crack addict. As I grew up and had understanding and knowledge of things, I look back at my mother and realized she's been doing it my whole life.

Tynesha remembered her mother as physically abusing her too, and so then CAS as being involved in her care. It was between age fourteen and sixteen she lived in group homes. At age sixteen she negotiated to live on her own with the income she received from OW; individuals as young as sixteen may receive OW if their parent or guardian is either abusive or will not or cannot care for them, and if the individual has no other means of economic family support (City of Toronto, 2017).

At age twenty-nine and single, Franco was undoubtedly the most gracious man I interviewed. After our interview in a hip, privately owned coffee shop, he walked me to the bus stop and waited with me for the bus, having learned that I was navigating a part of Toronto that I was less familiar with. Franco was of medium build, about 5'7" in height, and self-identified as Italian and "Newfie," being quite proud of the latter. He wore black lace-up loafers that were well worn and scuffed at the toes; a detail I remember because he made a point of drawing my attention to them to tell me that he had these shoes for year. Purchasing new shoes was not a luxury he could easily afford on his single-person income on OW.

Franco lived in a rooming house for men in treatment for substance use and was attending a trauma counselling group when I met him. He recalled relationships and events in his childhood home as harrowing and productive of his suffering.

> [T]hat's why I'm going to the trauma group.... [T]he neglect I had as a child with my mother.... I'd say to her: "Mom you're never around." "Well, you shouldn't feel that way...." So, as a child I would start saying, "Okay I'm not allowed to be angry. I'm not allowed to be this, because Mom told me that I shouldn't be." So, I started feeling that my feelings weren't matching reality.

Franco experienced physical abuse as a child and may have also experienced sexual abuse by parental-like figures in his life. He explained: "My sister was molested. I'm not quite sure if something happened to me. That's where we're going [in group] because I remember seeing some stuff, but there's parts of my life I can't see." By his mid-twenties, Franco was "falsely accused" (his words) of rape. Franco pinpoints the fall out of this event as when his substance use especially changed and escalated:

> I was acquitted, but it ripped me apart because it's something you can't talk about to people. People will judge.... I was on house arrest for three years.... That's when my alcoholism went to a whole new level. And that's when I went to crack because I couldn't talk to anyone about it. I can go to work but then I had to come right home ... like you're already in prison.... [O]nce I hit crack it had a dopamine rush on me that just took away all my problems. Then the feeling is I'm happy. Because I was just scared. I was terrified.

At the time of our meeting, Franco was sober and defined as being in recovery for about one year. Franco was certain that there was a connection between his experiences of traumatic events in childhood and young adulthood and his descent into repeated use of alcohol and crack cocaine.

The Trauma of Use Itself. Danni was the only person I interviewed who spoke about how she saw her use itself as traumatic. I feature this anomalous case for what I learned about use as trauma and to present the opportunity to explore stories like hers in future qualitative research and theorizing on becoming a substance user or developing substance dependency (see also Pearce, 2002).

Danni, age thirty-seven, had been on OW for two years and lived alone on the outskirts of Toronto. She made me a cup of coffee before we sat down in her apartment for our interview. Danni was an attractive white woman but seemed to me almost painfully thin. She commented that she was working on gaining weight, having finally become eligible for the $180 Special Diet Allowance through OW. She self-defined as clean for two years and in recovery from a heroin and fentanyl addiction. She continued to smoke cannabis to curb her anxiety and correct what she saw as the appetite suppressant side effect of her methadone treatment. Danni was also the mother of two young children that she no longer had custody of nor any visitation rights because of others' perceptions of her drug addiction (see also chapter 8).

Danni shared how her substance use changed her perception of reality and was harmful to her sense of self to the extent that she had been institutionalized a few times in her life.

> I've been in that paranoia, and it may have been drug-induced psychosis but it's the same psychosis. They were treating me for schizophrenia in the psych ward.... I don't remember two weeks of my life.... I know they had to chain me down to the bed. I don't go out easy. I'm just a drug addict. I'm not crazy.... Like crystal meth made me do that. I was injecting crystal meth for three months at one time.... I don't even know, my mind went. And sometimes I get flashbacks of what happened.... It's very traumatizing. I'm on two waiting lists for the trauma program at XXXX.... I was also raped in that two-week injection thing that I was doing with crystal meth.

Danni spoke like this, suddenly changing focus and introducing new information throughout our interview. Her experiences of trauma stem from her practices of use and how her use itself may be related to psychotic episodes. Being subjected to gendered violence, specifically rape, while using and feeling an impending death was in addition traumatizing. She further remembered: "A lot of people aren't in that position.... You really think someone is going to murder you and throw you in the dumpster that you're in front of. And thinking you're going to die is so traumatic." Danni's continued use following this trauma was partially shaped by it, though she was clear that her patterns and choice of drug changed over time and "ever since that happened, I've been really careful about doing drugs. Like I'll do them, but I won't do them to enjoy them."

I met Danni approximately ten years after these incidents in her life. Though she was alone in discussing the practices of her use as traumatizing, her experience is suggestive of the addiction cycle theorized in health studies, including medicine, psychology, and psychiatry (see, for example, Cleck & Blendy, 2008). In this cycle, initial use may create feelings of euphoria or "being high" as well as personal and psychological problems perhaps accompanied by harmful and sometimes violent consequences. Once no longer high or feeling the effects of the substance and instead experiencing withdrawal, however, people may use again to mitigate withdrawal or even any anxiety, depression, or stress that they experience when sober.

Behaviours, Interactions, Events

Some participants connected their initial substance use and later addiction to their experience of chronic or temporary pain. While medical researchers observe that persons who are prescribed opioids to manage chronic pain may develop opioid use disorder, there are few ways to determine which patients may develop an addiction (Klimas et al., 2019). Meanwhile, the prescription of opioids to manage pain has been on the rise (Wachholtz & Gonzalez, 2014).

I met Darlene, a white woman who was raising two children under age twelve on her own, at a downtown coffee shop on a wintry day. She wore a stylish toque over her blonde hair and fashionable but comfortable clothes. Though about eight years younger than me, Darlene's fashion style reminded me of my own: trying to stay somewhat relevant and yet still a parent, which often translates into looking "in style" but not necessarily carefully "put together." Defining herself as in recovery and no longer taking methadone, Darlene's drug of choice in the past was OxyContin. She connected her escalating use of the prescription drug to her chronic pain that was then exacerbated by two car accidents.

> I got told that I had fibromyalgia ... sixteen years ago. And then I guess probably about six or seven years ago, I got in another car accident, and it just made everything a lot worse. So, I was on pain medication then and I was having trouble managing it, I was taking more than I should and that's how I ended up going to CAMH [clinical care hospital and services].

A gregarious single white woman in her early thirties with long ash blonde hair, Carie was in methadone treatment and self-defined as in recovery. She lived with a roommate and did not have children, though she saw children as a possibility in her future. She was the epitome of the participant who becomes the "teacher" of all things related to the topic of the interview. When we sat down to chat, Carie's talk included stories about herself and her life experiences, but she also used the interview to teach me information about drug use subculture that she thought I should know, peppering her own experiences with stories of others that could be perceived as disturbing or titillating. Of all my participants, Carie embraced wholeheartedly my inexperience with drug addiction – she aimed to educate me.

Carie worked for years with a moving company and so would suffer from back pain, though she would not take medication for it. When her mother recommended that she take Percocet for pain, she told me "I never even used to take a Tylenol – no thank you, I wouldn't take anything." Once she broke her foot, however, she did agree to take what she was prescribed for pain: OxyContin. Carie reported her dislike of the drug for making her feel "drowsy and sleepy" and only temporarily relieving her pain. She convinced her physician to allow her to try alternatives, such as Tylenol 3, but they did little to lessen her pain and so she reluctantly took the OxyContin for eight months as her foot healed. After getting her cast off, she was supposed to return to the physician and get her prescription renewed. She refused, but soon felt the consequences of withdrawal: "I was feeling so sick, sweaty but cold. It felt like there was live wires in your [sic] arms and legs and they kept touching each other without you doing anything, your body would jolt. Puking, sitting on the toilet, everything just flushing out of you." Carie recognized herself having an addiction once she took her mother's offer again of Percocet to curb these feelings: "So, I took it and I was feeling a bit better. And then about twenty minutes later I started crying and she's like what? I go 'I'm a fucking addict.'"

Pat was several years older than Carie, at age sixty-four, but also attributed her escalating use of drugs to the physical pain she experienced. She understood her use of Percocet as an addiction by the time she was in her forties: "I was 180 [pills] every two weeks. And I'd sit down for breakfast with my coffee, my cigarette, and my Percs. I'd take three or four three times a day. So, I was very addicted." An attractive, single, white woman and mother of three adult children, Pat had been on methadone for about twenty years. She explained that started using street drugs and alcohol in her teenage years when she left home to escape her mother's physical abuse. Her exposure to Percocet occurred while she was incarcerated in jail (a provincial correctional institution) and through a "different circle of friends when I get [sic] out." She further explained:

> I was a waitress for twenty years ... carrying big trays. These big metal trays. And then I bartended for like ten years. I was in the bars for a long time.... And the lifting, the lifting, the lifting. I just started going in my job for ... for my arthritis. And that's how I fell on the Percs. And then they were working for you [sic].

Pat had stayed on methadone for so many years for the pain management it provided in place of Percocet. She was on a waiting list for a hip replacement when we met.

Growing Up Like the Joneses

"Keeping up with the Joneses" is an idiom that generally refers to people aspiring to emulate the "good life" of others they admire. For example, they can equate their own success and status in their communities with how they, too, have secured the trappings of the "American Dream" (or perhaps most aptly, the Canadian Dream, e.g., a home, manicured lawn and garden, and white picket fence). I met participants who seemed to live the "good life" in childhood and adolescence but became substance users and eventually understood themselves to be living with addiction. Hence my slight adaptation of the idiom for this theme that characterized these participants' stories.

Of the twenty-eight client participants I interviewed, just over ten of them (including Alexei and Darlene) perceived that they grew up in stable and supportive "working-class" or "middle-class" heteronormative nuclear family households not affected by substance use or violence. Danni grew up in a reasonably well-off nuclear family household with her sister. Her mom was a nurse and her dad a public service employee with the city in which they lived. When asked how she remembered the very beginning of her use, she said: "[I] saw drug addicts on TV and thought that that looked cool.... I started doing drugs with a girlfriend of mine. She went to a rave, she found a bag of coke, she brought it back and we started doing it. I was in grade 7 and 8." When she was asked to leave home for the first time at thirteen years old, it was not because she was doing drugs – which she was – but because "I was just a terror. I wasn't very nice to my mom. I was terrible." By age sixteen Danni was receiving social assistance as a minor while renting a room. She then seemed to move back and forth between the family home and friends' houses or shelters until she finished high school. Danni's eventual escalation of use took place throughout her twenties into her thirties and seemed partially shaped by her experiences of trauma during this period (see above). Mainly I wish to note here that Danni seemed to have a childhood ensconced in the dream for many. But for Danni, she did not see herself to fit in with this family environment and as her use progressed, she extricated herself from it.

I met Shawn at an A&W restaurant east of Toronto, and we sat and talked over burgers and fries. He was a white man in his early fifties with a lean build. He wore a ball cap over his sandy brown hair that was long in the back. Combined with his mustache, T-shirt, and straight-leg jeans, Shawn's appearance reminded me of the unspoken dress code of my father and his friends that I have observed at their classic car shows. Shawn's daughter was a young adult and lived with his ex-wife. When we discussed his first memories of substance use and experiences growing up, Shawn recalled his childhood and his relationship with his parents: "I had a normal childhood, I guess. We used to be down the street here, we moved to the street we lived in all our lives in 1969.... My parents were really good." Shawn clarified that his father worked for pay and his mom at home: "It was a single-income family, it was normal back then, a stay-at-home mother."

Shawn remembered beginning to use cannabis at about age twelve. His exit from high school before completing grade 12 was explained as follows:

I guess I was being rebellious or getting myself in trouble. I got shipped off to a different high school.... I didn't know anybody.... I went in grade 10 and I don't know, I just started thinking different things, I guess. And started thinking about working and having money and shit like that, and then I just started skipping and then it just went from there.

Shawn also remembered that his parents were not "too happy but basically it was 'if you're going to do that then you've got to get a job or whatever,' and I did. I pretty much worked since I was sixteen off and on." It seemed that Shawn's cannabis and alcohol use paralleled these events in his early adolescence and as he transitioned into young adulthood. He shifted to his preferred drug, heroin, at age twenty-one and while he was still living at home. He was still randomly using heroin when I met him and often methadone in place of it.

My Crowd

In adolescence, peer groups influence individual socialization and well-being (Lee & Lee, 2020). Sometimes the learning of substance use for recreational pleasure is part of this peer socialization (see also Hussong, 2002; Prinstein et al., 2011); I remember this even being the case in my own adolescence and depending on which group I was "hanging out" with. Several decades ago, Becker (1953) observed that cannabis use is learned from peers and, notably, stressed people learning of its pleasurable effects of use too. As shown in Chapter 2 considerable body of research continues to remind academics, other social actors like policymakers, and the lay public that people use drugs or alcohol for pleasure and/or leisure. Becker's contemporary, Edwin Sutherland (1947), also argued that illicit drug use is learned from others through communication, though his focus was more on seeing this as learned criminal behaviour. It was not surprising that some benefit recipients credited their first use of alcohol or drugs to using with their friends. Some even saw a connection between their recreational use of substances with their wanting to spend more time with friends and dropping out of high school.

Bianca defined herself as a proud Italian woman, single, and in her early forties. She was on house arrest in her married parents' home as she awaited her court date; she had been charged with trafficking drugs with her ex-partner. Bianca had lived common-law with him for many years, and they had four children between the ages thirteen and nineteen. Her nineteen-year-old lived in his own apartment, while her youngest daughter and two other sons were in the custody of her brother and sister-in-law. Bianca had been clean for over one year and on OW for over twenty when we met. During our interview, I learned that being with her friends and using drugs or alcohol was, quite simply, more appealing and pleasurable than going to school. Being part of a crowd and enjoying cannabis as part of everyday fun seemed an important backstory to Bianca's eventual transition to using other drugs later in life.

> BIANCA: It was a good childhood.
> AMBER: And your teenage years. Do you remember why, um, say you didn't finish high school? Things like that.
> BIANCA: I started smoking weed at that time (laughter). And my mom, poor thing, was so busy with work and stuff that she couldn't be on my ass about it. So, I just did what I wanted.... [T]here was this like billiards place behind our school.... [A]ll the fun things that you think are fun at the time.

Remembering his use of alcohol and cannabis beginning at age sixteen, Arash said: "So, it took me away from school and stuff because I wanted to have fun." Arash immigrated to Canada from Iran when he was a child with his mother, father, and sister. He was single and thirty-seven when we met in a cafeteria on a University of Toronto campus. He identified as in recovery from an addiction to alcohol and cocaine.

Arash was deeply introspective and philosophical, and most of his answers to my questions demonstrated his own thirst for knowledge and comprehension of it. Considering my social position and privilege as a university-educated woman and the personal bias I have towards higher education, I often felt I was talking to a colleague during our time together. When Arash seemed emotional during our interview, suggested by a change in his tone of voice and body language, I felt like I was talking to a friend. I retained these uncanny feelings of kindredness after we concluded our interview and set off chatting and walking together towards the subway to go our separate ways. Of course, we were neither colleagues nor friends: I was an interviewer, Arash a participant. And we would likely never see other again, a thought that still makes me feel sad even as I write this. I take the time here to be somewhat tangential about my interview with Arash to highlight how emotions can enter into the temporariness of the research relationship, sometimes producing an entirely unpredictable impact on the researcher.

Even after adolescence, the crowd with which one is part can have an impact on substance use. My first impression of Jesse was that at twenty-eight years old, he had seemed to live a hard life. He was thin, very pale, and very tall, and though he defined as Caucasian, he made sure to share his pride in his "Scottish, English, German, and Irish" ancestry. He was patient and seemed relaxed in his demeanour. He did not seem bothered as I shuffled my papers or fumbled with my tape recorder in my nervousness during our interview at a coffee shop. Jesse explained that the peer group through which he learned to use new drugs (e.g., heroin) and saw his use escalate was one he joined while in treatment: "when I first came into the program, I was only using Oxy-Contin, that was the only thing I'd ever used besides marijuana. And meeting other people and chilling with other people, I got into other things." Jesse was not alone in learning to use new drugs with new friends. Franco recalled that following his court case over his alleged crime of rape: "I cut myself off from friends and then the drinking went up. And then I started hanging around in the wrong circles, and then the drugs came in. I started with coke." In chapter 8, I will follow up on how people who use alcohol or drugs may find that they are soon using with different and new friends and sometimes because of their severing of ties with others they were once close with. These new friendships can be necessary when other family and friends are in some way harmed by users' behaviours and actions.

"Party Like It's 1999." Though I intend to dispel the association of substance use with only deviant subculture(s) throughout this book, some of the people I interviewed did suggest that there are unique "lifestyle" choices when belonging to drug-using peer groups. In using substances, some participants implied that one could become caught up in living and partying each day like it was their last – a way of living on par with Prince's imagination in his song, "Party Like It's 1999."

Cody seemed to embrace this way of living and began throwing raves and using and selling club drugs (e.g., ecstasy or MDMA) at the age of seventeen: "I started and that was a weekend thing. Having a good time. And then we started going to the after-hour bars downtown here." Cody saw his parents as quite laid back about his first experimentations with drugs at a young age, as long as his use was limited to "softer" drugs, like cannabis. His paraphrase of his parents' reasoning went as follows: "'[I]f you want to smoke weed go ahead, there's no harm in weed. Mushrooms, they're okay because they're a fun trip. If we find out you're doing acid, cocaine, heroin, any of these drugs, we have a problem with it.'" Now thirty-six, Cody was one year sober and defined as in recovery from a heroin addiction. He had been living with his father in his childhood home after exiting prison; his two children were in the care of others. An athletic-looking white man, well-groomed and with short hair, Cody was at his most disarming when he smiled. His slight nervousness about meeting me and vice versa seemed to put us both at ease: we agreed that though meeting for an interview with a stranger was quite odd, at least we were nervous about it together. We soon found we had much to talk about despite our differing life experiences. Our interview became a conversation full of laughter and us cutting each other off in our excitement to make a point.

It seemed that the sheer youthful excitement of living a life of partying had passed by the time Cody was in his twenties. Following a series of events, including a break-up and loss of custody of his first child, he transitioned into using heroin: "I just went out on a party, kind of self-destruct mode. That's when I picked up my break-ins." Cody was eventually sentenced to federal prison for crimes of break and entry theft that he committed while using drugs.

Similarly, it was Adam's work as a musician that immersed him in a party lifestyle.

> Running around the city playing countless rock n' roll shows.... Doing way too many drugs (laughter). Like way too many (laughter). I would go to like big parties ... and play for like seven-day festivals and stuff. You'd be on for like two hours but then the other five days, you could just do whatever you wanted.

A single white man, Adam was twenty-nine and had been on OW one year. When we met at a local coffee shop in his neighborhood, Adam was fashionably dressed in sneakers, jeans, and a comfortable and loose black blazer; it was a classic look. Adam saw his first using cannabis in his adolescence as a coping strategy for depression that went untreated. Though he still used it, he explained: "I use marijuana sort of the same way somebody drinks a glass of wine." While in his late teens and early twenties, he experimented with mushrooms, acid, and cocaine and cited the drug MDMA as a temporary problem for him. Adam defined primarily as a recovering alcoholic because he felt he easily gave up the drugs, like acid, "when I learned everything it could do... [U]nfortunately I haven't been able to do the same thing with alcohol."

While Cody and Adam's initial substance use and partying seemed associated with their belonging to club/rave culture or the music scene, Dante simply "partied" as an adolescent and attributed his substance use to how it benefited him socially. Dante was about 5'8" tall, average in build, and self-identified as a Caribbean Black man. At age forty-four, he moved agilely, talked with his hands, and genuinely seemed to like to laugh. I can still remember how quickly Dante would correct me and set me straight when I made wrong interpretations or seemed not to understand his answers, as several examples throughout this book will show. He sat us down at a large table in the common room of his apartment building for our interview, amid chalkboards, easels, and random children's toys. Dante explained that he was a good student in high school and impressed his peers with how he could get good grades and still really party it up. Dante made it clear that he was aware that others' reactions to him were shaped by the fact that he was a young Black man who grew up in a working-class neighbourhood but attended a prestigious private school where most of the student population was white. In Dante's perception, his substance use made him "stick out from everybody else ... because I was a bit of a nerd."

After high school, Dante attended college but left for an opportunity to apprentice as a mortician at a local hospital. He remembers it being a good job he had while he continued his party lifestyle. As he explained: "I was shooting coke up during the night and working the hospital during the day." When I asked him if he was able to manage his paid work at that time, he replied, "As long as I lived with my mother, I was able to manage. The second I moved out, it fucked things up. My mother kept me straight. She kept me in line." He had spent several years: using a combination of drugs; stealing to support his habit; moving in and out of provincial jail; accessing OW on and off; and/or engaging in paid work, most often construction. His drugs of choice were cocaine and crystal methamphetamine at the time we met.

A Tentative Typology

Typologies can be useful in how they facilitate categorical thinking and permit the sketching out of general "types" of a phenomenon. The risk in creating them, however, is in how they can promote reification of these same types; and they never accurately capture all experiences nor universally. I nonetheless conclude this chapter by sketching out the "types of becoming" a substance user to sociologically highlight the behaviours, interactions, and events through which many participants seemed to come to define themselves as having a problem with substances. Moreover, I craft this typology to deliberately refute stereotypes of alcohol and drug users of the moral and individualistic variety (e.g., all "addicts" are "bad" people) and stereotypes of the pathological variety (e.g., there is something innately and essentially wrong with the biological and physiological make-up of people who develop a dependency on substances). Finally, I offer this typology with the caution that it is entirely based on my interpretation (and social construction) of participants' stories; it must be noted that participants often fell within one or more types I discuss below.

Accidental

Becoming addicted to alcohol or drugs can be somewhat if not entirely accidental. We learn this from Darlene and Carie, who were both prescribed OxyContin as a pain reliever and then experienced withdrawal symptoms without a sense of how to respond to them. In Carie's case, her initial opioid use was to decrease the pain associated with an injury. Her subsequent and deliberate use seemed to begin with the desire to remove the pain, seemingly physical but perhaps emotional too, of withdrawal. While the pain-alleviating quality of using opioids had long since passed when Pat was working as a waitress or bartender, the pleasure-inducing effects of the drug might have spurred on her continued use. Though having very different life experiences, Smitri and Adam's use seemed to start and continue because using did something for them emotionally. In Smitri's case, she experienced horrific gendered trauma as an adolescent. In Adam's case, he professed that he suffered from depression during adolescence.

Participants for whom addiction seemed "accidental" were those who seemed to be using for healing purposes or perhaps even to reduce suffering. They either thought they were following a medical professional's advised healing trajectory by using primarily opioids, or they were engaged in self-coping strategies that could involve using alcohol or drugs. Along the way of this healing trajectory, they developed a self-identified problem with their use.

Surprised

For some participants, what was initially partying and "chasing a high" became a dependency on substances. These participants appeared to use to have a good time, but once the partying stopped, even for just a short time, they found that they could no longer abstain. That is, a lifestyle of random and optional use for fun eventually became mandatory use for survival; survival in the sense of staving off withdrawal and responding to cravings. Cody, Dante, and Adam, for instance, were surprised to find they had a problem with using substances. When Dante lived in his parents' house, he relied on his mother to support him in his meeting of his paid work responsibilities. When she no longer provided this support, he is clear in saying, "it fucked things up." It seemed a surprise to Dante that he could no longer maintain a balance between his substance use and the semblance of a scheduled day without others supporting the latter.

Considering a person's entire life course up until the time I met them, however, disturbs the simplicity of this or any of these categories. For example, it is awfully difficult to take stock of Cody's entire life story and maintain that his becoming an addict was only a surprise to him. While Cody might have been surprised to find he had a problem with using drugs once his stint managing raves ended, he reflected more deeply on his entrance into criminal behaviour and related his continued use over time to his anger and frustration over losing custody of his first daughter to her mother.

Ambivalent

Some participants (e.g., Alexei, Shawn) had mixed feelings about their use and did not share others' perceptions of it as a problem to the same degree. Though not introduced in this chapter, unravelling Clive's story throughout this book will show his ambivalence about his use of alcohol. In some ways, these participants could be thought of as "functioning addicts," at least in common treatment language, as they continued their daily routines in life, such as participating in paid work. Substance use was simply another routine in their day. Or, if one ascribes to the stages of change model advocated by Prochaska and DiClemente (1992) and popular in social work, these participants could be thought of as in the pre-contemplative stage. They did not define their use as a problem in need of change (see also D'Sylva et al., 2012).

Later in our interview Shawn shared that he was aware that others, specifically his OW caseworker, saw his heroin use as problematic. Shawn, however, used heroin when he wanted and was fairly satisfied with his ability to make ends meet through his receipt of OW and his casual employment as a handyperson. His mixed feelings about his use seemed most obvious when he acknowledged the inadequacy of his living accommodations. For instance, when we met, Shawn was living in a house in which he was completing renovation work for the owner; it had no running water.

Misunderstood

Participants in this category were those who were aware that their use patterns were not understood by others and sometimes caused problems in their personal lives. While they took responsibility for their use, they did not easily self-identify as living with addiction and did not see their use as creating harmful consequences for others.

Among the participants discussed thus far, Tynesha perhaps best falls in this category. She was aware that others saw her use as a problem: her children were removed from her care by CAS. Tynesha's life experience up until I met her illustrated another dimension of this category. She understood the consequences of her behaviour but not through the same moral threshold as caseworkers. Tynesha could clearly discern underlying reasons for using alcohol as a coping strategy, including a tumultuous childhood and sexual abuse by her father as a child and later violence at the hands of her ex-partner as an adult. Those who seemed misunderstood by others who labelled them as "addicts" could feel that they had every reason to use alcohol or drugs.

I have not yet introduced Jules and will spend time with her throughout the remainder of this book. Suffice it to say that Jules, too, did not identify herself as having a problem with her use in the way her OW caseworker did. As a lone mother of three children, one in guardianship of her own mother, she understood her past use of OxyContin to be problematic but temporary. Jules's use made sense to her in view of her experience of gendered trauma, specifically that of a miscarriage, but (unlike Adrianna who had some similar experiences) she did not define herself as experiencing substance use dependency.

To be clear, Jules and Tynesha were among the small number of participants who I place in this category. They were largely defined as having a problem with substance use by others and were targeted as such, for example, being assigned to a specific OW caseload. As we will see in chapter 6, though these participants did not agree with others' perceptions of their behaviours, they nonetheless conformed to caseworkers' expectations of them to avoid being cut off from the receipt of monthly benefits.

No One Reason

I began this chapter by noting that no one person I interviewed set out to become a person with a substance use problem. The various themes that characterized participants' stories further confirmed that there is nothing straightforward or simple about becoming a person living with addiction. Whether trauma related, to alleviate emotional and physical pain, or socializing with certain people because it was fun – and no matter what "class" one seemed to grow up in – participants developed some semblance of substance use dependency, whether they identified with this themselves or others perceived them as such.

It bears repeating that I see the themes that characterized participants' stories of "becoming" a substance user to represent often intersecting behaviours, interactions, and events that textured their lives over time and seemed, from my interpretation and their own, to somehow link to (not solely determine or cause) their development of a substance abuse problem. I saw people's stories of their unfolding and often escalating use to further imply that substance use dependency could happen accidentally or by surprise. Other participants told their stories to me to make clear that they did not share others' perceptions of their use as a problem. I therefore organized participants' stories of becoming into a typology. Though imperfect and not meant to be idealized, this typology loosely illustrates the many social relations involved in becoming a substance user. Participants' use as understood, labelled, and regulated by OW policy discourse and caseworkers, as well as participants' actual actions and behaviours while being on OW, are the focus of the next two chapters.

5 Being an Object of Welfare[1]

The discourse analysis that begins this chapter may seem a jarring break from benefit recipients' storytelling about their experiences of becoming a substance user. The shift in focus is intentional. I mean to locate, in a temporal period, how OW policy socially constructed addiction and regulated its experience by benefit recipients. This story is somewhat messy to tell, but it crucially contextualizes the subjective experiences of being a person living with addiction and accessing OW, a consistent focus in chapters in this part of the book. It makes possible an understanding of the problematic consequences of objectification and subjectification processes inherent in OW policy, including the risk of limiting lives to addiction.

Specifically, I move between uncovering living with addiction as an object of Ontario Works (OW) policy and revealing the subjectivity of benefit recipients produced by policy – endeavouring to consider the power–knowledge relations constitutive of them (Foucault, 1978). I begin with an analysis of the shifting discourses that have guided social assistance design and delivery and trace these alongside the emerging social construction of the target population of people living with addiction. I then reveal the relationships and experiences that materialize through caseworkers' application of policy, including the discursive constitution of benefit recipients' subject position, through the presentation of themes that cut across participants' talk and policy discourse.

---

1 Some content in this chapter replicates content presented in my earlier publication: Gazso, Amber. 2020."Dueling discourses, power, and the construction of *the recovering addict*: When social assistance confronts addiction in Toronto, Canada." *Critical Social Policy* 40(1) 1–21, 130–50. https://doi.org/10.1177/0261018319839158 (on-line 2019)

Shifting Discourses in Social Assistance Design and Delivery

Several discourses contextualize the changing conceptualization of eligibility for OW for people in general and then for people specifically living with addiction over the period 2009–17. These discourses have differently held sway and mutually co-existed. They are related to wider, global shifts in risks and rights that correspond with reflexive modernization and increasing individualization in Western post-industrial societies and shaping of Canada's neoliberal social policy context.

Shifting Discourses from a Crisis of Dependency to Poverty Reduction

In the 1990s, budgetary deficits, high unemployment, and loss of federal funding with the introduction of the 1996 Canada Health and Social Transfer intertwined with increasing social assistance caseloads and produced what was largely perceived to be a "crisis" in social spending across Canada. Many provinces responded to this crisis by engaging in an exercise of welfare reform (Béland & Daigneault, 2015). Concerning 1990s Ontario, neoliberal restructuring under Harris's Progressive Conservative government found an ally in the discourse of welfare dependency: rising social assistance caseloads could be blamed on lazy, fraudulent, and dependent people taking advantage of the welfare system. For example, in 1997 Janet Ecker, then Minister of Community and Social Services (MCSS), supported Bill 142, the *Social Assistance Reform Act* with the statement: "workfare will allow 'opportunities to break the cycle of dependency on welfare'" (Morrison, 1998, p. 43). Welfare dependency was both the scapegoat for Ontario's spending crisis and the discourse that catalysed reform strategies (Smith-Carrier & Lawlor, 2017) – and further interlocked with a newer "work first" discourse orienting social assistance eligibility, as I show below.

By the early 2000s, however, a different discourse of poverty reduction began taking shape across Ontario and through a different politics. Hailed as a momentous event (Degroot-Magetti & Blackstock, 2009), the province passed the *Poverty Reduction Act* in 2009 under the Liberal government of Dalton McGuinty. This Act stemmed from the province's recognition of the need to address increasing numbers of people experiencing poverty, to better integrate people into the labour market, and eradicate the "intergenerational transmission of poverty" (Benbow et al., 2016; Legislative Assembly of Ontario, 2009; Smith-Carrier, 2017; Smith-Carrier & Lawlor, 2017; Plante, 2018), though no publicly available government reports provided evidence of intergenerational transmission. Anti-poverty advocacy efforts of community organizations and social services, think tanks, foundations, researchers, and concerned individuals were also important to this Act coming to fruition (Smith-Carrier & Lawlor, 2017). The Act requires governments to develop poverty-reduction strategies through consultation and set reduction targets, and report on both.

The 25 in 5 Coalition Network's goal of reducing the number of children in poverty by 25 per cent over five years, for example, was made actionable in Breaking the Cycle, the $1.4 billion poverty-reduction strategy introduced for the period 2009–13 (Ministry of Children and Youth Services, 2009). Between 2008 and 2011, 47,000 children were said to be lifted out of poverty, but by 2014, the goal had not been met (Government of Ontario, 2014). According to the 2014 annual report of the Poverty Reduction Strategy, the province did, however, launch several other initiatives. These included increasing the amount of the Ontario Child Benefit, committing to a $50 increase in social assistance benefit amounts for single persons and investing $16 billion to create 1,000 housing spaces as part of the Comprehensive Mental Health and Addictions Strategy (Government of Ontario, 2014), a joint initiative of the Ministries of Children and Youth services, Health and Long-Term Care, and Education (Matthews, 8 May 2012). The report also outlined the second poverty-reduction strategy to be pursued until 2019, called Realizing Our Potential, which included a primary goal to "reform Ontario's social assistance system to remove barriers and increase opportunities for everyone to participate in the workforce" (Government of Ontario, 2014, np). As Smith-Carrier and Lawlor (2017) find in their analysis, however, Realizing Our Potential does not contain trackable measures of social assistance reform to create evidence of change in the economic security of low-income Ontarians. Moreover, the discourse of dependency did not disappear under the Liberal governments of McGuinty and later Premier Kathleen Wynne. The poverty-reduction discourse tends to subsume its idea that the responsibility for reducing poverty lies in the efforts of individuals themselves (Smith-Carrier & Lawlor, 2017). Its larger neoliberal shadow obscures the intersecting structures and institutions that (re-)produce poverty.

Notwithstanding Smith-Carrier and Lawlor's (2017) critical insights, the discourse of poverty reduction has meant some changes in social assistance up until 2017, the end point of this study. In 2010, the government appointed Ontario Social Assistance Review Advisory Council made up of advocates, community groups, public intellectuals, and academics, released its recommendation for a comprehensive review of the social assistance system. Besides growth in social assistance caseloads since 2008 (MCSS, 2011, p. 15), key concerns that pushed the Advisory Council's recommendation included the punitive enforcement of rules of assistance receipt, the requirement that recipients have no assets, and the stigma associated with receipt of OW. Based on the Council's early recommendations, earnings exemptions for small payments and in-kind gifts, and shorter periods of reduced benefits or outright suspension from the caseload were introduced (MCSS, 2012).

The government appointed Commission for the Review of Social Assistance in Ontario took place between 2010 and 2012 and directly consulted people to explore opportunities for improving social assistance programs in Ontario (both OW and the Ontario Disability Support Program). Its final report, *Brighter Prospects: Transforming Social Assistance in Ontario*, made several recommendations, including that people with multiple barriers to labour market participation who were accessing OW receive more intensive services (Lankin & Sheikh, 2012). Actual changes to OW brought about because of *Brighter Prospects* are documented in the 2013–14 and 2014–15 annual reports of MCSS. Some of these included increasing the monetary amount of income benefits for families (by 1 per cent) and single adults without children (by 3 per cent, or $25); improving earnings exemptions such that individuals could earn up to $200 a month on OW without receiving a dollar-for-dollar deduction on their total monthly welfare income; and increasing the amount of assets OW recipients could retain. In 2015–16, singles without children received $75 more than they had in 2012. Whereas a single parent with two children received an extra $120, a couple with two children earned $156 more per year (MCSS, 2017). The ministry continued to support the continuation of reforms as per the *Brighter Prospects* report in 2015 and as part of the poverty-reduction strategy (MCSS, 2016a). Indeed, in 2016 the province established the Income Security Reform Working Group to support changes to shift from a "complex system of social assistance" to a "client-centered approach" (MCSS, 2016b, np). Like the Social Assistance Review Advisory Council, the Group's agenda was partially informed by recognition that OW rules seem to punish rather than support persons with low income.

Social assistance reform as part of poverty reduction has not been without controversy. For example, in 2010, the special diet allowance was eliminated for OW recipients. It was re-introduced in 2012 largely as an outcome of an Order of the Human Rights Tribunal of Ontario (MCSS, 2011, 2012). More recently, the Wynne government's basic income pilot project was cancelled. This 2017 poverty-reduction initiative, historically contextualized by the 1970s comparable experiment in Dauphin, Manitoba ("Mincome") (Calnitsky, 2016), provided a sample of Ontarians living in Hamilton, Brantford, Thunder Bay, and Lindsay with a monthly income set at 75 per cent of the poverty line, or a "basic income." Recipients were allowed to keep earnings from employment, and their basic income benefit was to be reduced by 50 per cent of their earnings (Smith Cross, 2017). The ending of this pilot by Doug Ford's Progressive Conservative government, elected by summer 2018, was met with criticism because the program had the potential to make an important difference in people's economic security (CBC News, 2020).

Turning the focus to Toronto, its poverty-reduction strategy, TO Prosperity: Toronto Poverty Reduction Strategy, originated in 2015. Several recommendations were made as part of a twenty-year plan, among them assisting OW recipients to secure and maintain affordable housing. The subsequent *Year 1 Report* outlined initiatives undertaken and progress made (City of Toronto, 2016a). For example, pilot projects were implemented to explore whether case management strategies may change the experiences of OW recipients experiencing barriers to employment. How the experiences of people living with addiction figured into some of these pilot projects will become clear later in this chapter.

Canada is even winning its "War on Poverty" according to *New York Times* columnist David Brooks (2019). Statistics Canada (2020) data show that 13.6 per cent of families were living below the poverty line (the Market Basket Measure) in 2006 compared to 6.5 per cent in 2018. Whereas 15.6 per cent of Ontarians lived below the poverty line in 2006, this percentage fell between 2015 and 2017 (10.6 per cent versus 9.5 per cent, respectively) (Statistics Canada, 2019). Brooks (2019) attributes this change to Canada's multisector approach to combat poverty. Indeed, this is a key assumption of Ontario's poverty-reduction strategy, which includes the goals of partnering with the federal government, First Nations, municipal government, and community leaders and agencies (MCSS, 2017, p. 4). However, as I aim to show in this book, the "winning the war on poverty" rhetoric masks the multifaceted experience of living with addiction in poverty and how poverty is not limited to economic insecurity alone.

Shifting Discourses Work-First to Distance from the Labour Market

With the *OW Act* mandating participation in welfare-to-work programming as a condition of eligibility, individuals' market citizenship eclipsed their social citizenship as a basis of claim to income support. This "work-first" orientation – or discourse – of OW in the later 1990s and early 2000s (Herd et al., 2009) largely responded to and upheld the broader welfare dependency discourse. Both were unsettled by the

2000s poverty-reduction discourse. Moreover, embedded in the report of the Commission for the Review of Social Assistance in Ontario was another discourse that was tied to the recognition that there were sometimes varied pathways required to achieve poverty reduction if multiple barriers for individuals were present.

Brighter Prospects introduced the "distance from the labour market" discourse to guide service delivery and support income-insecure Ontarians' pursuit of employment. Some existing assumptions about eligibility were retained within it. For example, "in order to receive income support, social assistance recipients be [*sic*] required to participate in activities related to preparing for and finding work as set out in their Pathway to Employment Plans" (Lankin & Sheikh, 2012, p. 24). As well, it was written that everyone should be able to engage in paid work "to the maximum of their abilities" (p. 43). This assumption was further nuanced by the recognition that not everyone could immediately enter the labour market in the same way. People who experienced multiple barriers to employment, for example, could eventually "get closer" to the labour market with adequate and appropriate services and programs (Lankin & Sheikh, 2012).

According to annual reports of the ministry of Community and Social Services (MCSS), the Ontario government ministry responsible for social assistance, removing barriers that "prevent people from participating in the social and economic life of their communities" was a key priority between 2010 and 2013 and even until 2015. After 2015, MCSS priorities shifted towards provisions of short- and long-term support to help vulnerable people find work, become independent, and participate in their communities, and towards making existing services more efficient and accessible. By 2017, MCSS sought to further modernize service delivery, service integration, and strengthen community services. In its outlining of its four overarching pillars of social assistance reform, the 2017 annual report of MCSS carried forward the "distance from the labour market" discourse. For example, one of these pillars was: "Improving [*sic*] employment outcomes by enhancing supports and incentives to work, with an emphasis on clients more distant from the labour market" (MCSS, 2017 p. 6). Thus, by 2017, there seemed to be change in the conceptualization of benefit recipients' eligibility for OW, this change shaped by a shift from a static "work first" discourse to a more dynamic "distant from the labour market" discourse. Whether the regulation of benefit recipients' lives on OW as per a work-first discourse has disappeared, and how the distance from the labour market discourse has meaning for people living with addiction and accessing OW is explored in the remainder of this chapter.

Figuring in Addiction and Creating a Target Population

I pieced together my sense of how people living with substance use challenges figured into the policy design and administration of OW at the discursive level provincially and at the on-the-ground level locally in Toronto largely by combing through OW policy directives, reports from the provincial government, reports from sometimes disparate municipal government (City of Toronto) departments, and interviews with OW caseworkers. I therefore take full responsibility for any errors or omissions in my interpretation.

Information on how persons living with addiction experience OW is not only limited in existing academic literature. Across all annual reports of the ministry, there is rare mention of addiction. Though the ministry reported spending to support homeless people who suffer from "addiction issues" among other challenges (MCSS, 2011, p. 16), by 2014 addiction was absent and the tone shifted to referencing poverty experienced by Ontarians more generally. A review of the Hansard for the Legislative Assembly of Ontario yields a similar finding of rare mention of addiction as a topic of discussion and debate over the 2009–17 period of this study. At the time I was working through how to manage this impression, I learned about the provincial government's earlier introduction of the Addiction Services Initiative (ASI), in 2001. Adjusting my time period of analysis this one time and specifically to capture what happened in 2001 was fruitful. I soon came to understand the ASI as an effort to construct persons as living with addiction as a social policy target population (Schneider & Ingram, 1993) at that time. The ASI was designed with the purpose of removing addiction as a barrier people experience when searching for or maintaining employment and directed a shift to individualized support and the offering of a range of different services (Kanellakos, 2006; MCSS, 2006).

The ASI is linked to how OW employment assistance measures were revised to include screening, assessment, and treatment for substance addiction in the early 2000s (OW Policy Directives 8.4, 2009). If an OW benefit recipient pursued treatment for substance use, with treatment variously defined,[2] it seemed this was perceived as on par with meeting

---

2 Should OW benefit recipients pursue treatment for substance use in residential treatment facilities where they are to pay room and board, they can receive basic needs and shelter allowances. If they are in receipt of the cost of room and board from the facility, they may still receive three months of OW income before they may experience a lessening or withdrawal of this support.

"employment activity" requirements like those expected of by persons not working through substance use challenges. Policy directives make clear, however, that only treatment approved by the ASI can be counted as "employment activity" for persons living with addiction (OW Policy Directives 6.10, 2018b). They also make clear that paid work is not an immediate expectation of benefit recipients following their engagement in treatment (OW Policy Directives 8.4, 2009). Caseworkers are instead to encourage and support people in their eventual pursuit of paid work, such as through "pre-employment" readiness programming (e.g., completion of high school education) and to include evidence of engagement in this other pre-employment activity in their accounting of benefit recipients' employment plans.

While I have observed that ministry annual reports were largely silent about addiction since 2014, I note here that there were references made to "barriers" that can circumvent individuals' employability potential; I infer that these barriers may include drug and alcohol dependency. In a brief discussion of people "distant from the labour market" in the 2016–17 annual report, it is in addition implied that if barriers are overcome, an individual's employment outcomes would improve (MCSS, 2017). By 2018, the ASI was still in existence and directed specialized and intensive case management, including supporting access to treatment (Ministry of Children, Community and Children's Services, MCCS, 2018).

Addiction, OW, and Toronto

It seems that growing attention was given to people living with addiction on the city of Toronto OW caseload in the first decade of the 2000s. A vibrant woman and engaging in her demeanour, caseworker Merren shared her own sense of the construction of this target population at the time: "I came to the city, it'll be seven years ago in January [in 2009]…. And then all of a sudden, it came out a few months later, or a year later after I joined, that indeed they were going to be looking at an addiction caseload and they didn't really know what that was going to look like."

Municipal documents suggest that the experience of living with addiction was included in reference to people with multiple barriers and through the discourse of "distant from the labour market," much like in reports associated with the province-wide social assistance review and subsequent reform trajectory and later MCSS annual reports. The 2012 report, *Working as One: A Workforce Development Strategy for Toronto*, outlined how people experiencing multiple barriers may be "distant," "moving closer," "transitioning" towards, or "advancing" in the labour market (City of Toronto, 2012, p. 35). People were understood to require a diverse range of programming that preceded or accompanied their participation in any employment activity programming. In *Brighter Prospects*, the Social Assistance Review Commission even commended the city's offering of intensive services to those experiencing multiple barriers and fewer interventions for those closer to the labour market (Lankin & Sheikh, 2012).

About five years after Merren's hiring, Toronto Employment and Social Services (TESS), the city department responsible for administering OW, seemed to know what the addictions caseload was "going to look like." In 2012, 10–20 per cent of the total OW caseload in Toronto was identified as experiencing substance use challenges in their daily lives and were increasingly managed by specialized "addictions caseworkers." In 2014, the pilot Personal Recovery through Employment and Life Planning (PREP) case management strategy was launched. With corresponding case management software, this pilot was intended to better support people experiencing multiple barriers to employment, including substance use. Since PREP was not universally implemented across all Toronto OW office locations, only some addictions caseworkers became more formally known as "PREP caseworkers" under the pilot initiative. The naming of PREP was, in part, to cultivate a case management culture that resisted the stigmatization of addiction (M. Brait, personal communication, September 2017).

Sixty per cent of individuals on OW in Toronto were identified as having multiple barriers to employment (one of which may be addiction) in 2014 (TESS, 2015). By 2016, 85 per cent of individuals on OW reported at least one barrier to employment (TESS, 2017). Half of persons who received OW in 2016 reported that they were not ready to become employed (TESS, 2017). Both budget documents and annual reports noted that those who were "distant from the labour market" because of multiple barriers remained on social assistance for longer periods of time (e.g., 44 per cent for two years or more as of 2016) (TESS, 2015; TESS, 2016a; TESS, 2017, p. 6). Towards the end of my time spent interviewing benefit recipients in 2017, TESS outlined its new goal of delivering a personalized and holistic approach to employment, health, and social services (TESS, 2017). By 2018, it committed to enhance referrals to mental health and addiction supports and support benefit recipients' achievement of "life stabilization" in their employability and well-being (TESS, 2018).

In the remainder of this chapter, I turn to my interview data. I explore how the discourse of "distance from the labour market" is reproduced in "addictions" or "PREP" caseworkers' talk of eligibility-related expectations for individuals living with addiction, including those in line with ASI-relevant policy directives. I also explore benefit recipients' subjective experiences of policy discourse, how they "may work on themselves" (Rabinow & Rose, 2006) in relation to it and in their relationships with caseworkers. I begin by revealing how benefit recipient–caseworker relationships took shape.

Being Known as Living with Addiction

Most people I interviewed first accessed OW because they had no other way to financially meet their needs and, in some cases, those of their children. The reasons for their economic insecurity varied. Some benefit recipients had histories of precarious employment (sometimes including drug dealing) or unemployment, had poor physical or mental health, had exited prison or treatment, or had their intimate partnerships with others end. It was not unusual for participants to experience a combination of these reasons in their first accessing OW. For some women, receipt of OW enabled them financial independence from an abusive male partner, an escape from gendered trauma, or more simply, a home of their own when separated and their partner sought paid work elsewhere. In terms of the latter, Bianca explained that the first time she went on OW was because: "[I] had to support my baby. Yeah.... See when we, when I first had my kid, he was going back and forth to Portugal to help his parents with moving and stuff. So. Yeah. I just needed to pay the rent. He helped and all. But I needed, I needed my own money." Bianca's story of her entrance onto OW reflects the culturally informed gender norms of their relationship too; she had been living with her partner as a stay-at-home mother while he was the main economic provider.

In some way and at some time in their relationships with OW caseworkers, participants became defined as persons using alcohol or drugs, or desiring to change their substance use patterns. Benefit recipients did not always tell me how this occurred. Caseworkers, however, had their own ways of coming to know benefit recipients as living with addiction. Gale had over ten years of experience, more recently specializing in supporting people living with addiction as a PREP caseworker. She shared that her caseload materialized in:

> Two different ways. The client may come and actually be honest. They may say to the application centre that they do have an addiction issue and/or maybe they're in recovery, or maybe they're going to treatment

or whatever, and then that intake would come through. Otherwise it's a worker establishing that this client has an issue and then they will transfer to me.

Most caseworkers I interviewed understood their caseloads as largely formed through referrals from other caseworkers in their office. Zoe, a woman working in one of the busiest OW office locations added: "So my caseload is built up of all the other cases in the office and caseworkers sending me people that have declared that they have a substance use issue or an alcohol concern."

Amy also received referrals to her caseload but maintained, "There's no flag on the file or anything like that." I probed what she would see as an indication of a person's struggles with substance use. Amy gave the following list:

Serious drug use since teen years. Incarceration since teen years. Trauma. The women have children that are not in their care. And never worked, almost never worked. If they have, it's cash. So, no real ties to the labour market and very loose family ties. And concurrent disorders – always an underlying mental health, almost always there's depression and anxiety, personality disorders.

Caseworkers were aware, too, that there were likely many other people whose needs were not met because they were not on their own or others' addictions or PREP caseloads. Walter acknowledged that: "Usually they're coming to me right off the hop, right from the intake. If, of course, they express themselves. Now I know that there are probably five hundred cases just in this office that I don't have."

Case Management in Practice

When I asked how caseworkers perceived OW to define the target population of people living with addiction, Zoe and Walter provided answers that pulled forward the work-first discourse and its employable/unemployable binary that seemed to underscore the 1990s introduction of welfare-to-work programming. Zoe said: "I think from a caseload perspective it's unemployable." Walter responded: "I think OW would be very simplistic in their definition, which would be people that cannot sustain employment, cannot sustain shelter. I think it would be that simple." As a PREP caseworker, Gale seemed more attuned to the newer distant from the labour market discourse. She said: "The catchment phrase for that group of people is 'life stabilization' ... so they're the people who are probably the furthest away from the labour market and have a range of barriers that prevent them from going to an employment training program tomorrow and starting."

Gale offered the additional observation that addiction was not something that could be easily discussed by the caseworker and benefit recipients in the past:

> [O]f course, the policy really says you should be looking for work. And for years it was frowned upon to have an addiction.... I think some clients got a real pushback from the worker, because they would say, "Well you have to go to a training program, we want you to go somewhere." And they wouldn't go. So, then they would come in and then it would be, "How come you didn't follow through?"... Their [benefit recipients] perception is that you're reprimanding them. And they see a worker as an authority figure. So, you have to approach it differently, because then they certainly don't want to tell you ... they're afraid that what income they are getting is going to be jeopardized.... So, there's been a shift somewhat.

As per Gale's answer, the distance from the labour market discourse seemed to create room for conversations about the experience of addiction and low income to be safe and possible. In their answers, however, caseworkers also illustrated and (perhaps unconsciously) legitimized how some social actors, for example, politicians and government policy developers and analysts, have power *over* – in the Weberian sense – the construction and case management of persons living with addiction (see also Gazso, 2019).

Whether thought of as unemployable or distant from the labour market, the people I interviewed were then case managed as part of addictions or PREP caseloads. As Caseworker Walter reminded me at the time of data collection for this project (2016 and 2017): "PREP has been around since 2014 but it was only in one part of the municipality. I think it was in the east and it was just experimental, they were just trying it out. For me to be using PREP as a tool now, which we officially launched, has only been since January [2016]." Thus, some caseworkers I met specialized in working with people living with addiction but still did not have access to PREP software, such as Zoe. She explained how their office developed their own comparable case management practices.

> There was a pilot, and there was only four offices that had the official PREP.... So, we [our office] identified that there were people who had addiction issues so they [sic] put them on specific caseloads.... So, here's

the thing. So, I've been on the addictions caseload in this office. PREP has been here for maybe at least six years, maybe longer. We don't have the PREP tool ... of course, we're putting in all their updates and all their benchmarks in the other information fields because we didn't have the tool.

The changes in case management were perceived by people living with addiction too. Bianca had been on OW long enough to observe: "Oh, we were looked down on at one time. Bad ... like nobody knew I was an addict back then.... The last two workers I've had were wonderful." Bianca further shared that her caseworker at the time of our interview was fully aware of her struggles with heroin and she did not perceive their relationship as mired to the same extent in stigma.

Cody's on and off experiences of OW over time also point to the overall change in how persons living with addiction are case managed. He found his sharing about his addiction in the past to result in judgmental actions by caseworkers.

Okay, there's five or six times I've been on welfare, on OW.... They bring you in to do that quick questionnaire with you. I've been up front ... "I'm in addiction. I need a place to stay".... And I've asked: "What services are available? What can you guys get me?" At the beginning Social Services said "That's nothing to do with us. We'll give you your cheque but now that we know you're a drug addict ... we're going to give it to you in weekly instalments or biweekly instalments to discourage you from blowing your whole cheque on drugs."

Cody had been very forthcoming with his current caseworker and was having quite a different experience in his recovery when I met him, a story I will pick up on in later chapters.

Caseworker Chris further explained how especially people on his PREP caseload would be treated differently: "The PREP tool is employment planning, addiction planning, and life planning as opposed to just employment planning. So, they [clients] would notice a huge difference if they were in the other one and had employment, employment, employment." Caseworker Merren confirmed:

And the difference is on this system, there's a piece that speaks to life management.... Do they have ID, do they have housing, does their housing support recovery? Then the second section is around specific to their addiction. How long has their addiction been an issue? Are they in treatment, aren't they? Should they?... And it actually gives a numerical value to those things. And then comes education and experience, work experience … now it attaches three numerical values based on life management, addiction, and employment and when these [first] two are really low, those are the things that are going to be the priority.

Case Management in Practice

It was during my initial entry into the field, specifically my meetings with OW program managers and staff, that I began to worry about one of the primary research questions driving my study: what are the welfare-to-work experiences of persons recovering from addiction? This was because, quite simply, it seemed there were none. As I have described, caseworkers largely perceived people living with addiction as unemployable or distant from the labour market because of multiple barriers they experience. As explicit within Directions 8.4 of the ASI, participation in some form of treatment can be perceived as equivalent to other employment activity programming. One manager I met further confirmed that people living with addiction are not required to participate in education and training activities in the same way as people not living with addiction. So, I reframed my question to explore the experiences of persons living with addiction while accessing OW more generally.

The women and men I interviewed largely saw their caseworkers as having an absence of paid work expectations for them (see also Gazso, 2019). When I asked Darlene if she ever talked about paid work with her caseworker, she responded: "No, not really because I guess she has – I don't know exactly what it is, but I guess because of my pain and everything, and I guess addiction and mental health concerns, like I don't have to, I guess, do what regular people on OW have to do." Jesse explained that once he had graduated from a rehabilitation program via Drug Treatment Court:

> She [caseworker] doesn't bring it up, because she knows – I told her I said – we sat down and talked about it a long time ago and I said, "Listen Genevieve, until I get out of this program – I've got to take care of my mother. I don't have time for work….Yeah, I'm actually now doing my high school, my GED."

I met and interviewed Anais, a young single woman in her twenties, with a warm demeanour and quiet self-confidence, at a local coffee shop. My last memory of her is of her swishing long, long hair as she stepped out of my car when I drove her home following our interview. Anais had an experience similar to Jesse's in that she and her caseworker talked about her pursuing education as a first step towards exiting OW. Knowing that Anais was in recovery and had recently weaned herself off methadone, the caseworker recommended: "Think about where you want to go, pick a school and then we'll work it out." Also knowing Anais identified as mixed race and of Indigenous heritage, Anais said the caseworker "also brought up the status thing, if you [*sic*] can get that it could be really beneficial for school."

Since it might take some time before benefit recipients became known as working through substance use dependency, it was not surprising that some had experienced different paid work expectations over time. When Alexei's addiction was not known by his caseworker, he remembered that: "Sometimes the lady asking me to bring me every week some kind of signatures from the places I'm looking for a job. So, it's just really hard to explain that I can go and get the signature but what's the point of this?" When I asked if his current worker did not expect him to job search, Alexei replied: "Yeah, like I think he understands me at this moment ... he knew because I'm on methadone." Trevor had a similar story of how some workers were "so pushy, you know" about expectations of his employability but since he became known as living with addiction, his current caseworker "is not pushy when it comes to that."

Clive was a single white man, fifty-five years old, and soon exiting OW when I met him. He was awaiting his file transfer to the Ontario Disability Support Program for reasons I expected to do with his mental health challenges given a few guarded statements he made. His twenty-four-year-old daughter lived with his ex-wife. I met him at the Tim Hortons near where he lived. Though sporting a squashed-down baseball cap and a bushy beard, it was still possible to see the humour in his eyes when he talked. At first hedging in his answers, he soon opened up. I think my earnestness at wanting to hear his story entertained him. Clive saw himself as a functioning alcoholic and could recollect with precision what he saw as the frustrating ways that he was expected to seek paid work from other, earlier caseworkers.

> And my biggest problem was I'd get a young girl just out of school, twenty-three, twenty-four years old telling me I've got to do this and do that and they have no idea what I've been through. And for you to sit there and tell me that you're going to keep my cheque because I'm not doing this drives me over the edge. So, then I guess they decided that I needed a special worker. So, once I started seeing June [addictions caseworker], things got easier for me.

Caseworker Zoe confirmed that working with this target population is entirely different than working with benefit recipients not living with addiction: "You have other caseworkers that are wanting these people to get jobs, to do employment activities, to go to Employment Ontario agencies, go to job fairs. And they're not capable. They need to get their medication, they need to get ID, they need to be able to find a place to sleep."

I nonetheless persevered and intentionally asked caseworkers about the paid work expectations they did have. After some hesitation, I found that four of the seven caseworkers I interviewed shared case-worker Gale's approach, one she shared of assessing people "where they're at." Gale explained: "So it's really about working with the client where they're at and ultimately what their goals are. And that's part of the reason I have the whole range on my caseload, and I think it's really important that we understand as workers that that's how addic-tion works." Caseworkers' assessment of clients "where they're at" also seemed to suggest that benefit recipients were responsible for their own relationship with the labour market. Dante confirmed: "Well, if you tell your worker 'Listen man, I have a fucking drug problem.' Your worker will be like 'fine, no problem. Let's deal with that first.'"

Caseworkers may adopt the approach of meeting people "where they're at," but they also had to get the required work of case manage-ment done. For example, Chris told me how he had to find novel ways to appease people's anxiety as part of the process of completing his job requirements.

> So, what's happening now, the shift is OW is recognizing that we have to meet clients where they're at, and that's a whole part of this whole addic-tion thing. Sometimes my clients are so anxious they don't even want to come in through the door. So, I meet them around the corner, and I have coffee with them there and we have our catch up there, or our appoint-ments there.

Chris was unusual among the seven caseworkers I interviewed. Though he had only been working just over one year when I met him, he reported spending inordinate amounts of time at home and "off the clock" trying to develop knowledge about existing resources and supports in his community to which he could refer people living with addiction.

Meanwhile, the "where they're at" approach existed simultaneously with OW still being a program of temporary relief to persons in finan-cial need and still even retaining some of the work-first discourse of the

1990s. I soon came to understand that an approach of "where they're at" may be shared but could still clearly differ by caseworker. It could have the complementary subtext of "it depends." When I asked Merren about paid work expectations for people she worked with, she maintained:

> No. As a rule I haven't, but it depends on where they're at in their recovery. And the closer they start moving towards recovery and that they've been managing really well, then I say to them, "Yes, okay now it's time to move on. You're doing really well here, so let's start to look at do you need some training?" And that's when the essential skills program comes in. (see also Gazso, 2019, p. 138)

Of all seven caseworkers interviewed, Tamara was relatively new to specializing in working with people living with addiction. Nonetheless, she was confident in her overall approach concerning expectations of benefit recipients and that their paid work participation was the ultimate goal:

> So it just depends on where they're at with their addiction and this is something we can identify from the PREP tool.... But regardless, the plan is to move towards employment planning. So, it's just a matter of giving them more time to get there as opposed to "You're job ready, we need to get you started on working" and then we move in that direction and they're held accountable for that each time they meet with us. Whereas the addiction clients, we're more supportive in terms of the length of time it takes them to get there. So we're dealing with specific addiction, providing supports, getting them help regardless of how long it takes.

Dione provided other information that yielded my sense of the subtext of "it depends." She maintained "they [clients] want to work. So, right now in my caseload, I have in employment counselling, more than 25 per cent in employment counselling."

I came to understand that whether and how paid work became a topic of discussion, and expectation seemed to depend on caseworker discretion. Caseworkers often managed caseloads of just over one hundred clients a month by drawing on their education, training, and skill. They used decision-making tools constructed for them, like PREP software, as well as followed rules and regulations of their work (Maki, 2011; Pennisi & Baker Collins, 2016). They could, however, make decisions about applying these tools and manipulating rules. As I will continue to show in this chapter, caseworker discretion could result in achieving the maximum benefit(s) for a benefit recipient or the imposition of punitive sanctions, both actions Lipsky (1980) saw to be mediated by favouritism, stereotyping, and routinizing.

Treatment Expectations

Caseworkers' personal philosophies about treatment[3] shaped whether and how they expected it in lieu of other employment activities. Amy saw a difference between residential treatment and the seeking of outpatient support. She maintained: "[F]irst of all I do not expect my clients to go into treatment at all. I don't have that expectation. I think that would interfere with the relationship building.... I do encourage them to go into counselling just to talk to somebody." Merren had straightforward and immediate expectations for people that were more about improving their general health and well-being:

> Yeah, I'll say to them, "This is your job now. Your job is to look after your health and to do what it is you can do to get by for this next three months. Let's just see if maybe you can find a doctor. Maybe you can explore a couple of those places we talked about. Or maybe you can get to the ID clinic, and I'll make sure the money is there for you to get there."

Two other caseworkers were also quite reluctant to recommend a specific plan for treatment. Gale said: "Really I think treatment should be self-directed versus me sending them to you [the service provider] and I say, 'I've assessed you and I think you should do these things.'" Walter shared:

> My experience with treatment is that you put the olive branch out. Say, "If you have ever had enough and you truly want to quit, I have the phone number of every single treatment centre in the province of Ontario and I can get you in somewhere very quickly." So, we address it. I don't brow beat it. I don't do anything. Because there's nobody that, if they're not ready, there's nothing that's going to happen.... It has to be their idea.

Some caseworkers approached treatment expectations with the same "where they're at" and the subtext of "it depends" approach they had

---

3 Treatment can include participation in AA or the equivalent, attendance at a day program, an in-house stay at a residential treatment facility, or participation in one-on-one or group counselling with a counsellor in private practice or through an organization like the Centre for Addiction and Mental Health (CAMH).

concerning paid work expectations for benefit recipients. In example, Zoe said:

> It all depends on the client…. Number one, some clients want to move forward and they want to be referred to treatment or they want to be referred to out-patient or they want to be referred to withdrawal management. But there are some clients that they're just not there yet…. And I have some clients that are in after care and that have been sober for maybe a year or two but don't feel comfortable moving forward to a different caseload because they still want my support.

The caseworkers I interviewed seemed to orient to benefit recipients' individual agency about working on or overcoming their addiction. Caseworkers' listening and indirect or reactive guidance – in the vein of "I will give you some options but no pressure. I will help you more if only you ask" – can even be read as encouraging clients' self-confidence in their ability to take control of their substance use; an approach on par with empowering individuals (Augsberger & Swenson, 2015; Bolhaar et al., 2020). This approach seems to fit with the common-sense notion that an individual cannot manage an addiction unless they self-identify as having a problem and take actions to address it. However, this approach may not necessarily preclude caseworkers from exercising discretion in ways perceived as regulatory of benefit recipients' agency.

Benefit recipients were forthcoming in sharing how they understood their treatment as connected to their receipt of OW. When I finally met Charise after two failed attempts, I found her to be welcoming and open, especially once we realized we shared in having Hungarian ancestry. Charise was a white woman, age fifty-four, single, and with long brunette hair with highlights of auburn. Her adult son lived with his father, Charise's ex-husband, while she lived in an apartment she shared with a roommate. As we sat down with cups of coffee she made us, Charise explained that her continued use of crack cocaine made it difficult for her to plan her days, including making our earlier interview dates. Charise sometimes also had trouble maintaining her attendance at a group counselling program, but there were higher stakes associated with her missing this program.

> CHARISE: Yeah, I have that going on, every Tuesday.
> AMBER: Is that for CA [Cocaine Anonymous]?
> CHARISE: No. It's to talk about substance abuse and that, but I'm not getting it [CA] down there…. But I have to go anyway.

AMBER: Is it you're going as part of OW? Kind of an agreement that you're going to seek out this help?

CHARISE: Yeah.

Charise then pointed out that because she continued to randomly use crack cocaine, this suggested that her attendance at this program was clearly not by her own choice alone.

OW Directives 8.4 pertaining to the ASI outline sanctions for non-compliance with treatment expectations, such as withholding monthly benefit income, at the same time as outlining an awareness of individuals' potential relapse. These directives make clear that caseworkers are encouraged to work with OW managers to try to avoid deeming people ineligible for benefit receipt because of their non-compliance. I found that caseworkers exercised considerable discretion in enforcing sanctions. Amy seemed to avoid the use of them: "Yeah, they [OW] have compliance because you're supposed to be doing something. But if you're really kind, you're just trying to understand what's happening for you [the individual]. How come you're not reaching out to more things in your life? You [the caseworker] want to understand that."

Walter had misgivings about using sanctions but: "[A]t the end of the day it is the only time that you can get your client to come in and see you. It's the only time … it's a tool that I have to use in order to update [my records]." Zoe echoed Walter's perspective:

> So, I really hate holding cheques. I really don't like doing it but sometimes it's necessary. For auditing purposes they [benefit recipients] have to be participating in something.… If they're not attending appointments, that affects their eligibility, and if their eligibility is affected, that means it affects their payments. Because they have to have an active outcome plan. And for most of my clients it's they're participating in an addiction service program.

Walter's and Zoe's perspectives on using sanctions echoes my earlier discussion of the necessity for caseworkers to balance their discretion with their need to perform the actual work of case management.

Shawn shared an example of his personal experience of sanctions and why they occurred:

> She [caseworker] was off last week, so I phoned her Monday to say my cheque was short and she goes "XXXX [program] is calling me. Why are they calling me? Is there something wrong?" I said, "Yeah." I said, "You've got to be clean for three weeks or whatever." I said, "I wasn't even

supposed to go there." She said, "You were supposed to be there for three weeks." And I said, "I'm not going, they won't take me."

Shawn had attended a day program that prepared recovering substance users – in this program, recovery is defined as being clean and sober for thirty days – for employment through skills and training (e.g., goal-setting, computer literacy, interviewing and job skills). However, since Shawn was still using heroin at the time, he was deemed ineligible to participate by the program's intake caseworker. Thus, he stopped attending the program and his absence was recorded. In turn, a portion of his cheque was withheld for non-compliance. That his caseworker was surprised about his lack of fit for this program gives some insight into how difficult it can be for caseworkers and benefit recipients to share the same understanding of living with addiction.

Some caseworkers' reluctance to impose sanctions for non-compliance with treatment or "outcome plans" stemmed from their awareness of the barriers that benefit recipients faced in completing treatment. Case-workers named these to include transportation costs to attend, physical and mental health challenges, substance use patterns, histories of incarceration, and trauma. Even the push and pull of engaging in sex work or drug dealing in order to survive can make pursuit of treatment difficult. Caseworker Tamara provided one example: "I called a client yesterday and her drug dealer answered the phone. What do I have that I'm going to convince you to leave this drug dealer and be with me, [this dealer] who is meeting your immediate need at that time? It's really, really, really difficult."

Gale explained that should someone want treatment, there are also other systemic barriers:

> Wait lists are huge.... [I]n Toronto wait lists are really hard, so if some-body is looking for treatment it can be very difficult to get in.... Even then, some treatment programs will make you, what I call, "jump through some hoops" first. So, prior to actually going into a full treatment program, you have to attend let's say six weeks of meetings and interviews and what-ever. So, if they miss that's part of the problem. Because they have to meet all these benchmarks to get to the next level to get the next piece of help that they need. The problem is that the benchmarks for some clients are insurmountable.

And according to Zoe, the process of entering detox in order to qual-ify for residential treatment can act as a barrier too: "There is a central access line that they call. You pretty much have to call every hour and see if a bed is available. They're the point where you call out for all the other places. And you're basically trying to find a bed that does that kind of program."

Walter further explained: "So this is where it gets good, is because the central detox number will not talk to me. It'll only talk to them." That people are responsible for pursuing detox does suggest a lack of coercion on the part of caseworkers and an embracement of people's individual choice. However, Walter's misgivings about how he cannot speak to intake workers indicates his awareness that some benefit recipients would benefit from him directly supporting their plan to detox.

Given these barriers, it is not surprising that attempting and pursuing recovery requires considerable intellectual, emotional, and physical work, my focus in chapter 8. Here, I note that benefit recipients also identified these barriers named by caseworkers. For example, Bianca attempted to quit her heroin addiction more than once in the years before I met her, but the experience of withdrawal, coupled with her awareness that there would be few supports after she exited a program, were then deterring barriers.

> I went to XXXX [withdrawal program] about three times. I just couldn't do it.... It was hard, you go really sick, sick, sick, right? But then, I don't know. They didn't refer me to like [a] place, so I'm going to end up getting all sick and get better and then what? "Go home." You're not going to line [me] up with something? "Well, you gotta call and make arrangements." That could take months. I go, "I'm going to be using by that time." And sure enough. I didn't even clean up because I was suffering and my dealer was just down the street and I said "why?" I know I should have said "my kids." But when you're in the addiction...

Case Management in Practice

According to Caseworker Merren: "I have approximately 110 folks on my caseload, and that doesn't include family members." All caseworkers were required to check in with benefit recipients by meeting them at least every three months, though some of them were in contact with them by telephone or face-to-face meetings more often than that. Overall, it was well recognized by caseworkers and my manager contacts that managing this number of people could make "high-quality service" very difficult. It was therefore not surprising to learn from some benefit recipients that they felt they were "just a number" on OW and their caseworker's awareness of their own unique lives limited. Some benefit recipients implied that besides their name, caseworkers had no way of distinguishing them from other persons on the caseload.

There were three potential implications of this anonymizing potential of case management. First, benefit recipients could perceive that their unique needs were overlooked – or overwritten by computer software (see also Maki, 2011). Danni provided an example:

> It's stressful when you get a letter that says I need another transportation form because I guess their computer just pops them out.... So, when I get one of those forms it's "Oh my God." Because my rent is $804 and I get $969. So, if I don't get a certain thing on my cheque ... when I get a form that something isn't going to be on my ... then my heart starts beating really fast ... so I call Miss Jameson [caseworker] right away, and I'm always worried about the tone that I have after.

Danni also felt conflicted about resisting such a computerized letter because: "She probably has a lot to deal with as well from other people that are calling her all day long too, right? So, it's like 'what are my problems?'"

Second, the anonymizing potential could be used by benefit recipients to "play the system." Playing the system captures how people on social assistance can use their knowledge of policy by manipulating rules and regulations in ways that advantage their situation. The welfare dependency discourse continues to construct such strategic learning and manipulation as people engaging in welfare abuse or fraud. I am more inclined to see "playing the system" as people's resistance to the structural determination of their lives, an inevitable response to receipt of monthly income that perpetuates poverty, social exclusion, and stigmatization (see also Gazso, 2007). Indeed, some benefit recipients' awareness that they were but one of many on a caseload meant the risks of playing the system were outweighed by possible advantages, including having a roof over one's head and affording food, or even maintaining use patterns. When I asked Dante about his work for pay in construction and whether he reported his monthly income from this work each month (re: OW earnings exemptions), he replied: "Yeah, I don't do it, divulge shit.... Yo man, cocaine habit is expensive to feed. I don't want to go to jail. I don't want to steal anymore. So."

Franco provided the clearest example of how playing the system is made possible by learning the system from others on OW:

> There's nowhere that says on the [web]site I can get an air conditioner paid for me.... I had to find out through somebody else who fucks with

the system who said, "They'll pay for it. You get a note from your doctor." Why am I finding out this stuff through the people? I have to go to the scammers to find out what OW will cover or help me with. And it makes me feel like I'm a scammer too. But I'm not.

In his learning of how to get an "extra" while on OW, Franco also pointed to the third implication of the anonymizing potential of the caseworker–benefit recipient relationship: internalized oppression. Perceiving oneself as unseen and unknown by an OW caseworker (or the system itself) could then mean an individual compares their experiences with nameless others and takes on other, oppressive views or negative stereotypes of the marginalized group to which they belong (see also Baker Collins et al., 2020).

Caseworker Support

From the stories shared, it may seem that the caseworker discretion that I learned about was mostly the punitive kind Lipsky (1980) identified, for example, of reinforcing stereotypes. I also learned a great deal, however, about how some caseworkers showed favouritism or, as caseworker Amy saw it, simple kindness. Besides trying to avoid sanctions, she shared her own experiences of in some way "bending the rules" to support people she worked with:

> I try to give, if they have the courage to ask me, I'll try and toss you $30 for a haircut. If I gave you $100 last month, I'll try to give you another $100 this month. I'm not supposed to be doing that at all.... So, I could give six tokens over and over again. I've given double transportation repeatedly.

Although I perceived Walter as somewhat paternalistic in his approach to case management, he also conveyed respect for the people he worked with.

> I just basically say I've been doing this a long time. There is not one thing that can come out of your mouth that I'm ever going to shocked about.... It really starts from them not making them wait out in that waiting room when they come in very long. It starts by answering your phone messages when they call. I have clients that are going "My God, I can't believe you called me back."

Tamara, too, acknowledged the more supportive role of caseworkers for persons living with addiction. Merren, however, qualified that the giving of instrumental support that could be effective is constrained by caseload size: "I'm fine with my 110 [caseload] but if you're actually providing tangible supports in terms of being out on the street with them and helping them get housing and so on, you might want to look at about twenty people."

Jim was a single, white man in his fifties who self-defined as an alcoholic. I interviewed him by telephone. I had a difficult time interviewing Jim mainly because each time I spoke with him by telephone, even to arrange the interview, I found I was challenged by his wavering attention and sometimes confrontational style of conversation. This jarred with how he seemed genuinely pleased to be asked to participate in my study and had important insights to share, such as how he experienced kindness from his caseworker. As he put it: "Yeah, she bends the rules for me."

Other benefit recipients acknowledged these kindnesses from their caseworkers too. Clive found he could manage his receipt of income on OW as a single person only because his caseworker "[G] ot me a little, extra things. If I called her at the beginning of the month and said I need some razor blades she'd give me an extra $40. The next time I'd see her, my beard is longer." Here, Clive also hinted at the quality of his expressive relationship with his caseworker – they both knew he used the money on something other than shaving.

Trevor also experienced kindness:

And I know with Patricia [caseworker] when I was having problems on the street and that, she's like "Here." She said, "Hold on one second." She came back and she gave me a whole bunch of papers where I can go, like good places. And some of the places where I did go to, they were so comfortable. And she didn't just give me any kind of room or whatever. She put thought into it, "Where would she be comfortable?"

The intimacy permitted by the caseworker–benefit recipient relationship had the potential to be transformative of peoples' behaviours and experiences, a theme I will pick up on in a more fulsome discussion of benefit recipients' work on recovery later in this book too. For now, suffice it to say, it was clear that the instrumental and expressive support some benefit recipients received from a caseworker had the potential to be productive of their feeling they had the resources to meet psychological, social, and/or physical challenges (Dodge et al., 2012, p. 230), or productive of a sense of order and continuity in their everyday life experiences, what Giddens (1991) terms ontological security. Carie gave insight into these benefits of a supportive relationship with a caseworker in her sharing about respect:

> Yeah, and when you respect somebody, like I respect her, I don't want to let her down.... Yeah, I really like her ... and she don't make you feel like she's making you feel like you're in a psychiatry place. She doesn't look at you like she's judging you. If she knows you're lying, she'll lift up her one eyebrow.

Subjectivity Constituted: The Recovering Addict

Caseworker and benefit recipient accounts suggest that employability expectations for persons living with addiction do not exist, at least not initially in the same way as for persons without these challenges. And not being perceived as employable does not mean that people are not subject to other expectations, nor that these do not morph into employability expectations over time. Coupling the findings of my discourse analysis with my interview data leads me to conclude that benefit recipients experienced another expectation associated with their ongoing eligibility, most noticeably that of treatment. Moreover, I contend that the "distance from the labour market" discourse produces a particular benefit recipient subjectivity in the form of the "recovering addict." Benefit recipients' enactment and embodiment of the "recovering addict" subject position conditions their ongoing benefit receipt (Gazso, 2019). Caseworkers (re-)produced this subjectivity in their case management and even when they exercised kindness in their relationships with benefit recipients. Indeed, should benefit recipients not "work on themselves" to achieve this subject position, they could experience sanctions. If not outright sanctions, benefit recipients, especially lone mothers in my study, perceived that they experienced control and regulation at the level of their interpersonal relationship with their caseworker.

At the time I was to meet Jules for our interview, she was not at her apartment to answer the door, even though she had confirmed her willingness to participate in an interview by text message one hour prior to my driving to meet her. When I called her on the phone, she answered and told me she could not do the interview after all. But she said this just as she walked into the hallway where I was standing, and we met face to face. In the space of an awkward few moments, she explained that she had a cold, and this was why she said she was unavailable. Jules nonetheless generously agreed to sit in my car to chat for an hour. At twenty-eight years of age, Jules was a petite white woman with blonde hair and grey-blue eyes. Jules was participating in suboxone treatment and had custody of one of her children, her eight-year-old daughter. Her ex-partner had custody of her eldest, an eleven-year-old son. She was in the process of trying to regain custody of her youngest son, a toddler aged five years, from her mother when we met. When I asked about her experience working with her caseworker, Jules told me how she felt her caseworker viewed her employment potential as a lone mother:

> JULES: They don't promote us going back to paid work.
> AMBER: What do they promote?
> JULES: Their focus apparently, like her focus as that type of worker is to keep people clean. So, do people not reintegrate back into society? And every time I tell her I want to do this and this and this, she's like "You're kind of jumping the gun." I'm like "No I'm not! I'm a mom, I want to support my kids. What do you mean I'm jumping the gun? That's stupid."

Marnie had a similar experience with her caseworker, though I did not experience the same awkwardness meeting her. Marnie had just finished working out at a local gym and had already even bought a coffee by the time I arrived for our interview at a coffee shop in her community. A white woman, thirty-three years old, Marnie had ash blonde hair pulled into a high ponytail and warm hazel eyes. Marnie was raising her young daughter with the support of her parents; they all lived together in Marnie's childhood home. In suboxone treatment and in recovery for just over a year when I met her, her story of seeking support from her caseworker to pursue education echoed that of Jules's:

> And I like, I'll never forget, I called her, and I said I wanted to apply for the XXX program and she was like, "Well, why do you wanna do that?" I was like, "Ah, so I can figure out what I want to do with my life." "Oh, okay. Okay, fine."... I think maybe she didn't realize I was as far along as I was [in recovery].... I think maybe she looked at it and thought, okay, if you're in an addictions portfolio, why are you doing this?

That Jules saw herself as employable and Marnie saw herself as ready to go to school, but their caseworkers did not, illustrates how the distance from the labour market discourse could limit benefit recipients' subjectivity realized in their relationship with their caseworker (Bischoping & Gazso, 2016; Gazso, 2019). Jules and Marnie found their caseworkers' orientation to them as recovering addicts restrictive.

The discourse of distance from the labour market could also produce the subjectivity of the recovering addict for benefit recipients when caseworkers' discretion was mediated by their paternalism. In another difficult time of talk in our interview, Jim worked hard to make me understand that while I interpreted his caseworker as aware of his alcoholism and supportive of his recovery, he did not always entirely agree.

> AMBER: She's [caseworker] aware of some stuff you're going through. So maybe she's also just being really supportive.
> JIM: I don't know. Maybe she thinks she is. But I understand the system. And the system says I should be rotated out. And she's like, "No. I am keeping this guy." So, I'm like her fucking pet. Do you understand how degrading that is?
> AMBER: So, you don't like that.
> JIM: No. She's helping me. I get it. Guess what?
> AMBER: What?
> JIM: I don't want fucking help. I want to be my own person.

In saying "rotated out," Jim was referring to his view that he need not be on an addictions caseload and could transition to a caseworker who worked with preparing able-bodied persons for employment and exit from OW. Jim saw his current caseworker as both "bending the rules" for him and limiting his agency.

Some caseworkers more obviously conveyed paternalism and the regulation of benefit recipients' eligibility when they shared about when and why they thought people were ready to consider pre-employment or employment activities. When I reviewed her employability expectations for people, Zoe had responded that most "are not capable." While this seemed her honest assessment after years of experience, it had the possibility to lock into stereotypes of persons living with addiction. Considering people on his caseload in methadone treatment, Walter maintained:

> Well, first off, we have to get down to 40 mg of methadone before they're really considered functioning, before they're going to be accepted into any kind of skills training program. So, once we get to that, or even before that, we discuss volunteer placement programs. My feeling is partly it's the addictions but partly it's the morale and their self-worth. "Let's get some volunteer work, let's do this, get you out of the house." (see also Gazso, 2019, p. 9)

The discursive construction of the "recovering addict" subject position could create the experience of regulation, but its effect need not be entirely punitive. People living with addiction were assumed to eventually transition into non-treatment employment activities or pre-employment planning; as caseworker Tamara shared: "The plan is to move towards employment planning." Of all benefit recipients I interviewed, Tara provided me a small window into how PREP case management works. I interviewed Tara by phone in the afternoon, after she finished attending a college program. Tara was a single woman, aged fifty-three, a mother of three children with her younger twin daughters in the care of their father. She had a relaxed and open demeanour in sharing over the phone. I often felt like I was talking to someone with whom I was close, like a family member. She implied how being seen in recovery and closer to the labour market can also hold out the promise of transitioning off the addictions caseload.

> I really like the thing they do with the percentage thing. They have a new program for certain areas. And I'm going to school and blah, blah, blah. So, I'm at 89 per cent at that and then in another section, um, like for different areas that are going on? It's an overall sort of thing. And apparently when you get to 100 per cent you're not supposed to meet an addiction worker anymore.

Objectification, Subjectification, and the Limiting of Lives to Addiction

Discourses include statements and ideas that are employed strategically and encircle or transform social interaction and behaviour (Foucault, 1973/1994). Any discourse – so including policy discourse – is produced and governed by power–knowledge relations, according to Foucault (1978. p. 93), with power defined as an ever transformative and productive force. Foucault's genealogical analysis in the *History of Sexuality Volume 1*, for example, reveals the production of knowledge about sex – or discourse on sex – through its relations with power, including social actors, institutions and apparatuses, and procedures and practices. In deconstructing the discourse on sex, he further reveals its construction of objects such as that of the "hysterical woman," as well as her subjectivity. Foucault's theorizing of the objects (and subjects) of knowledge constituted by discourse is particularly salient to the points that I wish to make in this final section.

Earlier in this chapter, I have shown how "people living with addiction" were constructed as an object in and through OW policy, to be known and managed by OW directives institutionally and caseworkers practically. As McLaren (2002) observes, when objectification occurs through institutions and therefore discourses (as per the governments analysed in this study), and caseworkers' practice (including discretion), it involves "dividing practices," for example, the "addict" is different and to be targeted separate from the "non-addict."[4] Discourses in addition constitute subject positions or subjectivities (Mills, 2004). That is, in relation to objectification.

Foucault understands individuals' work on themselves to become the subject of a discourse; this is the process of subjectification (Bischoping & Gazso, 2016; McLaren, 2002). His notion of disciplinary power improves this understanding of the process of subjectification alongside objectification. In *Discipline and Punish: The Birth of the Prison*, Foucault (1977) writes that the prison panopticon produced the capacity for officers to survey prisoners at any time. Awareness of this structure encouraged prisoners to self-discipline and self-police their behaviour to avoid punishment and regardless of whether officers did observe them or not (Foucault, 1977).

I argue that so too does OW legislation and policy and enactment of it by caseworkers in their practice have this same reach of disciplinary power, and therefore achieves subjectification. Indeed, when benefit recipients living with addiction are objects of work, caseworkers pursue routinized and standardized case management that construes a subject position upon which benefit receipt is made contingent. I have tried to capture this by using participants' talk to show how the "recovering addict" subjectivity is constituted by the "distance from the labour market" discourse. My interviews with benefit recipients confirm that they can work on themselves to perform this desired subjectivity (Bischoping & Gazso, 2016) in order to avoid being misconstrued as otherwise and therefore experience harmful consequences, such as the loss of benefit income.

Opportunities for caseworker discretion (or even resistance), exercised through favouritism, stereotyping, routinizing, and paternalism (Lipsky, 1980), are still possible through objectification. On the one hand, caseworker discretion is suggestive of disciplinary power; for example, a lone mother's subjectification may be compelled in order to maintain her benefit receipt (Gazso, 2019). On the other hand, if

---

4 As a point of interest, a non-Foucauldian way to understand the construction of this target population is suggested by Gubrium and Jarvinen's (2014) concept of clientization. They argue that clientization occurs when individual troubles, such as troubles with bodies like that of addiction, are turned into problems to be managed and addressed by human services. Social policy sorting, such as that required to problematize and respond to living with addiction, can be thought of as part of the process of clientization.

caseworkers themselves are suspicious of the framing of the object of their case management, benefit recipients may perceive their caseworkers as supportive of their own agentic decisions based on their unique situations. Moreover, benefit recipients' agency and resistance are not necessarily curtailed by these objectification and subjectification processes, as surely seen in the ways they can "play the system" or pursue recovery in hopes of exiting an addictions caseload.

My main concern is that the objectification and subjectification that occurs through OW discourse and case management practices have the potential to limit – or can limit – the lives of people to their addiction. "Recovering addict" can become not just the subjectivity on which individuals know their receipt of benefits is contingent but collude with "addict" being their ascribed identity or "master status" (see also Hughes, 1949) in their relationships with caseworkers and others in the wider social milieux. Meanwhile, bearing and managing this weight is just one part of benefit recipients' lives when working through substance use dependency. Indeed, I turn to exploring benefit recipients' agency in their other everyday experiences of living with addiction while accessing OW, their resistance to being seen only and always as some kind of "addict" in the next two chapters. I offer one final point of foreshadowing here too. The possibility for benefit recipients to enact a recovering addict subject position *and* subvert it to their own ends, in deliberately claiming what recovery means to them and in imagining its possibilities, is not ignored in my final analysis and is explored in detail in chapter 8 on new beginnings.

6 Being a User, Sober, or in Recovery on Welfare

I began each interview by asking benefit recipients to tell me about the mundane and take-for-granted experiences they had living through each day. Those who identified as sober or in recovery had stories of their days that did not always seem so different from what I would expect of non-substance users. People wake up, they may have breakfast, they leave the house and go about daily tasks and responsibilities, they come home, and later may go to bed. If they have children in their care, they can engage in additional practices of caregiving, including exchanges of instrumental and expressive support (see chapter 7 for more on this). For those still using substances, however, little about a day could seem typical.

Participants' stories largely dispel stereotypical assumptions about the daily life of those who use substances or are overcoming their use of substances, such as their being irresponsible, selfish, lacking a moral compass and ruinous to communities, often taking on associations with race, class, and gender and even religion when concerning opioid use (Smith, 2010; Sobotka & Stewart, 2020; Szott, 2017). Moreover, people living with addiction experience poverties, not just poverty-level benefit amounts but the lack of supports or resources, this lack inhibiting their economic mobility. This chapter reveals participants' daily lives as not limited to that of only and always addiction, not centred only around a "recovering addict" subjectivity via their relationship with Ontario Works (OW), but rich in experience, nuanced in terms of relationships, replete with obstacles – and, ultimately, boundless in opportunities and hope.

A Typical Day of Managing Substance Use?

A typical day in the life of participants was not solely about, but could be shaped by, their choices around use, sobriety, or recovery.[1] Participants who shared what they saw to be a typical day in their life were those who defined as sober or in recovery. There was nonetheless considerable variation in their daily living and whether they saw there was any semblance of routine beyond waking, eating, and sleeping.

At one point, Jesse and Smitri had similar typical days in that they had both participated in Drug Treatment Court; their participation obligated them to engage in a daily treatment program in lieu of jail time (Public Safety Canada, 2022). By the time of our interviews, Jesse had successfully graduated from the program and Smitri was in the process of deciding whether to continue her participation. Both were experiencing the somewhat liminal space of feeling they no longer had a set schedule for their week but knowing that they were expected to do something in pursuit of their recovery. Jesse, however, was beginning to see his day as mainly centred around providing care to his mother in the afternoon and evening.

> My normal day for me, I go to sleep last night, I wake up in the morning about 7:30–8:00. I go and I take my dog for an hour walk or whatever … go back to sleep for an hour, maybe an hour and a half. Then come out have breakfast, stuff like that, maybe lunch. Go out walk the dog again, take her to the park, throw the ball around. And about 3:00 I have to go and see my mom at East General Hospital to pick her up. Then we usually go back to her house and have dinner or something like that. So, now I'm getting to about 6:30–7:00 and my day is pretty much done almost. So, I end up coming home and taking my dog for another walk, go to the park or whatever, go home, go to sleep, play some video games.

Smitri perceived that her typical day included little activity but the continued effort to attend programming.

> I don't do much with my time. I get up, I walk my dog. I'm not a breakfast person. I was smoking a lot of weed. I've recently cut down. So, my life

---

1   Whereas sobriety in this project refers to abstaining from use for some time, recovery is defined as active engagement in maintaining sobriety or practising harm reduction, within the context of an overall holistic approach, of working through mental and physical health challenges to the betterment of health and well-being. I learned from participants through their stories, too, that recovery assumes individuals' ongoing efforts to overcome their suffering associated with their use and to achieve healing.

really doesn't consist of much. I'm with the boyfriend 24/7. He does run his own business, but it's on a call base, he's a contractor … he's at home too, he's on OW also, and he took a business program with OW. So, his is a little different than mine. He has to do more reporting and whatnot. But it really consists of sitting in the den room, smoking cigarettes out the window, watching TV, cleaning, doing nothing with my time, coming to program, coming home to do the same thing.

Steve was the only person I interviewed who had the unique experience of participating in a residential program run by the Salvation Army for persons committed to recovery; we spoke while he was finishing his day of work in a laundry; taking part in the program involved his engagement in this work to build his employment skills and contribute to the community. I remember our telephone interview fondly. Steve was a "talker"; he had a genial spirit and peppered his talk about his life with humour and deep introspection. As a white man in his early fifties, Steve had led a rich life in the past, working for pay as a high-rise window washer and while living in a rented apartment. He had had various relationships and enjoyed a lifestyle of partying alongside his engagement in paid work. His drinking and substance use patterns, however, culminated in his inability to continue his work, and he eventually lost his apartment and became homeless. Steve drew a comparison between his daily life while participating in the program and the mental struggle he faced trying to consider and act upon recovery while living on the street.

Well, now that I'm in, ahh, this program here, it's, it's pretty much almost full time. Which is nice because I, I really have a respect for weekends again. Umm, and ahh, ya know, when you, and you put in your eight hours or whatever, and then ya factor in laundry and sleep and cleaning up, and, ah, so they're [my days] actually pretty full now. But, but prior to that, just the shelter and the OW, you're just looking for a place to go sit down, ah, read, ah, look in some programs if possible. Um, it's actually, ah, quite, ah, boring. Umm. And it can bring you down a lot and too much time on your hands.

My interview with Adrienne occurred in the middle of a typical day of her being in recovery. Adrienne co-parented her seventeen-year-old son with her partner and son's father, Eddie. She had temporary custody of Chase and an ongoing relationship with the Children's Aid Society (child welfare) when we met. Both Chase and Eddie were in and out of the home the day of our interview. Our chat was punctuated by random phone calls, Adrienne calling to her son in the next room, Eddie and her discussing his upcoming doctor's appointment, some of which accidentally recorded when I could not hit stop fast enough as events unfolded around me. Adrienne reflected on how a typical day used to centre on her planned substance use.

> It was, um (pause) that was pretty much all I cared about really. I didn't care about, you know, cleaning the house, doing laundry, buying grocer-ies, whatever. It was just about I need to budget and space out the money to buy the pills and do it in a way where I wasn't gonna go through the withdrawals. I put more care into planning how to be a drug addict then probably how not to be a drug addict at that point in time. Yeah, so, I would spend my day doing that.

In recovery and in suboxone treatment at the time of our inter-view, Adrienne maintained that in the present: "It's either I do it or I don't." Like Adrienne, Tara had worked on changing her patterns of crack cocaine use several times by the time we met over the tele-phone. Tara did not share an abstinence approach with Adrienne, nor was she in a suboxone treatment program. Though she consid-ered herself sober when I met her, Tara made clear her day involved continuous work at this, saying: "Harm reduction, you know, it's a process."

The typical day for other individuals involved in methadone or sub-oxone treatment for opioid addiction could sometimes seem to unfold around the ingestion of their "drink." Most of these women and men took their dose of methadone under supervision at a clinic. Trevor had even created a personal schedule around his methadone ingestion and, by implication, to achieve a sense of purpose each day.

> So right now, for the past little bit, I just get up, um. Then. Um. Get my drink. And I have a coffee. And then I go, I do my grocery shopping. I, uh, so I spend a couple of hours here [at Tim Hortons] on my computer. I look around for like, you know, things like, types of jobs that are out there. You know. You know, just mess around on the Internet. Um. And then I go do my grocery shopping. By the time I get home, it's maybe like 4:00. I try to kill as much time out as I can.... I don't want to like waste away at home. And then when I do get home, I like prep my din-ner for the night. And then I just like watch tv usually. Or like go on the computer or like. Or usually something like that, that's like a calm-ing thing. Things change. Things happen. I'll meet with somebody you know or go out or whatnot.

Marnie was one of the two participants who received weekly "carries" of suboxone, meaning she had been prescribed suboxone to use at home and not under clinical supervision. Her typical day tended to be organized around taking her dose as well as her young daughter's time spent at school, engagement in self-care and pursuit of self-growth, and participation in programming or one-on-one counselling.

> Um, a typical day. I wake up and I, I like do my, my coffee and breakfast and everything, and then I get my daughter's lunch ready and then I wake her up and I take her to school. And then, after that, I'll usually hit the gym. Or if I don't have the gym, I'll go home and do like some yoga or some meditation. Ummm, and then I like try and do, just do a lot of self-development and like listening to podcasts and, um, reading books and things like that. I go to, um, I go to some programs still.... I meet with my, I'm on suboxone. So, I meet with my suboxone doctor once a month.

Days that unfolded "typically" for some time for participants in recovery, however, could suddenly and dramatically change in the face of triggers: cue-induced cravings that must be acted upon (Dennis, 2016). Season worried about how she could pinpoint her triggers but could not seem to overcome them, observing that she could too easily use her triggers as excuses for behaviour that was harmful to herself and her children.

> You know what, it's just compulsive.... Like everything will be done. I'll make sure all the bills are paid and whatnot and it's just like this – I think a lot has to do with my child's father too. When he's not consistent in coming by to see my kids and me, and that's what throws me off ... it's just flashbacks. It's just certain things that I see, hear, or smell that were really bad from that place [time in foster care] and it'll trigger, and then I just want to freak out about it. So that's when I usually go and use. But it's excuses, I think, to use.

Season identified herself as mixed race and age thirty-eight when I met her. She cared for six of her own children as a lone mother. Her eldest daughter was also a lone mother and lived with Season. Though Season was quite introspective in this excerpt from her interview, hers was an interview that I did not think would happen because of mistakes I made. I arrived late to her home, and I handled my anxiety over being late by quickly reminding her what we would be talking about as we stood in her kitchen. Season abruptly cut me off and told me that I was "speaking way too loud" and then informed me that her children were in the living room next door to the kitchen. Mortified that I had revealed way too much about her life (and, yes, loudly) in the first few minutes of meeting and in the presence of her children, I asked if she would like to re-think her participation in the interview. I reminded her that she could choose not to consent to participate in the interview. Season surprised me by agreeing to participate but told me assertively her terms: I needed to be careful in how I worded questions given how her youngest children (two children under age six) may come in and out of the kitchen and they did not know she was on OW or that she used drugs. I agreed and we proceeded through her grace. Our code word for talking about OW was "work"; my questions were re-phrased in the moment to ask Season how she felt about her experiences at "work." We somehow talked about her patterns of use by miming in body language and also speaking about "health." By mid-interview, I felt that while I was likely a person she would not choose to have another social interaction with, I was nonetheless perceived as a vessel through which she could share the stories that mattered to her and her journey.

Individuals who randomly used alcohol or drugs, and who did not define as sober or in recovery, did not always pinpoint anything typical of their days when I asked. Among benefit recipients who seemed quite uncomfortable or anxious about their use, this was especially the case. According to Charise, who was attempting to become sober through participation in treatment: "[S]ometimes I get picked up go to a meeting, sometimes I relapse and I'm out using, and I just go back and forth." For Dante, too, there seemed little that was typical.

> DANTE: These days? I don't know. My life's like torn up. I've been in hibernation mode for like, from like January, since after Christmas, I've been like basically watching TV and ... ah, Yeah. Yeah, the odd, after program I go to…. Weed almost every day now. I'm, since Christmas, because I met a woman, the crystal meth started for a bit. But I'm trying to wean that off.
> AMBER: Do you still use crystal meth every now and then?
> DANTE: Maybe once a month. But here's the thing. That once a month, it lasts for a week. That's the problem. And then it takes two weeks to recover after that. So, it takes like a whole month. You know? Fuck.

While Dante seemed to recognize that there was little typical about each day, he did perceive his breaks in his use of crystal meth to coincide with those he was using with.

> DANTE: I went over to my buddy's house, and I hung there with him. But here's the thing. We just finished using for a few days.

AMBER: Okay. And then you're going to see him again.

DANTE: Yeah, but here's the, the good thing is that he had to go back to work today too, so he just wanted to just do nothing. Oh good, perfect. "Come, come, come. Make lunch, make supper. Don't bother me. And clean my house for me." Today I actually helped him clean.

Each time I re-read this excerpt, I clearly remember Dante's performance of his friend talking; I smile again at his ability to make me see that, in the midst of their shared use patterns and what might seem to be a power imbalance, theirs was a strong friendship. It involved elements of physical and emotional support of one another and provided Dante with some sense of peace in existing together in a shared space, not using, and completing the routine activities of living. Indeed, among some people who used substances like Dante, there might seem little typical about their day, but what could seem consistent were their patterns of use and their feelings about their use, for example, whether they were somehow managing it in some way.

Alexei, who also still used heroin, had his own sort of typology of "typical days": Day 1: responsibilities determined by his father; Day 2: musings about his use and attempting or potentially attempting sobriety; and Day 3: hustling for his drug of choice, heroin, often requiring criminal behaviour.

ALEXEI: This really complicates me, when my father tells me what I have to do for a whole day. I only do one thing at a time. It's fine, I'm just saying – I do go to meetings and one thing at the time will help me more than just put myself into, to have to think about everything I have to do. So, what's the first question?

AMBER: So, things you do during the day?

ALEXEI: I spend time at home. When I'm sober and not trying to plan using drugs. It's usually going to be more sleeping because if I was using drugs for a week, I'm going to be tired. So, I just stay home thinking how to maybe change my life or something. Or why I'm doing this? But mostly after, just I try to, I don't know, go and hustle some money.

AMBER: And what ways would you do that? Do you work under the table?

ALEXEI: Steal. Get some, lots of criminality – maybe how you see this.

Shawn was also a daily user of heroin when he could afford and access it. He was on a low dose of methadone daily but, in his case, to avoid withdrawal. He had been using heroin for over twenty-five years and worked for pay while using for the same employer for twenty years. Between the ages of forty and fifty, after he was laid off from his job, he had been consistent in his seeking of "under the table work" in landscaping, construction, and home renovations. His typical day began as follows: "I usually get up and get a coffee or go get my drink [methadone]. I'll either try to have some work lined up or I'll go out and find some and make some money or whatever. I try to work every day, just so I can eat or if I need to get something." When I wondered aloud if Shawn would define himself as "basically a functioning addict" because he would work every day while he used, he replied: "Functioning addict, yeah. It's just like today – I still use, it's there.... I know at some point in the day I'm probably going to go get something. But I get up normal like you do and plan your day. You get up, 'okay what am I doing today?'" Thus, Shawn was perhaps clearest of all participants in making clear that substance use could be part of a typical day too.

Everyday Lives of Multiple Challenges

The behaviours, events, and transitions that seemed to shape participants' substance use and/or their recognition of their use as an addiction are related to their applying for and receiving OW. For example, some participants' experiences of past trauma, including gendered trauma, might have shaped their substance use but also could partially shape their turning to OW for a semblance of income security. Participants in addition experienced other and sometimes multiple barriers to participating in employment programming or paid work. In this section, I pull forward some themes from earlier discussions in this book to show how the everyday experience of being a user, sober, or in recovery on OW is one that is compounded by the challenges of low income, emotional and physical pain, and criminalization.

The most obvious examples of the poverty single participants experienced included the total amount of money they received each month through OW coupled with their lack of affordable, quality housing. A few single participants engaged in "under the table" (cash) work in order to alleviate some financial strain, such as Shawn and Dante, and did not report this cash as income as per OW rules. Others simply did their best to survive on what they received each month. Pat explained how a single person's income insecurity is perpetuated by OW policy itself. She was careful to differentiate between the basic needs amounts and shelter allowance she received each moth (see also City of Toronto, 2020).

You only get, not even $400 for rent. You get $370 for rent. So, you can't even get a room for that right now. Rooms are $500, $600. Well, I pay $450. And you only get $300 and something for food and all your extras. So, you're just getting, just over $600. It's crazy. And you know, they wonder why people live like they're on welfare? Like, oh my God. They treat us like we are.

I asked Pat how she managed to afford rent and everyday costs. Her reply was telling: "Well, I don't eat a lot." She had lost a great deal of weight over several years. Since she participated in a methadone treatment program, it seemed further problematic that her overall health and well-being was compromised by insufficient income to afford food. Danni also attested to the stressfulness of living in poverty in her story of a potential budget shortfall governed by the anonymizing potential of case management. And Anais made clear that she was alone in her struggles, saying she cannot ask for help from family.

The repercussions of low income for participations could include a loss of a sense of belonging or social inclusion. Smitri and Pat both hinted at their dissatisfaction with how much time they spent doing nothing. Pat told me: "I really don't do anything.... I walk the dog. I clean the house. Like that's it. When my kids are in town, I spend time with them. That's it." Tara was pursuing further change in her life by attending a bridging program at a local college; the program allowed her to apply previously earned post-secondary credits towards the completion of a degree. Her social interactions in this program, however, were sometimes inhibited by her low income.

> You know the limited amount of money that you get [from OW] now. You know, a big part of it is especially when you are trying to do something? You know, like, and I'm at school? I mean it's hard some days, I mean, when you can't afford to buy a coffee.... I take my one coffee with me in the morning. And they have the water thing ... or whatever at school. But you know. I mean you still get to socialize. But you know, you can't go off campus. Like you can't say "hey, let's go down the street to McDonalds or...." You know.

Among the lone mothers with children in their care that I interviewed, grappling with their household poverty was a daily challenge. Season observed that even including the child support payment she received from the father of two of her children, this was not enough money to help her afford shoes, clothing, or recreational activities for all six of them: "$200 for two kids and then for three kids is nothing. I get $400 a month, $200 for each." Jules was not receiving her full income support payment from OW for reasons of alleged welfare fraud. She shared about her income for the month in which I met her: "I'm not getting it [welfare]. I got $2.50. How are you going to do that to a single mother?" I asked her if she had received her child tax benefit for the month. She replied "$280. That's supposed to what, cover my rent? Which is way more than that. And food, clothing." She was in the process of appealing the charge of fraud and in extreme poverty, relying heavily on the financial support provided to her by her boyfriend.

Finding and maintaining affordable housing when experiencing low income was a challenge for all benefit recipients. Though Steve had worked for pay for several years, he remembered:

> Like if you're functional [while using], which I was for many years, ah, I'd make a decent buck, but you know, I still didn't have a car, I still didn't take a vacation, really, you know. I was just, I was just functioning, right? So, I was just ah, I, ah, I was just, ah surviving, not really living. Umm. Because a lot of my money would go for, you know, ah, towards addiction even before food, so.

Steve saw the main challenge to continue to participate in the residential treatment program would be staying long enough to save money to afford an apartment of his own.

> If I stay six months, that's six thousand dollars saved. You know, that's, that's a pretty good, ahh, start for, for a place. Yeah. I mean, I would love, the biggest challenge is, ah, it's like the patience for getting a, a place, ya know. Because there's, ah, there's ah, I think, sixty guys on each floor. No walls, ya know what I mean, like – it's like, it's like an army barracks.

Adam saw his own problems with acquiring and maintaining affordable housing as negatively affecting his overall sense of health and well-being. His loss of housing coincided with a very difficult period wherein he perceived his alcohol use becoming uncontrollable.

> Yeah, that was, the lease holder for our house ended up moving out. Ah, and so we like lost the lease for our house. Ah. Our landlord then tried to, like, up the rent to get us out of there and stuff. At which point we took a month away from the house. There was a big deal with a bunch of issues in the house. Like bed bugs, cockroaches. And that was, like, a nightmare. And then coming back to March, we sort of came up with an agreement, um, about raising the rent but not as much as he had wanted because it was just crazy. He was trying to raise like 25 per cent or something, which is like nuts. Um. But then when we made him aware that he can't really do that with a building built before 1991.

Primarily through his relationships with his roommates and their knowledge of Ontario's landlord and tenancy regulations (e.g., *The Residential Tenancies Act*, 2006), Adam was eventually able to live again in the same location.

Like Adam, Charise shared how maintaining an affordable and safe place to live was tied to her overall health and well-being. Charise saw where she could afford to live on an OW income to affect her mental health and to create too many opportunities to continue to use drugs rather than pursue recovery.

> [I]'m not going to speak for anyone else, but for myself it [housing] makes a world of difference. If I have peace, if I know peace, if I live peace, I might not want to do crazy chaotic things, like start smoking drugs and mess up my whole night. Because I'm at peace already, why do I want to disturb my inner peace? So that's a biggy: housing, housing, housing.... That's first and foremost, shelter. I've been without, and that and hunger are the two worst things I've ever experienced in my life.... That's what I said to Ben [her caseworker], the amount that you're giving me, like not you yourself but the system, is asking me to go out and be an addict again because you are a product of your environment.

The experience of pain not only informed some individuals' becoming a substance user but also their unemployment and, hence, their need for a welfare income. Here, I want to highlight physical and mental pain as a challenging part of the everyday experience of being on social assistance and living with addiction for some people.

A single white woman in her fifties and the mother of a twenty-four-year-old daughter who lived on her own, Theresa had lost the use of her legs through her prolonged drug use in earlier years and was confined to a wheelchair. She did not see herself as in recovery and was transparent about her use of alcohol. "I drink," she said when I asked how she spent time each day. I quickly learned to delight in the way in which Theresa used deadpan humour to tell stories about her experiences. I also soon learned that besides drinking, Theresa looked after her cats, made tea, fed herself, and most notably, engaged in self-care to achieve her physical health; Theresa was adept at changing her own catheter, for example. She acknowledged that her main source of physical pain each day stemmed from years of using heroin. As she explained: "I have also, from using needles in the legs, I have dead feet, I have very bad [inaudible] physical damages." The physical health risks of using drugs, especially those associated with injection drug use, is well documented in research across disciplines (Adrian & Barry, 2003; Long et al., 2014).

Pat and Clive also saw their physical pain as associated with their initial substance use and texturing their experience of being in recovery or still using substances while accessing OW. Alexei provided another example of the challenge of managing pain, in his case dental pain, when experiencing low income: "My father helped me to pay for a root canal last month. Or I have to pull the teeth. They pull a few teeth in the detention centre for me, because there was no other thing to do." Alexei was not alone in citing dental pain as a challenge. Adrienne told me about how she could not afford to correct some of her dental problems and was working with her caseworker to try to figure out a plan to address them, a challenge made more complex by the way in which Adrienne would not accept being prescribed opioids post-surgery.

So, too, was managing mental pain a daily reality for some participants. Cody had been diagnosed with bipolar disorder, a disorder characterized by extreme mood swings between "highs" (mania) and "lows" (depression), in years past. A strong recovery trajectory was made difficult by his changing mental health and well-being and corresponding treatment strategies.

> Well, the bipolar is really tricky. So, you feel like a lab rat at first because there's so many different meds. And trying to find a doctor that can work with you steadily, like once a week … and [understands] that addiction feeds into it.… And then you bounce back, you have your manic day and you think "I feel way better. I don't need these meds no more." So, you jump off and you've got a month and then kind of start sliding. The hardest thing to do is go back in and say what's happened.

Tynesha also experienced mental health challenges that were diagnosed. Tynesha, however, questioned why her emotional displays seemed to be seen as suspicious by her therapist when, in her view, it would be more suspicious to not react emotionally to the loss of her children and to not fight for improved visitation with them.

> I got diagnosed with situational depression and anxiety … and borderline personality disorder. I'm like "okaaayyyy." She [her therapist] said because of all these things that are happening, I'm like emotionally unintelligent. I'm like, "I disagree." I don't think I'm emotionally unintelligent, I just think that I'm emotional because I miss my kids and I want my kids. I can't be a robot. You can't expect me not to cry or get upset when I have three people in my ear telling me what's best for my kids.

Besides caring for her six children and trying to continue to focus on recovery while sometimes relapsing, Season struggled with managing her memories of her adolescence, including of the child welfare system. As she explained it, she could not necessarily provide what she saw as good instrumental and expressive support to her eldest daughter and her grandson, with whom she lived, because of mental health challenges: "I'm supposed to be watching my grandson while she [her daughter] goes and finishes on her education. But I was diagnosed with post-traumatic stress and anxiety, so even though I want to do things I just can't mentally do them." When I asked her whether her counsellor had reasons for diagnosing her as having PTSD, Season responded: "My childhood. And all what stuff happened to me in [foster] care." The way she explained it is that at age eleven, her mother dropped her off with child welfare services because she perceived Season as out of control. But, for Season, there were other reasons: "basically I just told my mom I was tired of her having multiple men in her life and a few of them abused me."

Arash was participating in a day treatment program when I met him and working on overcoming his depression and substance dependency.

> I'm pretty depressed right now, but I go to the gym every day, which makes me feel good.... I put an ad out and I got a couple customers. And I went and put a business plan together. And I went and I got confidence, and I started doing that actually – had a few clients. But I still had some personal issues, depression and stuff like that, and interpersonal issues.... I started using again. And in the beginning of using, after four years of sobriety, and you know how to use it differently now, it's much different. It's a whole new world. It actually helped me a little bit, it knocked down my inhibitions and stuff. I would make cold calls [to prospective clients].

Arash's four years of sobriety followed his release from prison after he served a sentence for armed robbery associated with his drug use and dealing. He completed his high school diploma while incarcerated and had gone to college to specialize in physical fitness training upon release. Elsewhere in our interview, he implied that his worsening mental health and return to alcohol and drug use was associated with an intimate relationship ending and his knowledge of the pleasures of use.

Other participants had past experiences with the criminal justice system. Besides Jesse and Smitri participating in Drug Treatment Court in lieu of jail time, Alexei referred to his past experiences of provincial detention centres and Cody spent some time in federal prison, to name just a few. Indeed, among all participants I interviewed, ten were forth-coming with their stories of their past criminalization, six men and four women. In all cases, their contact with the criminal justice system was linked to their substance use, whether they were sentenced for crimes of trafficking drugs, were engaged in physical altercations under the influence of drugs or alcohol or over drugs or alcohol (e.g., assault), or committed crime to procure money to afford their habit (e.g., theft). Sea-son, for example, was incarcerated in prison for two years: "I had quite a number of charges ... robberies, guns, forcible confinement. I did a lot. The robberies were to help me with my addiction."

The women and men I interviewed spoke about how difficult it was finding employment with a criminal record, a challenge to exiting social assistance that is recognized by OW caseworkers and manag-ers in Toronto (Herd et al., 2018). The crimes for which Cody went to prison were covered quite extensively by media. As he explained: "So the criminal part is the part that's holding me up the worst because a lot of people.... Yeah, if they type my name in on the Internet, the first article to come up is the story, so that kind of really deters a lot of employers from me." Cody remained optimistic, however, because he was taking part in a program that provided him with training that would enable him to navigate this challenge by becoming an entrepreneur.

Season, however, made it very clear that there are greater challenges for women with a criminal history.

> Okay, when a man comes out prison he can do construction, carpeting, roofing, whatever. When a woman comes out of jail with a criminal record what really, as a woman, what job can I do? Other than a sex trade or sell-ing drugs? It's a cycle. Are you bondable? What's your answer going to be? Where I can't be doing construction on roofs and stuff like that – that's not a woman's job.

Season was acutely aware that the gendering of occupations would shape her paid work future that was already compromised by her holding a criminal record. As she implied, certain trades overlook a criminal record for men, suggesting that their future opportunities in paid work could be more plentiful than those of women with depen-dent children (see also Gazso, 2019). Her observations echo the work of colleagues in Ricciardelli and Peters's edited collection *After Prison: Navigating Employment and Reintegration* (2017), who show that little job experience and a criminal record, among other challenges, inhibit ex-offenders' employment opportunities in Canada; another American study finds this is especially true for women with children (Curcio & Pattavina, 2018).

Surviving violence was the last challenge to negotiate as part of the everyday experience of living with addiction and being on OW that I learned about. Having experienced gendered violence as an adolescent, Smitri had not escaped it as an adult. Her current relationship with her intimate partner was a tumultuous one. She had left him several times because of experiencing mental and physical violence at his hands.

> There's been times where we've had arguments and I've applied their advice of shelters and whatnot. I did the whole shelter thing. Yeah, I did that three times in the last four or five months. And I'll last a day and come right back. So, I'm trying to get used to the shelter thing. The problems at home fluctuate. One week it'll be fine, totally. The next week not. You know what I mean?

Research consistently shows that women experiencing low income face still further challenges to leaving violent intimate relationships. Sometimes to leave means they face greater economic disadvantage and the risk of homelessness (Daoud et al., 2016; Fernández-González et al., 2019; Tutty et al., 2013). As Barret and St. Pierre (2011) observe, noting these challenges is by no means intended to pathologize or disempower survivors of violence. As their quantitative study shows, Canadian women who have experienced intimate partner violence engage in a wide range of help-seeking behaviours that involve informal and formal supports and may include but are not limited to dissolving a relationship. Indeed, though Smitri was aware that she could enter a shelter and stay for a longer period of time and so dissolve her relationship with her partner in the process, she appeared to still be assessing whether this was the decision she would make. Smitri seemed aware that there are costs of entering the shelter system, including some limitations on length of stay, regulation of behaviour, inadequate conditions and crowding (Ngabo, 2019; Webb, 2021), as well as a change in her lifestyle compared to when partnered.

Tynesha was not experiencing violence from her ex-partner at the time of our interview. However, she still had to maintain an indirect relationship with him through her meetings with CAS and lawyers, her own and his, to re-negotiate custody of and visitation with her children. The process of leaving abusive relationships and navigating them, including their end, subjected some women participants to heteropatriarchal power dynamics that certainly challenged their everyday efforts at trying to achieve sobriety, pursue recovery, and make ends meet. Indeed, that mothers who have survived violence must engage in emotion and identity work to achieve improved health and well-being (as further detailed in the next chapter), is woefully overlooked in understandings of the everyday life realities of people living with addiction on OW.

Multiple Poverties

Many academic studies of poverty assume the concept of relative poverty, operationalizing poverty as low monthly income relative to a measure of the average standard of living in the society in which one lives. Low Income Cut Offs (LICOS) (before and after tax), the low income measure (LIM) based on median household income, and the market-basket measure (MBM) – now Canada's official poverty line (Heisz, 2019) – are all examples of common relative measures of poverty used in research. I mention all of these because they share an assumption that lack of income and inability to meet costs of living is the definition of poverty.

Inroads have been made, however, in conceptualizing poverty as more than just lack of income. For example, multidimensional poverty, as defined by the Oxford Poverty and Human Development Initiative (2020), refers to lack of money and experiences of poor health, lack of clean water and electricity, poor-quality education, and lack of non-precarious work. While currently operationalized quantitatively and largely within the discipline of economics (see, for example, Duclos et al., 2018; Zedini, 2020), varying conceptualizations of multidimensional poverty have considerable application in comparative analyses of countries in the Global North and South. Halpern-Meekin (2019) has offered another way to think about poverty too. Based on her analysis of the experiences of couples participating in a relationship education program in the American state of Oklahoma, she argues that poverty should also be conceptualized as a lack of social resources in and of themselves, what she calls social poverty; this poverty is not subsequent from income poverty. Couples in her study were economically marginalized but also experienced a lack of social connection. While I appreciate Halpern-Meekin's argument, I find the general idea of multidimensional poverty resonates most with the experiences of benefit recipients in this study centred in the city of Toronto, Canada. Indeed, my intent in this final section is to conclude that the findings revealed in this chapter give credence to a *qualitative* understanding of multidimensional poverty.

Broadly speaking, benefit recipients experienced poverty as the lack of some material and/or intangible thing that could facilitate their meeting of individual needs. Undoubtedly, lack of income is a primary source of concern for the women and men managing substance use that I interviewed. People on OW I interviewed in 2016 and 2017 were receiving incomes below the MBM, LIM, and LICOs each month (Tweddle & Aldridge, 2018). Given their poverty-level incomes, participants were challenged in their efforts to afford reasonable food, clothing, and shelter. I have noted how Pat simply did not eat very much to cope with the monetary amount she received each month from OW. She told me how her children observed her decreasing weight, from size 12 to size 5, in a two-year period before we met. I remember Franco pointing to his black tie-up loafers, scuffed and cracking, as we walked to a bus stop, and him telling me that they were the only shoes that he had owned for years. And certainly, lack of income shaped participants' access to poor housing. Participants could not afford the housing they would prefer, and many single participants lived in rooming houses or shared accommodation with roommates they would rather not. If singles could afford a bachelor or one-room apartment, oftentimes their cost of rent ate up over 75 per cent of their total income they received from OW. If mothers or single persons accessed subsidized housing, their stories highlighted how their residences were often substandard and in communities they saw as characterized by crime (see also DeKeseredy et al., 2003a, 2003b).

The challenges that people living with addiction face while on OW further illustrate *lack* in its multiple meanings, such as those articulated by the Oxford Poverty and Human Development Initiative. The people I met went about their daily lives, caring for themselves and others, while also knowing first-hand and in varying degrees the financial inadequacy of total monthly benefits to meet needs, including housing, when living in Toronto; weakened physical and mental health, and so overall health and well-being; *and* insecure and unsafe intimate relationships. To be clear, the challenges benefit recipients face when living with addiction and in low income are, in my view, more aptly termed pover*ties*.

The interrelationships among the poverties experienced and their implications for benefit recipients' lives were exceedingly complex. For example, affording housing could mean not spending money on food and clothing. Lack of income could mean that participants could not afford transportation to travel to neighbourhoods wherein they may be eligible for programming to support their efforts at recovery. Lack of income for transportation, in turn, could negatively affect one's ability to create and sustain a social support network. Participants who experienced weak support relationships could especially experience a lack of social inclusion. In turn, being isolated from social relationships with others could inhibit the continued development of the self.

I want to make it clear that I do not view participants' experiences of multiple poverties as reflective of their individual personalities, capacities, or potential. Instead, I see these poverties as largely structural and systemic. That participants seemingly experienced personal or individual lack is too simplistic, as their stories surely attest. As well, in the way OW is administered as a program of "last resort," benefit income is set and dispersed each month with the intent of not incentivizing any one person to remain on it. Hence, the below poverty-level amount. So, the system of OW itself suffers from lack.

Meanwhile, the current mental health and health care system in general in Ontario is overburdened and people in need underserved (Anderssen, 2017). Gaps in services continue to exist for persons with substance use and mental health disorders (Urbanoski et al., 2017). There is a paucity of mental health programs for young adults in Toronto (CTV News, 2017), a shortage of beds in residential treatment facilities (White, 2017), and a shortage of detox opportunities. Though efforts have been made to correct this latter shortage in Toronto quite recently (Ngabo, 2019), too many people have been and continue to be lost amid the ongoing opioid crisis, confirming that detox and other resources and services, as well as emergency response, have remained weak overall (Young, 2016). Indeed, the women and men I interviewed could not afford private residential treatment and could not pay for private counsellors, psychologists, or psychiatrists. If they were not connected to services like the Centre for Addiction and Mental Health (CAMH) or other non-profit organizations in their communities, they were not connected to supports that could make a difference in their health and well-being. For especially participants who identified as experiencing gendered and/or racialized trauma in the past or present, or ongoing anxiety or depression, the lack of mental health treatment was a troubling problem. For participants who were in physical pain, treatment for problematic conditions required waiting that was conditioned by the unavailability of appointments with specialized physicians.

And still, daily life moved on in other ways. And lack characterized other facets of daily life too. To name just another two: (1) people's increasing experiences of food insecurity meant that in 2017 when I was completing this study, the need for food banks was higher than years immediately past and back to levels during the fallout of the 2008 recession (Daily Bread Food Bank, 2017); and (2) affordable, accessible, and licensed childcare was also limited in supply (Mac-Donald & Friendly, 2017).

Benefit recipients who participated in my study could seem to live daily lives that were "typical" like so many people do. However, they lived these days as textured by multiple poverties, and so with needs that stretched across multiple domains of their existence. Needs that could not be always adequately met in the current neoliberal, political, economic, and social policy context. I contend that if we understand the multilayered lived experience of poverties, there is not just the need to overturn the double stigmatization of low income and addiction, there is a need to think through how to begin to change the poverty of our systems – income support, mental health and addiction, health care, etc. And if not a dramatic rehaul of the entire systems themselves, we need to at least start with shifting the discourse, to re-imagining and conceptualizing a different way forward in supporting persons working through substance use amid multiple poverties, an argument I centre in the final chapter of this book. Understanding participants' daily lives as not limited to addiction and challenged by multiple poverties is also not enough. Still needed is a stronger understanding of the experiences that individuals caring for children face. It is to these I now turn in the next chapter, including especially the emotion work of shifting or maintaining identities, say, from that of addict to mother, all while continuing to care for children and despite interactions with policy systems and discourses that may try to ascribe identities otherwise.

7 Being Part of Families and Social Support Relationships

When I read Dassieu et al.'s (2020) article about substance users with chronic pain, I was struck by their observation that participants' double stigma in the eyes of health care professionals could "reinforce both their isolation and the invisibility of their pain" (p. 7). I wondered how the stigma substances users face could make other social relationships invisible too. I was therefore inspired by their argument to explore and make visible specifically the family and social support relationships of people living with addiction and accessing Ontario Works (OW).

In the first half of this chapter, I share mothers' and fathers' stories about their family dynamics and support relationships and see these stories as in addition revealing of their identities and subjectivities as parents. In so doing, I reveal parents' caregiving for others and their work on the self as magnified, accentuated even, in view of how it is performed in relation to the "recovering addict" subject position constituted by OW discourse and caseworker practice (see chapter 5). Moreover, I develop a broader argument that parents living with addiction engage in emotional labour and identity work in response to broader, societal "feeling rules" that are interactionally, ideologically, and discursively produced and constrained (Hochshild, 1979, 1983) and that coincide or conflict with their perceived master status of "addict" in the wider social milieu. In the second half of this chapter, I turn my focus to the social support relationships that meaningfully shape the lives of all benefit recipients living with addiction, no matter their parental status.

Parental Caregiving and Support

Only six of the mothers I interviewed were actively living with and caring for some or all of their children. Like so much other Canadian research on lone mothering in low income has shown (see Breitkreuz et al., 2010; Gazso, 2007a, 2007b, 2012; Pulkingham et al., 2010), raising children requires adopting several strategies to make ends meet and ensure family survival. Darlene confirmed: "It's a struggle. As far as grocery shopping goes, checking the flyers and sales and stuff like that, and price matching. Yeah, so I do that all the time basically. And just buying things on sale."

When I asked these lone mothers about their overall "typical day," I found that although their mothering was challenged by their patterns of substance use or ongoing efforts at recovery, these women persevered: they mothered. And just as most other custodial mothers do to the best of their ability in any one moment and in each day. For example, any activities or programs Darlene participated in, including doctor appointments or counselling sessions, had to take place when her children were in school and she was not immediately responsible for their care. She met her children immediately after their school day ended:

> Sometimes I enrol them in programs through Parks and Rec. So sometimes we'll have a program to go to after school or after dinner or something.... I guess just make dinner when we get back, then we're pretty much – in the winter time we're pretty much at home after that. Some nights if there's time we might go skating or something like that. We like to go to the outdoor rinks.

Darlene seemed proud to share that she had worked hard to create a reciprocal support relationship with her children, to some extent: "Yeah there are little things that they do, but it's a bit of a struggle to do it at times. But they do help out with some things." Excluding the time her daughter was in daycare, Marnie's day was similar to Darlene's in that it seemed to revolve around meeting her daughter's needs: "Like, I'm a very hands-on parent. So, when I'm like, when my daughter, as soon as she's home from daycare, we're doing something."

Besides mothers' ongoing provisions of love, affection, and nurturing (the giving of expressive support), they had to make tough decisions about how to spend money to support children's needs and wants (the giving of instrumental support). For example, Darlene was aware that she could not afford to fully support her son's ideal choice for sport and recreation, hockey. So, she tried to support his interests elsewhere. "He likes hockey. He's never played ice hockey, although it's something I would love for him to be able to do but, just money wise, it hasn't been an option. But he plays things like ball hockey, and he's also interested in computers."

Compared to the other mothers, Season was clearest in acknowledging how she managed her addiction alongside caring for her children: "I wake up, I go get my methadone. I come back. I tidy up the house and I do my errands, cook supper, and get ready for the kids to come home." Season was also adamant that a woman cannot mother while actively using drugs. Her view seemed to be informed by her own experience of using and temporarily losing custody of her children in the past. According to Season:

> You can't be an addict and be a mom. You can't. No matter how much you want to be – we have the right intentions, but we make bad choices. When should I come home? Even phone calls and text messages and stuff, just to let them know I'm here, I haven't abandoned you. But they know what I'm up to. They know.

The Children's Aid Society of Ontario (CAS) seemingly agreed with Season's self-assessment. Like other lone mothers with custody of their children but working through addiction, Season had an ongoing relationship with CAS. When our discussion turned to how CAS was involved in her life at the time of our interview, Season further explained how her addiction affected her children's well-being:

> [W]e have a monthly [visitation from a caseworker]. But my daughter had a breakdown at school that led up to some – she has a black eye and stuff, and they were concerned because of what she had said, like "My mom hasn't been home." And she has a lot of stress. She feels that, a lot of the adult responsibility's on her when I go [away to use]. Which is true. I'm not gone every day, but when I do, it's for a period, anywhere from a day to three. So yes, I have daycare, but it's still a lot.

Season was aware that she burdened her eldest daughter with caring for her own infant son and her younger siblings when she left their home to engage in a period of drug use. CAS was becoming increasingly aware of these family dynamics.

CAS was also involved in other mothers' mothering. Adrienne's temporary care of her son Chase was through her involvement with CAS. Her son's father, Eddie, was directly involved in their life but lived apart from Adrienne; theirs was a sort of "living apart together" relationship (Funk & Kobayashi, 2016). Eddie even arrived at Adrienne's house to visit halfway through our interview and seemed to be genuinely pleased to learn that Adrienne was sharing her story so that others may understand her journey of recovery and learn from it, as well as learn about the quality of her life, including her relationship with him and their son. Adrienne explained how her relationship with their son was somewhat tenuous at the time of the interview:

> We still have the temporary care. So, um, he, he's staying here, but on paper, he's living at a foster home on Children's Aid. Yeah, so, that, that, that's what the temp care, he's temporarily, like, in their care thing. So, we're doing a transition for the summer with them still being involved, at least on paper. Just in case that's, you know, for all purposes I'm not sober, then they can just swoop right back in, you know, basically.

Adrienne could and did feed, clothe, and provide shelter for her son and with support from Eddie. However, she had too often made false promises to Chase about her sobriety and so had strained their emotional relationship. Thus, Adrienne saw the involvement of CAS in their lives as facilitating her son's perception of being cared for and supported.

> I think it helps with him actually ... 'cause again, like I, I, I've been the boy that cried wolf with sobriety quite a bit of times. So, if they [Chase and Eddie] don't believe me, I, I c –, I don't blame them for not believing me. If I am sober until, like, I don't know what more else to do to prove to them that I am. I, I, from them just seeing my actions and my choices. Because I, I've promised up and down, swore on everybody's life, and everything that was ever holy that I was sober – when I wasn't. So. It's, I'm, I'm okay with them [child welfare] still being, like, around. I'd rather them not, but I, I do understand that it's better for him to have, um, that cushion if you will. In case I ever do go back to, you know, to the way, whatever. Until he feels completely, um, safe. I guess, to say, to be home.

While we were still discussing caring and relationships, Adrienne's telephone rang while Eddie was still at home too; he was in the other room for most of the time we talked. She answered the call and after hanging up said: "That's his [Eddie's] doctor, like – I do everything. Yeah. For him." By this time, Eddie had re-entered the room and Adrienne gave him a quick update on the call. I said to Adrienne: "You support him." To which she replied: "I run his life." Eddie laughed. And agreed. While working on her recovery, Adrienne also offered instrumental and expressive support to Eddie too.

About seven years before I met Darlene, she had been raising her two children with her husband, though they did not share a residence: "We weren't really living together at the time, but he was there basically. He was there every day, but he wasn't really sleeping at this apartment." Darlene explained how CAS became involved in her life:

> They [CAS] were involved because of a situation with my ex-husband.... Like basically he got arrested and that's why they became involved. So, you can probably take a guess what it has to do with, or what type of – he got arrested for luring a child over the Internet at the age of sixteen.

Darlene made it clear that her ex-husband, the father of her daughter, was currently incarcerated for his criminal behaviour. While re-telling, tears began to fall from her eyes. As she quietly wiped them away, I too was overcome with emotion as I became caught up in her re-living of the memory of first learning this news. It was clear that Darlene had been gob-smacked by her ex-husband's behaviour. Up until his arrest and conviction, she had perceived their familial relationships in a positive light. Her astonishment about his behaviour and incarceration soon turned to anger and then sadness. As she saw it, it was highly unlikely she would allow her daughter to have any relationship with her father, at least not until her daughter was an adult and could make her own decision.

Children in Care of Others

Eighteen participants defined themselves as single and not part of an intimate relationship but also as parents and had children in the care of others. These parents' levels of involvement in their children's lives, and so their provisions of instrumental and expressive support, were connected to the ways in which their children came to be no longer in their care. Most of the single men who were fathers that I interviewed lost custody of their children following divorce. The single women who were mothers usually lost custody of their children when child welfare officials intervened because of perceptions of their problematic substance use. What I want to stress here is that while these parents no longer resided with their children and so did not engage in activities such as preparing food or getting children ready for school or bed, they still parented in some way and to the best of their ability and capacity. Even when providing what might appear to be limited support, parenting identities and practices did not end when a relationship with a partner dissolved (just like for many post-divorce parents), or when their use of substances seemed to supersede them.

Since Smitri had recently participated in Drug Treatment Court in lieu of jail time, her choice to become sober was perhaps not so much of her own volition. However, by choosing treatment over jail, she recognized she also had the opportunity to try to become more involved in her children's lives. Achieving this greater involvement was challenging for Smitri because she had lost custody of her children to her mother with whom she experienced conflict.

> Initially in 2009 when she [my mother] took them, she wrote that I can have them every Christmas, every Mother's Day, every week.... I went and messed up on my own.... [T]his particular time I got arrested again for trafficking in 2013. She [mother] actually came around and bailed me out ... she didn't talk to me from 2009 to 2013, but she was dropping the kids off every weekend.... But because they [the children] were in one of the [police] raids, she decided she's not going to contribute to that anymore. And to this day she doesn't know what I'm doing. I've tried to talk to her and tell her how good I'm doing – she just, "well, what do you want?"... The [current] boyfriend screwed that all up for me. I tried to gain all this trust from my kids and her, and recently he had an altercation with one of my kids on their visit. So now I'm back at square one again. Now I see them once every two months. It went from every weekend to once every two months because now I have to meet them at a mall. The little one doesn't even want to come anymore.

That her relationship with her live-in boyfriend exacerbated tensions among her children and her mother meant that when I met her, Smitri felt she could provide very little in terms of even indirect expressive and instrumental support to her children. Smitri's attempts to provide support to her children were also thwarted by her poverty. Since her mother had made her visits with her children conditional upon them meeting at a shopping mall, Smitri had to plan these visits carefully in order for her to be able to shop with her children or treat them to lunch. The culmination of these challenges created mental and emotional anguish for Smitri.

It was her ex-partner and child welfare officials' perceptions of her problems with alcohol that seemed to lead to CAS removing Tynesha's three children from her care.

> And that's what [alcohol] I used to cope my whole life. But it's never developed into an addiction. Because I've seen people addicted to alcohol and I'm not even close to that point.... When I was growing up, come weekends, I was like "Yeah, let's go out." So please get out of here, I'm not dependent on alcohol, that's never been my problem. But they've [CAS] classified it as an addiction.

When Tynesha's young children then went to live with her ex-partner as part of their custody arrangement arranged with CAS's involvement, she maintained that she still supported them instrumentally as their mother: "When I gave them to him, I was still receiving the child tax, but I was still maintaining everything that they needed. I paid for every single thing. Clothes, diapers, food, whatever. I paid for it."

Tara, by contrast, described how it came to be that her ex-partner gained custody of their twin daughters and without any involvement of CAS: "I took care of them, and I had care of them and then my drug addiction and what not got to a point where I was just like 'I can't do this.' And I called their dad and said 'Okay, it's your turn.' They were about, the twins were seven and Cara was about twelve." When we discussed how her relationship with her children's father was at the time of the interview, she explained that it was amicable. She had found that she could still provide care to her younger twin daughters who were still living with their father.

> TARA: They're in their last year of high school. They both work. They are lifeguards and swimming instructors. Like their life is really together. And, like, their dad is awesome.
> AMBER: Okay. And do you have a good relationship with him now?
> TARA: Their father? Yeah. Like I call him. And I know everything that is going on with them because I call him. And so "What are the girls up to? How are things? How did school go?" Um, they're in soccer. So, I call and ask him, you know, "So how's their tournament going? Did they win?" You know. So, yes, he keeps me in the loop.

The cognitive process of wondering was another way in which women could engage in mothering despite their children being relinquished from their care by CAS. That is, in wondering about how children in the care of others were faring, some non-custodial mothers engaged in caring too, though this care was certainly not the same as the direct practice of physically caring for children or even the expressive support implied in Tara telephoning her ex-partner and asking about her daughters. Danni, however, described the indirect care that wondering involved:

> I want to be here for my children.... I don't want my children to find out one day when they're trying to find me that their mom died of an overdose and never know me.... So, the things that I wonder is how they feel about me. Do they miss me? I don't want them to feel like that. I want them to know their mom is okay. So that's how I'm feeling. Before when

I was sicker, it was like I miss them, I want them close to me. Now that I'm better, I'm out of myself and I'm saying more things like, I'm thinking more things like, how are they thinking? What are they going through? What do they have to do in their day?

In her wondering, Danni in addition managed her feelings of love and affection for her children – and how she thought she should feel these – since her addiction meant she lived apart from them. Danni and I sat and cried together when she told stories about the loss of custody of her children, first through their removal by CAS. Though not having experienced Danni's pain first-hand, I thought of my own young child and could feel through her energy how the loss of her children was a depthless feeling. This feeling persisted for Danni even when she acknowledged how her drug use conflicted with how she wanted to mother and how others thought she should mother too. My sadness about Danni's loss was also mixed with sincere admiration for how she worked at moving through her own emotions during our conversation and, by her account, in her life.

When I asked about the biggest challenge that she faced each day, Tynesha answered in a way that echoed Danni's story of wondering. She replied:

The biggest challenge is just not being able to see them [my children] and wondering. I'm missing out every single day.... The homework and that, it's those things. And I'm not going to get this time back. And it's just in my brain. Unless I go there and I try to knock it out of my brain, because I don't want to be upset all the time.

In their wonderings and accompanying work on their emotions, Danni and Tynesha had arrived at the same conclusion: with children no longer in their direct care, this wondering had to come from a place of feeling selfless – to wonder for the good of the children. For Tynesha, to "knock it out of my brain" meant that, like Danni, she recognized that missing the present with her children was not healthy for her or her children. Tynesha, too, implied that mothers no longer caring for children directly must transform their own meaning of mothering from direct, immediate, and intimate practices of care to wondering, and to then to wonder in ways that were not selfish.

Season shared about a time in her life when she did not have custody of her children. This was when she was eight and a half months pregnant with her fourth child and had entered a residential treatment program. Her own mother took on the guardianship of her children. Her recollection of that time shares some plotlines with Smitri's experience of losing her children and solidifies how, besides wondering, parents can and do find alternative ways to provide support to their children, even when others hamper their efforts.

> She [her mother] would only allow me to see them [her children] at church. So, my [eldest] daughter was actually talking to me about that – that she really appreciated the effort that I made. Even though I was sick and they weren't with me, I still went every single Sunday to that church just to see them.

Some single men with children in the care of others found ways to continue to father even if in ways far different than the past. Clive had one daughter, Arlene, from a previous relationship. When he and his wife divorced, Arlene lived with her mother. According to Clive, Arlene was not aware that the divorce was acrimonious because of the extra-marital affair her mother had. When I asked Clive about his relationship with Arlene and how often he saw or called her on the phone, he replied that he saw her "not that often," only a few times a year, and that he talked with her on the phone "not that much" because "she's twenty-four years old, busy with her life." In his view, however, they were close. Since Arlene lived in another town, she also travelled to see Clive. In many ways, it seemed the relationship was what it was because of Arlene's efforts. Clive made no effort to present himself as a father try-ing to make up for any challenges their relationship had suffered fol-lowing the divorce. However, he seemed to relish how Arlene provided him opportunities to be a father even if his fathering just meant being available to visit, to talk and listen, when she came to town.

Shawn retained an identity of being a father but was more vocal than Clive in seeing how much it had changed over time. He had lived with the mother of his daughter from about age twenty-two, when Janie was born, until his mid-thirties. When he and Janie's mother separated, he moved in with his parents, who were aware of his using drugs but were accepting of it: "I think that was my mom, okay? She'd rather keep quiet about it and keep me there." It seemed that his parents even made possible and supported Shawn's parenting of Janie. Shawn explained:

> Yeah, she's in XXX [city], but really the only time – like my parents moved out to Brooklyn about five years ago, at that time I was living with my parents and Janie was coming over every weekend and stay with us. So, since that kind of went out the window, my parents moved, I haven't seen her as much … she always had her own room there.… She had her own room and I had my own room and that kind of thing.

At the time of the interview, Shawn's parenting practices of then nine-teen-year-old Janie were limited not only because his parents moved away but because he was experiencing housing insecurity, and: "[L]ike I said she's of age and she's doing her own thing or whatever, so I don't see her a whole lot anymore."

Parents' Identity and Emotion Work, Discursively Shaped[1]

In their stories, I heard more than mothers' and fathers' descriptions of their parenting practices and the meanings they gave to them or the feelings they had about them. Given my analytical strategies, I also heard mothers and fathers tell stories about how parenting children in their care or the care of others is intermeshed with wider discourses and ideologies and their corresponding feeling rules. Thus, I turn my attention here to how parents living with addiction engaged in parenting *and* emotional labour and identity work in relation to broader discourses about family relations, addiction, and poverty.

I have made clear earlier in this book that the discourse of welfare dependency entrenches moral judgments about people accessing social assistance in general. This discourse constructs poor parents as not just "dependent" but ill-suited for the demands of rearing children; they are "bad" parents (Gazso et al., 2020; Weigers & Chun, 2015). In turn, the discourse (re-)produces feeling rules (Hochschild, 2013), specifi-cally others' feelings of pity or anger towards parents for their poverty; otherwise known as the stigmatization of poverty. Some mothers and fathers I interviewed implied that they felt the power of this discourse and worked against it. For example, I read into Darlene's story of being unable to afford to pay for her son to play hockey her emotional work to reach a point of compromise. I can imagine that she felt sad and perhaps angry that she could not afford her son's sport of choice and yet aware that she could be satisfied if not outright happy in being able to afford for him to play a similar sport. In saying to me that she would "love for him to be able to play," she also worked to convey that she cared for her son and in this way was a "good" mother. Darlene's emotional labour also invited me to empathize with – not pity – her decision, nor judge her past.

---

1 Contents of this chapter also appear in a slightly different form in the journal article: Gazso, Amber. 2023. Managing more than poverty when living with addiction: Par-ents' emotion and identity work. *Journal of Family Issues*, 44(1), 46–67. First published online September 2021. https://doi.org/10.1177/0192513X211041981.

Alexei's relationship with the mother of his son ended when his son, Peter, was an adolescent. He explained that he and his son had a strained relationship even before the divorce. In his recollection, he engaged in drug use while raising Peter but kept it hidden from him. When I asked Alexei if Peter knew he used drugs during his childhood, he was not sure. However, he was certain of Peter's perception of him by the time we conducted our interview. Our conversation went as follows:

> AMBER: Does he know now at twenty-one?
> ALEXEI: Yeah. Because he learned from my ex, she was screaming I'm a drug addict, this and that.
> AMBER: So, when you do talk to him, do you think that gets in the way, like kind of he's worrying about that?
> ALEXEI: He doesn't respect me ... he thinks that I'm a lower person or whatever. Even if I try to tell him something, what to do, he says "Who are you to tell me this?"

As Alexei implied, his efforts at parenting Peter were stymied by Peter's anger towards him for his poverty and drug use lifestyle, a viewpoint aligned with the discourse of welfare dependency. For Peter, Alexei's identity as an addict surpassed that of father. Hinted at in Alexei's relationship with his son, a strong case can be made that the stigmatization of the poor via the welfare dependency discourse in addition involves the reproduction of the cultural trope "deadbeat dads." Such fathers are perceived perhaps the most ill-suited to raising children – they do not pay child support to mothers or guardians and/or disappear from children's lives (Mandell, 2002).

Cody's relationship with his eldest daughter, Mandi, involved his emotion work to tolerate and "work around" what he perceived as her anger that he, her father, was becoming a deadbeat dad. In his telling, Cody thought that Mandi believed that he had left her stepmother, Christine, and their child (Mandi's stepsister) in the same way that she understood him to have left her and her own mother as a child.

> CODY: So, she [Mandi] kind of got her nose out of joint, she was like "I don't understand what you're saying to me. Why would you just leave her [Christine] like that?"... I was too scared to say I'm a drug addict. She was only twelve at the time.
> AMBER: So, she was mad at you that you left.
> CODY: Yeah, mad that I left Christine. She was like, "You did this to me when I was a child." I said, "No, there's more to that." So, all she hears from me is "Oh there's more to it, but I can't tell you right now." There's a few things in people's lives that are better discussed at a later date.

Cody's emotion work was particularly intense, because he felt trepidatious about talking to Mandi about his substance use in the past and his work on recovery in the present. In his view, Mandi was not quite ready for him to explain that her perception of his abandonment of Christine and her stepsibling needed to be replaced with the knowledge that his and Christine's co-enabled drug dependency eventually led to their union dissolution. Cody was also reluctant to admit that it was his past struggles with addiction that had ended his relationship with Mandi's mother. In his relationship with Mandi, Cody was working to acknowledge the anger and stigmatization an individual – in this case Mandi – is to feel towards a deadbeat dad. He was also working at managing his own self-anger and self-stigmatization while somehow maintaining his identity as a father.

When Season argued that "addicts" cannot mother, she unconsciously invoked social constructions of motherhood. Indeed, the discourse of intensive mothering is particularly salient for the mothers I interviewed whether they had children in their care or not; based on an extensive review of literature, Christopher (2012) even maintains that scholars generally agree that intensive mothering is an "ascendant ideology." Feeling rules associated with intensive mothering include selflessness and unconditional love (Hays, 1996; Leigh et al. 2012), demonstrated, for example, by mothers' unlimited time, energy, and money spent on meeting their children's material and emotional needs. That mothers who epitomize this "good" mothering are not "deviant," not partaking in the uncontrollable use of illicit substances, is taken for granted.

No wonder Season then struggled with how she felt as a person who used substances (less bound by conventions of time, routine, and responsibility) and about the consequences she created when she did not live up to her own as well as society's expectations of good mothering.

> But still when you are an addict, in fact even when I go out and I do not do it in the home, I do not come home when I'm under the influence. Never. But it's like you just can't.... I don't know how to say this (pause). Because when I'm not here, I still affect my children. I could be out. I'm still doing it away from them. But I'm still affecting them because they're here and they know that mommy didn't come home. Which I hate it. I hate it.

Other mothers, notably Tara and Danni, seemed to respond to this conflict between what they felt and perceived they should feel as "good" mothers by relinquishing the care of their children to others earlier in their life course. Indeed, sometimes it was not just the matter of child welfare officials intervening in their lives but mothers volun-tarily stepping away from their mothering. For example, Tara came to understand her drug use as inhibiting her ability to care for her three daughters. I also read Tara's account as implying that she felt conflict between her two identities of "addict" and mother to the extent that she asked her ex-husband to care for their children. Though Danni had incredible remorse about the loss of her children and questioned the extent to which she really consented to their removal by CAS, she had somehow, too, begun to see their eventual transition into their fathers' care as best meeting their needs.

By contrast, in Tynesha's view, child welfare officials had wrongly removed her children from her care and placed them with their father, who eventually gained full custody of them. This arrangement was somehow connected to child welfare officials defining Tynesha as hav-ing an alcohol addiction. The mixed emotions that Tynesha continued to feel about losing her children attest to the work she engaged in to manage the feeling rules of intensive mothering. On the one hand, Tynesha did not agree with how she saw child welfare officials to use her alcohol use as a reason to remove her children from her care. On the other hand, Tynesha cared so much for her children that she felt she could not testify against her ex-partner in court about his violence towards her. She was concerned that if she told this story, she would still not gain custody of her children, her ex-partner would go to jail, and this would then escalate the risk of her children officially entering foster care and potentially being separated from one another.

> Like okay, they [child welfare] weren't going to give them back to me at that moment.... Yeah, so I didn't testify, and they withdrew the charges against him. What was I supposed to do? I'm like "Okay if they take my kids, they're going to separate them first of all, which is going to trauma-tize the shit out of them." I thought I made the best decision. Sometimes I feel bad and I wonder if it was.

As Tynesha shared about the abuse she endured from her children's father, how she knew she over-used alcohol at troubling times in her life, and how she associated this use with losing her children, her men-tal pain registered as tears of anguish in the moments of our interview. In imagining the experience of these events through her eyes, I empa-thized with her emotional pain and her alcohol use as a coping strategy. Now, as I write this over a year later, I am further struck by how her alcohol use would be seen as violating the norms of selflessness associ-ated with intensive mothering and, correspondingly, how CAS would see removal of her children as in their best interests. Of course, I remain aware that I heard only some stories about some moments in Tynesha's life, not sharing the same knowledge that perhaps CAS had. And yet, given growing research on the systemic inequalities in Canada's child welfare system and Toronto in particular (Adjei et al., 2017; Clarke, 2011; Phillips & Pon, 2018), I am also convinced that there were likely ways in which racism intersected with classicism, and insensitivity to cultural differences in child rearing, these intertwined processes some-how productive of Tynesha's story of losing custody of her children as a woman of colour.

Often associated with gender ideologies conscripted in the transi-tion from modern industrialization to post-Industrial (Western) or late modern societies – notably the nineteenth-century ideologies of true womanhood, cult of domesticity, or familialism (Boucher, 2013; Roberts, 2002) – is the discourse of family as a safe haven. Feeling rules attached to this discourse include that individuals are to feel love and to cherish their (nuclear) family members, or to live by the adage that "blood is thicker than water." I focus on only Marnie's experiences as a single mother here, as they best illustrate the work associated with responding to the feeling rules of this discourse.

Marnie was the only lone mother I interviewed that shared accom-modation with her parents. Existing household dynamics exacerbated underlying tensions and produced new ones in her relationship with her parents.

> [E]ven in the beginning when my, when I was living with my aunt, my mum is like: "Please come home. I promise I'm gonna stop smoking and drinking if you move back with the baby." And that never happened. I feel like I got conned.... Mom still drinks … when I was addicted to opiates, I was getting them from him [her Dad] … even now, they're struggling. Like they're always doing, like, payday loans and things like that. And I mean, my mum's main concern is to make sure she has enough, ah, money for rum and cigarettes.... And my dad, I think my dad has like, a gambling problem.... [W]e have a big deck in the backyard, my daughter will go out there, and my mum will be like smoking right beside her like it's noth-ing. It's so frustrating.... That is the goal, getting outta there, yeah. But then now it's frustrating, 'cause my, like my daughter loves my parents.... [W]hen I talk about like, us living somewhere else, she's like, "Well, what about grandma and grandpa?'... And then part of me also feels guilty. 'Cause I feel like, if we leave like, right now, I feel like, that's all, like my daughter is all my mum really has to live for.

These tensions suggest that Marnie felt somewhat boxed in by the discourse of family as a safe haven. Marnie had moved home, I surmise, because her parents promised to help her raise her daughter – and they did. Marnie shared how much her daughter's receipt of instrumental and expressive support from her parents meant to her elsewhere in our interview, and as I discuss below. And yet, the contradiction between how Marnie thought her mother and father would behave (e.g., not having problems with alcohol, nicotine, or gambling) once she moved in, and how they did behave, created mental and emotional turmoil. Not only did Marnie have to engage in emotional work to continue to reproduce her identity as a sober mother, she had to manage her feelings of being torn between seeing her childhood home as a safe haven for her and her daughter and as a place she would like to leave.

Social Supports Including and *beyond* Kin

No matter their parental status, people living with addiction and accessing OW were involved in social support networks made up of informal and formal supports to varying degrees. Informal support can be defined as instrumental (e.g., financial or physical aid) and expressive support (e.g., affection, closeness, guidance) exchanged not just with family members but with friends and even neighbours (Connidis, 2001). Of the six lone mothers, only two could rely on partners who did not live with them for informal support, specifically that of caregiving for their children. Adrienne was clear in saying Eddie was financially and emotionally supportive of her in her efforts to mother and regain full custody of Chase. While appealing allegations of welfare fraud, Jules was anticipating the celebration of her daughter's birthday on the very day I interviewed her. Our conversation went as follows:

> AMBER: What are you doing for her birthday?
> JULES: Well, you know, I didn't get a welfare cheque and Christmas is coming. I don't know what the hell I'm going to do. We got her a gift, luckily because I have a good boyfriend.

Indeed, it was because of her relationship with her boyfriend and his instrumental and expressive support that Jules was able to provide a gift as a gesture of her care for her daughter.

Like Darlene and Season, Marnie's ex-partner and father of her daughter did not provide her any form of support, financial or otherwise. As I indicated above, Marnie recognized that her parents were a crucial source of instrumental support to her and her daughter in place of her ex-partner's lack of support. Again, although Marnie was frustrated with her mothers' smoking and drinking habits at the time we met, she was simultaneously grateful for the care her parents provided her daughter too.

> They'll watch her, like they're, they're amazing with my daughter. Um, I am concerned about like, when she starts to notice, like, "Oh, grandma's like, a bit off." Things like that. That bothers me, but I think I'm a little bit dependent on them just for like, the childcare aspect.... And I mean, I'm driving a car right now. But it is, like, it's, it's their car. It's just a car that they don't use.... So, it's like it's got its pros and its cons.

Justice could rely on her mother Season's support to care for her infant son. Her son's father was in no way financially supportive of her and the baby. Justice was the eighteen-year-old eldest daughter of Season whom I interviewed by phone for only half an hour and several days after I had met with Season. The way in which Justice seemed guarded in much of what she said in our interview and its overall shortness is why I make my reference to her experiences being on OW in only this chapter. What I did manage to learn in our short chat is that Justice randomly used cannabis and drank alcohol and had been placed in foster care by Season for a time before being allowed to return home. The only time in our interview that Justice spoke at length was to make clear that despite their fractious relationship, Season was a large source of instrumental and expressive support in her life and, by association, her son's: "She does little things, like, she listens to things that I want help to do, that I liked to talk about. And then she'll do them. She knows the small stuff. Which is nice."

Adult children provided significant informal support to some benefit recipients. For example, Pat had a close relationship with her one daughter and stayed in touch with her other daughter and son. She could count on this daughter's consistent expressive and instrumental support even though the two of them did not always agree about the best way for Pat to achieve improved health and well-being while managing her pain and past opioid addiction. Pat explained their support relationship as follows: "Well, Tessa isn't supportive of me being on methadone. She wants me off. But you know, my kids are good with me.... Tessa always does [help me]. She went to Jamaica yesterday. And she gave me $100 for groceries. Before she went."

Several benefit recipients named one or two close friends as sources of support. Bianca maintained she counted one woman as a very close friend: "I have a couple of good friends, but I talk to one regularly. Yeah.

She doesn't do drugs. She doesn't. Yeah. We used to go to the clubs together." While they lost touch with each other for about ten years while "she was wrapped up with her boyfriend and her problems and I was going through my own," they found each other again on Facebook. They have since maintained their friendship for almost another ten years.

Adam provided perhaps the best example of how friendship, and its mix of instrumental and expressive exchanges, can mean so very much to a person living with addiction especially if a friend has had their own struggles with substances in the past. Talking about one friend in particular, he said:

> Our issues were a little different so he's, so it's fun to talk to him and be honest and joke around with him. He came to me in direct help for, like, my type of addiction because mine's based on being alone. But then again, it's good to have friends to joke around with so that's not as serious. Because especially when you're dealing with something serious like addictions, sometimes you just want to make fun of it.

People's provisions of caregiving to others were not just limited to caring for children. Four participants participated in family dynamics that were characterized by caring for older dependents. Besides picking his mother up from the hospital after her dialysis treatment, Jesse provided other forms of instrumental support to her.

> Right now, my mom, she's got in the last year I'd say, she has COPD.... Yeah, I was helping her the other day. I had to go to the grocery store for her because she doesn't get around too good now. In the past year, she's on oxygen tanks now, and she also has to go on dialysis three days a week, so I take her there and back, everywhere she goes.

Jesse was concerned to provide this care because his father (still married to and living with his mother) was an alcoholic in his assessment and so unreliable.

> JESSE: That's why I have to be there most of the time.
> AMBER: Because your mom needs help and you can't always probably predict where he's [your father] at?
> JESSE: Yeah, exactly. It's not like he wakes up in the morning and he has to have a drink. He wakes up, goes about his day. And then 6:00–7:00 at night when you'd normally, I guess get off work, have five or six beers, seven beers. But every day.

In contrast to informal support, formal support includes financial, or material, assistance provided by agencies, services, professionals, and workers on behalf of state programs or community organizations (Connidis, 2001; Gazso et al., 2016). Of course, all benefit recipients received formal support from the provincial government in the form of OW itself. And I have already made clear earlier in this book how benefit recipients could perceive their relationships with caseworkers (representing "formal support") to include caseworkers' provisions of expressive support too. Here, I briefly note that food banks were the other formal support that benefit recipients relied upon most, beyond kin and fictive kin. People's reliance upon food banks, however, seemed infrequent at best; food banks were only turned to when really needed. The minority of participants who did not access foodbanks attributed this to the quality of the food they would receive, or even their inability to benefit from them. Shawn shared an example in terms of the latter. Shawn worked odd jobs as a handyperson and his residence at the time of our interview was a house under renovation. "[T]here's no washroom, there's no fridge, no stove, no nothing," he told me. He did not pay rent conditional upon the renovation work he would complete. So, while Shawn had a roof over his head, the below-standard quality of the home he lived in meant that it was not logical for him to continue to visit a food bank – he had nowhere to store or prepare the food.

Only a few participants told me stories about how they relied upon non-profit community organizations in their communities for food (e.g., soup kitchens), a warm place to hang out for a few minutes, or other drop-in services like clothing banks. Theresa's support received from community, however, was perhaps the most unique since it did not necessarily involve a community organization per se. I met Theresa at a Tim Hortons in her neighbourhood for our interview. When I walked into the restaurant, I saw her dozing off in her wheelchair in the open space in which people would line up to place their orders. Her occupation of space and her confidence in doing so, even while dozing, was admirable to me. Theresa was clearly her own person and was using her time to wait for me to arrive how she pleased. None of the staff seemed to find her presence unusual; it appeared that this was a space where Theresa was known. Indeed, while she lived alone and did not name any particular people as friends, it was through more or less "hanging around" in her neighbourhood that she made clear that she maintained a sense of belonging and perceived her receipt of especially expressive support. She provided another example.

I just go to the liquor store, buy a beer, and come out and drink it. Then just kind of sit around people watching. And other people come, they're in the same kind of predicament, they want to come out and just have somebody to talk to, something to do, something to see.

I also heard stories of the lack of informal and formal supports that a minority of benefit recipients experienced. Compared to the other lone mothers with children in their care that I interviewed, Darlene appeared to have the weakest social support relationships with others. Darlene did not receive any support from her ex-partner and did not want any given his criminal conviction for child luring and subsequent incarceration. However, in contrast to Marnie and the other lone mothers, Darlene did not seem to have kin that provided other helpful support to her and her children, aside from mentioning that she and her children would very randomly visit her parents and their grandparents.

The absence of a support network contributed to some benefit recipients' social isolation and even exclusion. This seemed an experience shared by Darlene and some other single participants without dependents. Indeed, social isolation is not uncommon, particularly for single individuals on OW (Herd et al., 2018) or for low-income lone mothers (Gingrich, 2008; Weigers & Chun, 2015) when monthly income is not enough to afford food, shelter, and clothing and there are zero dollars for leisure or recreation time. Despite naming her children as sources of support, Pat also made clear that her poverty prevented her from feeling like she belonged in her community. Specifically, her relationships with people she considered friends and even her ability to purchase clothes were curtailed by her low income and what she saw as her less-than-understanding OW caseworker. Pat explained: "I visit a couple of friends sometimes. I never have bus fare. So, it's very hard for me.... I get money to go to the methadone clinic and that is it. Like I wanted to get money to go shopping. They [caseworker] won't give me nothing."

Charise also received very limited support from family, friends, and community. Years earlier Charise had divorced her husband. Her son, now over age eighteen, was still living with his father, her ex-partner, who was ill. Charise explained that she would prefer to live on her own because even though she considered her roommate a friend, he used to be her client when she was a sex worker. Since she was still using crack cocaine off and on during the time we met, she reasoned that given her use patterns and her receipt of very low income on OW as a single person, renting the room from her friend and ex-client was the best she could do at the time. As she acknowledged, her friend also provided her emotional support, stating: "He's the only one actually." When asked whether her son provided her any support, Charise replied: "Yeah, on the phone. If I'm depressed or whatever, he'll say 'What's wrong mom?'

And we'll talk. He tries to make the picture prettier than what it really is. You know there's a light at the end of the tunnel. And I don't see that light." Charise was aware, however, that her son could not offer her any instrumental support because he was not working for pay and that even his availability to provide expressive support beyond a telephone call was limited by his caring for his ailing father.

Among all participants, Trevor's complete lack of social support was atypical. Most participants had at least one other person, a friend or family member, that they counted on as a source of instrumental or expressive support. Trevor had experienced the loss of several family members before I met him, as well as the end of an intimate relationship. He was actively working on his recovery – but alone, except for his relationship with his OW caseworker.

> AMBER: Anyone you can think of that's, like one of your friends, or even a
>   family member that's really supportive of your recovery?
> TREVOR: No.
> AMBER: Okay. So, no one where you're like, you know, someone who's
>   like "yeah, you can do it."
> TREVOR: No.

Meaningful Relationships Made Visible

Some people living with addiction who participated in my study were also parents who spent their days parenting as others do, whether indirectly or directly caring for children. Their work of parenting, however, was challenged by their experience of multiple poverties. This work of parenting in low income was even further layered in with other work they performed upon themselves to manage or overcome dependency on a substance, or to manage their emotions and identities when responding to feeling rules constituted within broader discourses about family relations, addiction, and poverty.

Many single participants without custody of their children shared stories that were exemplary of their emotional work involved with (re-)producing their identities as mothers or fathers. Work made necessary as they grappled with their own self-awareness of their "addict" identity, the way in which they were defined and seen by OW policy and caseworkers as "recovering addicts," and the feeling rules associated with especially the discourses of welfare dependency and intensive mothering. Another few single participants without custody of their children, however, seemed ambivalent about adopting or wrestling with having only an "addict" identity; other facets of their self remained intact over time. Clive, for example, knew that he drank a good deal, but he knew he was still a father too. Among all benefit recipients, lone mothers seemed to be invested in emotional labour to the greatest extent to (re-)claim and (re-)produce themselves as mothers in their own eyes and the eyes of others (read caseworkers for OW and child welfare services). Adrianna, Marnie, and Season were effectively deconstructing what was others' ascription of their identity as primarily that of "addict" and engaging in a process of renewal of their identities as mothers in ways befitting the discourse of intensive mothering, and in especially Marnie's case, in relation to the discourse of families as a safe haven too. How these mothers could also subvert the "recovering addict" subjectivity constituted by OW discourse in their work of recovery will become clearer in the next chapter.

To summarize, the first half of this chapter explored the parenting practices of the women and men I met more generally and then shifted to how mothers and fathers comprehend discursively constituted feeling rules and manage their emotions in relation to them, thereby consciously or not sustaining or creating a coherent sense of self. Based on my findings, I contend that parents were partially compelled to engage in this emotional labour to (re-)produce, reify, and create their identities as mothers and fathers to transform OW policy and caseworkers' construction of their "recovering addict" subjectivity, or ascription of "addict" as only ever their master status (Hughes, 1945).

The second half of this chapter illustrated the ways that not just parents but all people living with addiction participate in social support networks, inclusive of and beyond kin relations too. Participants were part of socially supportive relationships with family members, friends, non-profit service providers, OW caseworkers, and members of their community. It was unusual for a person to have very few to no supports, as was the case for Charise and Trevor. It was clear that people who depended on substances could experience changes in their support networks over time; their behaviour while using could fracture or completely end their relationships of support with others, something discussed at the very beginning of this book. However, I also learned from some benefit recipients that even when they used substances and despite any risks associated with their use patterns, they still were part of social relationships that had the potential to be transformative of their lives, for better or worse. Moreover, I gained the impression from my participants that if they met people who resisted societal pressures to stigmatize them – people who offered empathy and mindful presence in their lives – their life courses had the potential to unfold all the richer for these relationships, a point I will return to in the next and final chapter of this book.

The findings presented in this chapter in total lead me to invite others to de-stigmatize addiction for a very simple reason. As powerfully illustrated by benefit recipients who were parents and part of social support networks, an identity of substance user or recovering substance user is but one aspect of the self – it need not be *the* master status through which one experiences the social world. An identity of substance user or recovering substance user, even if self-imposed, should not make invisible other facets of individuals' family and social relationships. Indeed, if identities are seen as malleable, emotionally and discursively constituted, and the self multifaceted, people's lives unfold in tandem with an ever-evolving self. In making visible the parenting identities of the women and men I interviewed, as well as their family dynamics and other social support relations, I substantiate the argument I have been making throughout this book: a person is not their addiction.

8 Beginning Anew, and Recovery

To want to surpass cravings for a substance of choice, to learn to practise harm reduction, to be determined to change one's self-concept – these were only some motivations implied by benefit recipients not simply "starting over" but beginning a life somehow new, from a different space and place, part of a larger trajectory of self-actualization (Maslow, 1943), and driven by an imagined future. In this chapter, I focus on these new beginnings and the ongoing mental, emotional, and physical work of some benefit recipients in recovery. I explore how these participants claimed a "recovering addict" subjectivity for themselves. Thus far, I have been concerned with demonstrating how participants' subjectivity can be regulated by Ontario Works (OW) policy discourse or caseworkers as a condition of income support. Here I am interested here in people's own stories of how they moved towards a deeper understanding of themselves as agentic and resolute in their work of recovery – and how they reflected on and re-produced and/or subverted a "recovering addict" subjectivity in the process. I also contrast the emergent actual, or anticipated, life course trajectories of participants who defined themselves as in recovery with those who remained ambivalent about their substance use. Lastly, I consider the social support networks participants perceived as necessary to their new beginnings and how employment – the desirable outcome of OW and seen to facilitate an exit from it – factored into this. I conclude with a discussion of the resoluteness required to create and maintain new beginnings when one lives with addiction amid multiple individual and structural – sometimes systemic – poverties.

Moving Forward

So, our caseload is probably the most challenging caseload in the office, especially because they have multiple issues.... [W]e're dealing with people who are homeless, we're dealing with people who are in and out of incarceration ... people who have an active street life. So, all of those things really come into play. When I have an active client who every day needs to feed their habit, they're going to do a whole bunch of other things than just see me, just to maintain that addiction. And I think there has to be a realization from that point of view.

Caseworker Gale

When I adopt Gale's point of view, the implication for me even as an outsider is clear: the first step in beginning, in changing one's substance use patterns, is huge. The sheer magnitude of research on recovery and the growing addictions and mental health "system," "industry," or "market," from non-profit organizations and associations to for-profit residential treatment centres in North America, further attest to escalating responses to honour and support the giganticness of this step towards change (American Addiction Centres, 2019; Munro, 2015).

To be blunt, I learned from benefit recipients that "a lot is going on" at any one time, in a person's mind and in their social interactions, and is shaping of their actions about recovery. Those who identified as in recovery, however, shared stories that suggested that people are ready to move forward, sometimes into treatment, for some specific reasons. So, maybe including their meeting of a supportive caseworker who perceived they had a problem with substance use, the people I met shared that they are ready to move forward when: (1) they are determined, (2) they are tired, (3) there is a specific reason to change, and/or (4) a major life event happens. Benefit recipients often spoke to one or more of these factors as shaping their change in substance use. An encompassing characteristic of all participants in recovery seemed to be a change in their self-conceptualization.

Anais shared about her act of quitting Percocet as one of determination. She participated in a methadone treatment program but only for a short period of time, as she was dissatisfied with its process. According to Anais: "I just made the decision and stopped." When I mentioned that I understood from others that it was hard to wean oneself off methadone, Anais replied: "It is. But if you want to do it you can do it." Often participants who saw themselves as in recovery explained their change in use to require deep introspection, coming to terms with seeing it as problematic, and then subsequently determining to become sober or to reduce the harm of their use. Adrienne, for example, had engaged in a great deal of reflection to reach a place of determination to abstain entirely from using substances.

> I know real reasons why I do what I do, and I know the reasons that people think I do.... But at the end of the day, I'm also a believer that ... these are my choices.... I spoke to a lady down at CAMH, a doctor there before, and her method was, she saw people progress better as a social drinker than just quitting entirely.... It's either I do it or I don't. The same thing with the opiates and everything.... And that was, I guess, my addiction of choice ... there's no in between for me.... It's just, it's just I'm gonna do it wholeheartedly, I'm gonna do it best of, or the worst of, my ability. And then I'm not gonna do it at all. So same, so I see the same thing with alcohol.

Besides determination, deciding to move forward to something different could also stem from a feeling of being tired of using (see also Pollini et al., 2006). Benefit recipients' tiredness of substance use could be shaped by the lifestyle, time, and loss associated with their use. Danni explained this tiredness as follows:

> [W]hen I first went on OW it was more, "I'll see".... But now I'm in my recovery because I want to be here. I have the want to, want to stay clean now. I never had that before. I'm at a point in my life now, I'm thirty-five years old, I've lost my twenties to drugs and Hepatitis C, I've lost my thirties to drugs and Hep C.... I'm tired of living this way. I'm so tired of it. I'm tired of living like a crack head. So, I've been really trying this last couple years to get a little bit better and think a little bit clearer and build a place so eventually I can have my children in my life. I know I'll never have them back, but I can have them in my life.

When I asked Pat why she quit her use of substances, both alcohol and drugs, and then eventually transitioned into methadone treatment, she replied: "Because I got tired of it. Ah, like kind of the lifestyle, like kind of everything that was involved?" I was curious as to whether she sought out other forms of treatment to support her choice to live differently.

> No. I took myself off of it. I believe in "If I can't do it myself, then no one else can do it for me." I have to do it. And I did.... I can't remember how old I was. Probably in my forties. Late forties.... Enough is enough. I had enough. You know.... [W]hen you take pills every day, you kind of gag after a while because you don't want to take them.

Marnie seemed ready for change when she realized she was not mothering as she wanted, because specific events in her life happened, and she was tired of her patterns of use.

> I can't like, live with this, like, with what I'm doing to, like, my daughter. I can't be away from her like this, and I just knew that I couldn't live like that anymore.... I ended up losing my job at the oral surgeon's. So, that like, that was kind of like a little, like a, like a, a really low point.... I think, I didn't tell my parents for like, a week or two. Instead of, like, going to work, like, when I was going to work, I would just be going out with him [her ex-partner and father of her daughter] and using, and I was just (pause), I don't know, I guess I was just, like, sick and tired of feeling so sick and so gross, and, like, just awful all the time.

Besides Danni, the other mothers I interviewed, whether children were in their care or not, generally spoke of their determination to move forward in order to have a relationship with their children. For example, when I asked Bianca what gave her the strength to move forward in her commitment to recovery, she said:

> My kids. I can't wait to see, like I really want to see a clean future with my children.... All of us back together. I would never tear them out of that family they're in because they're happy.... And they've [my relatives] done great jobs with them. And hopefully they don't leave, go down that road of abuse, right? But just to have a relationship with them.

To the same question, Pat replied: "My kids. Yeah, if they weren't here, I really wouldn't give a crap.... I brought them into this world. I'm not, you know, going to just give up on everything." To be clear, I do not see mothers' determination about getting clean as *for* their children. Rather, mothers seemed to want to change their use so that they could maintain or re-develop their own identities as a mother – who deeply cared – and garner a privileged place in their children's lives.

A major life event or "fateful moment" was another reason why some other benefit recipients began the process of changing their substance use patterns. These life course events prompted people to dramatically alter their ways of being in the present and future (Berger, 2008; Giddens, 1991; Webb & Gazso, 2017). Substance use could change in response to an unexpected event, such as Marnie pinpointed earlier: the loss of a job. However, participants' use of substances could also literally change in a heartbeat – a near death event. Jesse told an exemplary story:

> Well, something happened to me about fourteen, fifteen months [ago]. Like I said before, I was only using OxyContin and I got to learn heroin, learned how to use needles and stuff like that. One day I was at my friend's house and my friend hit me up or whatever and the next thing I know, I'm at the hospital. And that was the last time I ever used…. My sister just had her kid. I'm only twenty-eight at the time. I'm only twenty-eight years old, so my whole life, man.

Ten months prior to our interview, Adrienne was in the hospital undergoing gastric suction or a "stomach pump" for alcohol poisoning. "I got sick in October, and they had to pump my stomach. That was the last day. That was the last day that I actually drank."

Treatment

Some benefit recipients decided to move forward specifically through treatment. Treatment can be a condition of OW benefit receipt, intertwined with "the recovering addict" subjectivity constituted by the "distance from the labour market discourse." But treatment was also some participants' choice because they were determined to change their use, they were tired of using, or they saw different events in their life to lead to it. Some participants shared about how a change in their thinking prompted them to determine treatment as the way forward. Trevor perceived his choice to enter methadone treatment as associated with a crystallization of his negative perception of self while he was using:

> But you know I wasn't long, I wasn't long on that [heroin] because that's what opened my eyes to like, "I got to get the hell off of this." You know, once I started seeing myself using needles and track marks on my arms…. And then you know, once I saw myself hiding my arms and stuff, you know, and like that's when I was like "I need to get off of drugs."

Arash shared how he felt a kind of spiritual pull towards a different life that no longer involved his use of substances. This occurred after he had had a confrontation with a police officer who shared what he saw as an outcome of Arash's "bad" life choices and chances:

> So, they [police] let me go. I couldn't believe it. One of the cops, he looked back at me, and I'll never forget his words, he said "If you keep doing

drugs, you're fucked." And then something went off and I felt I'd better do something about this. So, I kind of found my way to, I believe a higher power, somebody liked me there. It wasn't me – not that it wasn't me, but some deeper connection with something else that led me there [residential treatment].

Other participants pinpointed the experience of treatment itself as the turning point in their relationship with substances. Adam first began to understand his own use as linked to his depression through participation in one-on-one and group counselling.

[I]'ve already figured out after being in the program, maybe it's sort of like a big turning point actually, is that I'm probably dealing with depression. It's sort of just been re-teaching me how to think about these things.... [I]t's better for us to just get even more comfortable talking about it as well. Ah, because when you meet up with someone on a weekly basis and you're in this situation with other people who are going through similar things, ah (pause), you just start breaking walls you build up in your mind. Maybe without even realizing it.

In many ways, Adam was learning firsthand the extent to which substance use disorders can occur simultaneously with mental health disorders. According to psychiatric research, comorbid psychiatric and substance disorders are related to genetic and environmental factors (e.g., childhood traumatic events). Some scholars find that individuals become dependent on substances as a way to self-medicate when diagnosed with anxiety, depression, or PTSD, among other things (Hasin & Kilcoyne, 2012; Smith & Book, 2010; Wu et al., 2010). When I asked Adam what gives him strength to continue to pursue his recovery, he said: "Um, just feeling like myself again. Feeling happy. And even putting that work into working towards something is better than feeling nothing or getting nothing." Of all participants, Adam was the most observant of all the "work" (e.g., mental, physical, and emotional) involved in changing patterns of use.

In total, eight participants were taking part in methadone or suboxone treatment or pharmacology therapy. Methadone or suboxone, however, were not a panacea for all users. For example, by the time I met Pat, she had been on methadone for almost twenty years. Despite many attempts made, she found she could not lower her dose. Shawn and Alexei were even transparent about their use of methadone as a replacement for their drug of choice, heroin. The timing of their use of either drug was carefully planned. Trevor, a past heroin user too, even spoke quite passionately about the importance of intention as it related to methadone use. In so doing, he also and unintentionally confirmed that Shawn and Alexei's use of methadone would be circumspect to others (and could be to themselves too), saying, "Because a lot of people get on methadone. They take it when they don't have drugs." Trevor felt that there was no point in being on methadone unless one was determined to recover from addiction to heroin.

Carie, however, was certain of her resoluteness to overcome her addiction through methadone treatment. Like some other participants, she also struggled with establishing a dose so that she would no longer have cravings. Her pride in receiving her first "carry" seemed to confirm her determination to chart a new beginning or a different way to live her life.

> Right from the beginning I wanted to be clean. And I did use in the beginning, and they know everybody does because they're not at their comfortable point yet.... [A]bout a year, and I was comfortable. And all of a sudden, I'm like "Oh my God I got my first carry." And it felt so good. Like I don't have to come down here every day. It's [methadone treatment] like a job. Like, you cannot have a job.

It was also not unusual to hear about participants' experiences of relapse and repeated efforts at treatment, a finding echoed in the broader literature on treatment (McQuaid et al., 2017) and especially among persons receiving methadone and still using other opioids (Naji et al., 2016). Some participants discussed being determined more than once to move forward in establishing a recovery trajectory. For example, Bianca's desire to have a relationship with her two children who were in her sister's custody motivated her overcoming her crack cocaine addiction. But then she relapsed and developed a heroin habit.

> Had to give my kids up … it just took over me … for two years, and then after that I made the decision either I'm going to pick my children or never see them again – because I never would go see them messed up. Right? And I was hardly seeing them. Or "You stop this crap and get your shit together." So, I picked that one. And I haven't touched it [crack cocaine] since.... But then, then I did (laughter), I did heroin. Do you know what? With heroin, you can function.... I hid that for years.

Bianca had laughed at what she saw as the absurdity of going into residential treatment to stop her use of one drug to then, eventually, turn to another once she was outside of treatment, what is known as addiction replacement in the wider literature. When we met for our interview, Bianca had been sober for three months and was determined to develop and maintain a recovery plan. Her latest turn towards recovery was spurred on by: "Trouble with the law," specifically her arrest for drug trafficking. In fact, she was on house arrest in her childhood home and under the supervision of her aging parents. Bianca looked at her arrest as a turning point that inspired her most recent efforts at recovery.

> [I]t was kind of like I needed it to wake me up. Do it now. Now I can ask for their [parents'] support because it's out in the open again now. And I did. And I cleaned up. And I'm going to try and stay that way…. I finally said if I ever get to the point that I wake up normal every day, I will not ever touch it again. I am waking up. I don't have to do anything to be normal. Why would I go back now? I know addiction is strong. But I can't. I can't do that. I got too much to lose all over again.

I interviewed Bianca at her basement suite in her parents' home. Even despite her many attempts to quit her drug use, she maintained they were always "there" to support her. I shared in her delight over her one way to "be normal" and to keep moving forward in recovery: the art of crocheting. Throughout each day, Bianca would "watch her shows" and crochet (learned by watching YouTube videos). She explained that she liked the busyness of using her hands and she felt excited and a sense of reward when she held a final product she had made. The day of our interview, I also met her mother and father. I got the impression that her parents were checking in with her while I was visiting. I saw pride in her father's face when she explained to him that she was being interviewed by me about her substance use and her experience at changing it in order to help out others.

It was not unusual for benefit recipients to speak about how their earlier determinations to move forward by participating in treatment could be thwarted by the structural and social environment of treatment itself. In specific cases, their stories implied how easy it was to continue to use or change their substance of choice because of the social relationships they developed within treatment. Indeed, some participants' stories underscored how loss of control over use can occur simultaneous with an individual's "on-the-face" actions oriented towards sobriety. Finally, these participants' stories can also be read as suggesting how, perhaps, a subconscious lack of determination to change substance use patterns can enter participants' treatment with them.

There was a certain ease by which people could continue using substances when attending especially AA meetings and group counselling sessions. It was through attendance at a day treatment program that Jesse eventually learned to use heroin:

> Since I've been in the program, it was really hard to try and get off of it because they put you together with all these other people.... I was just doing opiates and had to learn to use a needle and this and that.... I never, before I came into this program and met people and went over to their house, and just because they're doing it, I'm doing it.

After Marnie participated in residential treatment for alcohol use, she reconnected with friends she made there: "when I got out, that's when I tried cocaine for the first time, 'cause I met all these girls in rehab who did cocaine." Dante was transparent in saying that he sought out a dealer through a relationship with another patient when he entered residential treatment in lieu of serving the remainder of a criminal sentence. Through his social and intimate relationships with other patients, he continued to use alcohol and even began to use crack cocaine.

> I went to the therapy. I immediately met some guy, asked him to get us some drugs to buy from. He got caught using. He told on me. They [the program staff] said: "Listen, you were supposed to go back to jail. But we're going to let you report yourself back." So, I went home. Actually, I tried.... I wanted to go back to another rehab. Well, hence why, how I ended up here in Bellwoods.... And while I'm there, I ran into a chick. Again. She finished the [program]. I was two weeks away from finishing. And they kicked me out.... I kind of didn't want to be there anymore, there, I wanted to be with her.... And um, I was drinking with her. I had never smoked crack before Toronto. Couldn't find any coke. Crack was everywhere. And that's how that became that.

Cody had served time in a federal correctional institution in British Columbia (BC). Part of our interview conversation turned to our memories of prison, mine of working as a correctional officer and his of being incarcerated in one. By all appearances, Cody would be seen by many as moving forward and becoming clean and sober because he was incarcerated and had no access to substances. However, I remembered one of my responsibilities as a correctional officer was to conduct random searches of inmate cells for contraband. So, I asked Cody if he was able to maintain his drug habit in jail. He replied: "Not quite as much but you can still maintain it. Things are pretty expensive. I made my own booze." When I probed further to ask him if he saw himself as sober upon his release, he explained:

> When I got out, I turned around and I had to go on a methadone program because when I got out, I had to find something just to get better for the day. And then after I got better, not to be sick [withdrawal], then I'd go out and now I could get high.... So, the doctor that was in prison, she also had an office outside and I went to her. I told her "if you don't put me on the methadone, you're going to see me next week [in prison]. I can't continue to live like this or I'm going to be back inside, please help me." And she put me on the methadone program.

Like others, Cody's social relationships within an institution that may have facilitated his recovery instead facilitated his use.

The Work of Recovery

The meaning of recovery can be different for scholars and the lay public alike (Anthony, 1993; Deegan, 1996; Roberts & Boardman, 2013). Adrienne implied these debates surrounding its meaning when she shared her conceptualization of recovery versus her partner Eddie's:

> His [my boyfriend] thing is I'm not a recovery addict. It's "Either you're an addict or you're not. When you draw the line and you stop being an addict and you stop drinking or you stop doing the drugs, then you're no longer an addict." I believe in recovering ... I think you're either functioning, you're an addict, you're a functioning addict. Or you're a recovering addict. Something like that.

I take my inspiration from Adrienne and do not see recovery as meaning only abstinence, as in some addictions literature. Nor do I see recovery to mean only harm reduction, an approach favoured in some mental health circles (Bartram, 2021). I instead conceptualize recovery as an ongoing process of individuals' renewal of their health and wellness, which can include the absence of substance use or controlled substance use and its effects on themselves and others. The emphasis on self-improvement and growth that underscored some participants' talk of recovery tended to coalesce into a common theme: the work of new beginnings, a different path in their life course, or the work of recovery.

When I asked Franco about the biggest challenge he faced every day, he echoed what Adam implied about the sheer amount of mental and emotional work involved in being in recovery:

> For me, it's a feeling of being stagnant. Realizing that sometimes stay-ing still is moving forward. I have to realize that.... I believe I am stuck between old views, old values, and today. And accepting who I am now versus who I was then. And that's a lot. And I've forgiven my past mis-takes but that doesn't mean it changes the effects that's occurred because of that [sic].... So, the hardest part is sitting there and going, "okay. It's okay."... [T]hat the track I'm on is the right one for me.

Thus, just like the initial decision to change substance use patterns, some participants spoke of the intention and then determination that was part of the work of recovery. Adrienne explained:

> So, if you choose to stay away from the opiate part, and you're dedicating, and focus on the treatment part, then it will work. But you have to be in the mindset if I want it to work.... I want to identify. I want to, I want to address. I want to identify. I want to mend, and I just want to move on.

Marnie implied that being busy with something else can also make the work of recovery seem to stick: "Different programs. Just, um, staying active. Staying, like, healthy, and positive and, um, just like I said ... I know in my head it's done. Like ... it's something I can never go back to." And yet, not every participant could be as active as Marnie or even feel like there was enough to do each day. Indeed, since Pat and other single participants implied that being on OW can be quite boring and isolating given their poverty, their work of recovery included having to answer: "Recovery for what?"

The work that must go into recovery could also be stymied by with-drawal. Pat explained how she had not yet been able to complete the work of withdrawal from methadone specifically: "But I can't get off it. I've tried. I go into, like, depression. I get, you know, the jitters." One of Cody's experiences of withdrawal from heroin was made worse by the environment he was in at the time – solitary confinement in a pro-vincial jail – and because his was withdrawal that was not voluntarily intended, "It's a very different world, especially going through with-drawal because you're right there in it. It was sixteen days – sixteenth day they put me back on the range. That was when I finally could stand up." I asked if any doctors or nurses checked on him when he was withdrawing in his cell, something I remembered as obligatory at least once in twenty-four hours when I worked the solitary confinement unit in federal prison. He replied, "No, not nurses. Just the guards do the one-hour check in the slot."

Since not every person I interviewed was seeking to change their substance use patterns, working on recovery seemed therefore irrelevant. Some people seemed comfortable with their decisions about their use. Clive was transparent in saying that after his relationship with his wife dissolved, he "took up drinking seriously." He liked to drink and even wished he could drink more. Our conversation that enabled him to arrive at this conclusion went as follows. It's also a good illustration of Clive's character:

> CLIVE: The alcohol kind of controls me. If I go out and get drunk, the next day I'm so sick that I'm not going drinking. I'm not doing nothing.
> AMBER: Yeah. Are you okay with that? Or are you like "This is my life?!"
> CLIVE: I wish my stomach and liver weren't so screwed up so I could drink every day.

Shawn, like Clive, was not working on recovery and similarly saw his substance use as simply something he lived with. In explaining his heroin use pattern, he said: "Yes, I do use basically every day, or whatever. But I don't let it ruin my life. Put it that way. I've gotten used to it now. But like I said I don't let it dictate what I do every day. I don't think about it. I just do what I have to do and carry on. Just like you do anything else." When I then asked him if he thought he would get to a place where he would want to quit, he said: "I think so in time. I'll get fed up and I'll wean myself down. I do what I do, but I've got to live too. I'm not totally happy but I'm okay."

Alexei was transparent in noting that he had not yet reached a place of intention to quit his drug habit: "I think I have to come to the point where I have to do it myself.... If I go there [residential treatment] thinking 'Let me just save up some money for a month and I will make a big party,' it will not change. You understand?" Alexei did note, however, perhaps more mixed feelings about his use and tried to limit his use to continue to receive both instrumental and expressive support from his father: "He [my father] comes here very often, with his work or business. So, every time he comes, I try to not upset him. So, when he's here I try to be sober. Like kind of because every time I get upset, I get less support from him. So, it's a kind of, one of my support."

Harm reduction was part of the work of recovery for some participants, meaning ongoing symptoms of substance use could be part of their recovery (Bartram, 2021). Some participants saw their controlled use of substances as better than their using other, harder drugs more frequently, and better than outright abstinence. Steve, for example, was learning to reduce the harm of his alcohol use and to view any time he used heavily and compulsively as but one moment in time. Steve adopted this tactic because he had begun to understand how his feelings of guilt or self-loathing could perpetuate his continued use.

> I haven't been perfectly clean for six months … every once in a while, ah, I step off the road. It hasn't been severe yet and I talked to an addictions counsellor who's at the shelter and I do my meetings and stuff like that. One of the things that keeps yah going is yah, ah, yah feel so lousy once you start using, ah, when you sober up. Yeah, just ah, you know, you kinda hate yourself, ah. And if you keep that mindset going, the depression and everything, you'll just keep using to numb that ah, feeling right?

Many benefit recipients used cannabis as a form of harm reduction, their use preceding its formal legalization in fall 2018 and reflective of wider cultural tolerance of cannabis use (Duff et al., 2012; Hathaway et al., 2018). The following excerpt demonstrates that I was slow to understand Dante's cannabis use, and his joke too:

> DANTE: Right now, I'm on the marijuana maintenance program. Have you ever heard of that one?
> AMBER: Well, I know you can get, of course, legal weed prescribed.
> DANTE: No, no, no. Marijuana maintenance program. Basically, instead of doing all the hard drugs, you smoke weed instead.

When I then asked Dante if he had entertained a program like NA or AA, he replied:

> Fuck no. I tried. Been there. Done that. No…. It's more of a cult I find. I'm totally not into it. Um, until I heard of harm reduction, I was like: "What? Absence? I can't quit weed. I can't quit the occasional drink…." Harm reduction makes sense to me.

Besides Dante, other participants identified other harm reduction actions as part of their work of recovery. Adam explained his chosen practice of harm reduction as follows: "It's kind of like just keep reading and be like, 'Oh, I'm going to get to this next chapter.' And even if I spend three hours reading, then I might have a beer. But then it's like midnight and I've had one or two instead of seven or eight." Tara was a firm believer in and advocate of harm reduction.

> If you just keep telling them abstinence, they probably won't get straight. Harm reduction, you know, it's a process. You take it as you can, right. A little bit here, a little bit there. You know, like I said, I've been doing drugs and that since I was seven. I'm fifty-one years old and I'm just getting straight now. And part of that is because of harm reduction. Not because of abstinence. I slowly started out. I cut out this. And then I cut out that. And then, you know?

Ontario's ministries of Health, and Children, Community and Social Services, have supported elements of harm reduction in programming directed at adults and youth since the late 1980s, largely as part of the national drug strategy (Zilkowsky, 2001). Hyshka et al.'s (2017) analysis, however, shows that harm-reduction policy is underdeveloped across Canada and stigmatization of substance use persists even in government documents on it, to say the least of polarizing (often moral) views about the efficacy of harm reduction that surface in the broader social milieux. Notably, Ontario does not have a stand-alone provincial-level harm-reduction policy. Only needle and syringe distribution were named as specific interventions in 2017, a stark contrast to the several harm-reduction interventions in other provinces and territories (Hyshka et al., 2017). I was therefore not surprised to learn from caseworker Miranda that one challenge of her job has been to convince people accessing OW that there is space for them to identify and continue their controlled practices of substance use and while still orienting to the rules and regulations of OW.

> And I'm working with … a local community agency and I go out once a month to their Harm Reduction Drop-in Program. So, I've built a relationship there now. So, they will refer clients, clients will self-refer. I have clients who've actually referred clients. And it's because they have a trust now, so they feel like they can tell me anything and we're still going to continue to move forward and we're going to work with them where they're at, and that's very helpful.

Transitions of the "Recovering Addict"

It was clear from interviews that some people had quite specific dreams and goals for their futures that included and pushed along their commitment to recovery. From a life course perspective, stories of this nature can be thought of as participants' actual or prospective transitions, of events and trajectories to continue or orient towards anew. They can also be thought of as stories of hope (Kimball et al., 2017; Stevens et al., 2018). Based on their research with participants in an AA program, Frings et al. (2019) even argue that narratives of recovery are more accurately tales of hope, especially if these narratives touched upon a person's future in general or specific aspirational goals. Indeed, a great deal of interdisciplinary research emphasizes the place of hope in recovery (Deegan, 1996; Stevens et al., 2018; Weinberg, 2013).

The undertone of hope in participants' stories of recovery especially invites my continued nuancing of earlier arguments made in this book. I wish to show that while a "recovering addict" subject position can be produced through the "distance from the labour market discourse" infiltrating OW design and administration for people living with addiction, this position need not be felt as static nor deterministic. In focusing on family and social relationships in the preceding chapter, I showed how this subject position was constantly laboured over. Placing benefit recipients' stories of recovery in conversation with findings of my discourse analysis of policy (see chapter 5) specifically prompts this understanding: a "recovering addict" subjectivity can be transformed by those who re-work it for themselves and for others in their recovery and as they transition to new beginnings. The next and last chapter of this book further explores hope as being not just integral to individual change, but paramount to societal, collective change that will overturn the stigmatization of addiction.

Assuming this hopefulness of recovery, my concern in this section is twofold, to explore: (1) how actual or anticipated transitions, or new beginnings in general, are contingent on social support relations; and (2) participants' feelings about paid work. I make clear how what participants receive, want, and need as social support in general, and specific to their potential employability, are part of their recovery process.

Social Support

Instrumental and expressive support from friends, kin, and fictive kin (i.e., people who feel like family) (Gazso & McDaniel, 2015) seemed essential for participants who worked on recovery and sought new beginnings. Some participants had friends that supported them no matter how many times they relapsed, and then worked on recovery again. In these cases, friendship and its possibilities for reciprocal exchanges of support seemingly shaped some participants' perception of self and facilitated their development of ontological security (Giddens, 1991).

For example, Charise, though she still randomly used crack cocaine, shared that in each of her efforts at recovery through residential treatment, one friend provided the help she needed: "He's a really good friend. My son knows him, my mom and dad know him. Because I don't drive, he's done so many wonderful things. Like he's the one that's taken me to rehab every time I needed to go. He's awesome. I call him my angel."

In the process of changing substance use patterns, however, friendships may also be lost, and so newer relationships of intimacy must be created. When Carie had lived on the street when her use of OxyContin was at its worst, she experienced friendships on the street as like family, saying, "When we're tight, we call each other fam, out there. It's not like friends … if someone calls you fams, you're in the good books." In leaving the street, however, she left behind these relationships and had to work to re-invigorate friendships that she had before she was homeless or develop new ones. She also had to put trust in someone else to afford a place to live on her limited monthly income from OW as a single person (around $700 in 2017) (Income Security Advocacy Centre, 2020). Carie thought of her roommate as a constant friend who supported her efforts at recovery and someone who could even help her navigate her own prospective intimate relationships with other men.

> We've known each other my whole life.… [H]e's like, "I need something [a roommate] and I know you're clean."… We don't look at each other like that. I feel pretty comfortable with him. Like when people say you can't have a guy friend, that's bullshit. Yeah. It's good to know that you have a guy friend. "What does it mean when he says this?" You know what I mean.… There was only a couple of people I would have moved in with and he was one of them, so I was like, "Thank God."

Some participants received steadfast support from parents even amid their changing patterns of use. According to Arash:

> My dad is supportive. He's supportive in every way.… I've never asked him for money, this last time, just for groceries or something. And I'll pay him back.… As far as, well, my dad supports me with moral support and is a sounding board I can talk to easily.

Arash was aware that his sister, however, was weary of having an intimate relationship with him, hedging her closeness with and support of him on his actions and behaviour and how it affected her: "My sister is supportive as long as I'm consistent … we became really close, and then

I left again. So, it kind of broke her heart and she can't stand – it's hard to see somebody that you love hurt themselves, because that's all we do, we hurt ourselves." In switching to a mix of first and third person in his last sentence, Arash's words powerfully illustrate his and other participants' awareness of and responsibility for how they hurt those they love and themselves with their substance use.

Marnie pinpointed her desire to work on recovery for reasons of feeling "gross and tired" and wanting to mother her daughter in ways she saw to fit with contemporary norms of mothering. She further explained during our chat that she was indebted to her brother in helping her see a way forward. On one occasion, his support made a profound difference in her life.

> Um, so I guess he came home for a Thanksgiving break, and I had just gotten wasted. Um, I don't know if it was a little bit of him saying, like, "What the fuck are you doing with your life? Like, you have this beautiful daughter" and me just like breaking down, and just being like, "Look. I need help. I can't – I can't. I need help, like now." He ended up driving me to, um, XXX [hospital] ... [a]nd like, he walked me through everything, and like he was there while they checked me in.

Formal sources of support, including instrumental and expressive support received from government and community programs and so the people who work for them, also facilitated participants' recovery work. Despite the anonymizing potential of casework, I have already made clear that several OW caseworkers shared examples of the support that they provided benefit recipients. I narrow my focus here to how some caseworkers saw their provisions of support as especially important when working with benefit recipients pursuing recovery. Gale did her best to create relationships with benefit recipients characterized by various supports and not immediately centred on employment.

> I think, they've [clients] certainly told me that it's made a huge difference for them, a positive difference in that I've had more time for them, in actual time. That we actually are able to discuss some of the actual problems that they're having ... they know that I have more flexibility on my caseload, and I tell them that. That if something happens out of the blue and you need to come in, just come in and I'll see you.... Flexibility is big. Just not feeling like they're being pushed to go into employment or training.

Chris felt more involved in people's lives than the usual caseworker–benefit recipient relationship that materializes with people not living with addiction: "And I have clients who come see me, like some see me every single day, some come in once a week." Merren was clearest in naming the specific instrumental supports that she could provide OW benefit recipients.

> Ontario Works definitely would provide the transportation for them to go. As soon as they are linked into a program, we can give them some clothing and grooming money. So, if they want to get themselves a couple new outfits or whatever, they've got the money to do that.... Certainly, what I find about Ontario Works is they allow us [addictions or PREP caseworkers] the flexibility to ensure that whatever we can do to help those clients move towards treatment, or to manage in this life.

Some benefit recipients acknowledged the character and quality of the support that they received from caseworkers and what it meant to them when they felt they were in a place to move forward. Bianca explained:

> I did disclose that [my addiction] to him [my caseworker]. I, ah, said, "I've been clean since January." And I said, "I have a drug issue and I want, I'm looking to getting help." And he [Caseworker Scott] just took it from there ... my last worker said that to me too. And I like that. Because they understand us. They don't judge. And they know what to do when you need the help. When you are ready for it. Because you got to be ready for it.

Charise's experience with a PREP caseworker who seemed to easily volunteer information and made it clear that she would be eligible for some financial support for her education made a difference in how Charise looked towards the future.

> I do, I want to go back to school actually, but I'm putting that on hold for now. But he [caseworker] knows I want to get my Certificate, Culinary Arts ... [s]o he's already given me the pages and stuff I would need to do.... And he told me things that I don't even know, like they pay for my knives and my outfit. I didn't know that.

Cody was participating in an employment program at the encouragement of his PREP caseworker. The combination of his caseworker's knowledge and the knowledge he gained from an assessment of his vocational aptitude enabled him to feel supported as he moved further along in his work of recovery and began the process of choosing a career.

> That's something Metrics helped me with. Breaking down if I did [work], what would I do? And I went from graphic designing to cooking, sewing, I always wanted to sew, to social work. And [my caseworker said], "If you do graphic design, you're going to have to run your own business, with the competition and stuff." But she says there's a huge market for social service. And she said with my experience, I could help others.... It would be like, "I've been through this," and I want that job, and they embrace it. So that's more feasible for me.

Benefit recipients also offered their assessment of the types (formal and informal) and kinds (instrumental and expressive) of support that they still needed from an addictions or PREP caseworker. In general, benefit recipients conveyed that they need caseworkers who were nimble in their expectations of people living with addiction and varied in their provisions of support to aid recovery, not caseworkers that adopt a "one size fits all" approach. Adrienne had this to say:

> It's not all about rehab. And I like the fact that Wesley [her caseworker] is not forcing me to that or whatever. Cause I don't think rehab does it for you. Rehab just, in my opinion, just keeps you away from it for like thirty days, sixty days, and they try to do it "Out of sight, out of mind".... Unfortunately, you can only afford to live in certain neighbourhoods.

In her reference to neighborhoods, Adrienne was also making the point that when rehabilitation ends, people most often return to homes in neighbourhoods they can afford while on OW – and where peer groups who use or sell legal, prescription, and illicit substances are readily available.

Benefit recipients also shared that they more generally need to feel that their own unique concerns, life course paths, and current social and economic situations are understood and respected by their caseworker. Danni and Carie's experiences of withdrawal hinted at how when help is desired, it is needed *now*, not later. Tara was particularly blunt in saying that when help is sought and one is accessing OW, lack of money for transportation should not hinder its receipt.

> When you're an addict, you don't want to be going here [and there]. If you could go to one place and do something or do a few things, you'll go. But when you start making me "Okay, you know what? You got to here, you

got to go there, you gotta go here."… [W]hen I first started my AA and NA meetings, ah, I lot of time I wouldn't be able to go because I didn't have bus fare.

Franco maintained that a "one-stop shop," where health and social services were networked and offered in one physical space, could best support his work on recovery. His belief in the importance of this style of service provision was informed by his own experience of seeking help and having to wait to receive it, and thereby experiencing doubt about his determination to pursue a new beginning.

One-stop shop, yeah.… So, if I ever went to XXXX, which I have to, to get certain procedures done, they share the same information [as OW]. So, I don't have to bring this file to this guy. Because in [the city], that was los-ing a lot of time. And the reason I bring this up is because time brings up doubt. The longer it takes to process things, the more you think nothing is happening.… You want immediate gratification when you're coming down, when you're coming off drinking or drugs.

Concerning Paid Work

In my interviews with caseworkers and benefit recipients, I also explored what may happen if benefit recipients are perceived as enact-ing a "recovering addict" subjectivity and moving along a recovery trajectory to the extent they are seen as employable. I found that some-times the transition into paid work for benefit recipients seemed quite straightforward, with participants transitioning from the addictions or PREP caseload to another concerned with employment. Caseworker Merren explained: "I was talking to one of my guys yesterday because I said, 'This is a good thing, you've graduated from me, you're doing really well'.… [He went] to the employment caseload." Tamara gave another example of someone who easily transitioned off her caseload and would soon likely leave OW itself for employment.

I just had another young lady, she got a job in communications through a taxi company. So that's full time, so she'll be working there. So, likely she won't be on assistance very much longer because in her discharge I will make sure she stays connected to addiction supports, in case she gets stressed out at work or whatever may happen, so she can maintain her job.

Considering the benefit recipients I interviewed and even includ-ing those working on recovery, none were in a position where they no longer had an addictions or PREP caseworker. Many participants working on recovery nonetheless planned or hoped for an eventual transition onto the employment caseload and into paid work. Season, for example, had dreams about her future employment but carefully tempered these given her criminal record and low income.

> I would love to own my own business. Nails, makeup. Something like that. Or outreach work. I think I'd be amazing at it because it's not theory, I have stories to tell myself.... That's the only thing we [women with criminal records] could do is open our own business because then we don't have a criminal check, need a background check. But who has funds to do that?

Dante was less committed to working on recovery but was already thinking about how he should no longer view construction as his primary option for paid work. As he said: "Fucking getting old, man. And doing all this heavy labour? For much longer? And I was thinking, maybe, um, doing addiction, um counselling classes. Slowly ... I was hoping for next September, but I don't know man." By contrast, a handful of other benefit recipients seemed to be nearer to a transition to the employment caseload. These were people who defined as being in recovery and seemed "closer" to the labour market (as per the "distance from the labour market discourse") – and so were being funnelled into welfare-to-work oriented programs. Cody's experience in employment programming, reviewed earlier, was a good example of this.

Some other benefit recipients anticipated a different transition than from an addictions caseload to the employment caseload. They implied that they thought their addiction to substances made them less able to work and therefore eligible to receive benefits from the Ontario Disability and Supports Program (ODSP). Among all benefit recipients I interviewed, two were awaiting a review of their application (e.g., Jesse, Theresa), and three were considering the submission of an application (e.g., Franco, Shawn, Charise). It is likely the case that some participants' efforts to transfer income support programs would be in vain since addiction is not recognized as a disability (see Section 5(2) of the *Ontario Disability Support Program Act*; D. Sokolovski, personal communication). Caseworker Tamara provided an account of these unlikely transitions.

> [T]his particular gentleman that I'm watching, he's disclosed to me that he's schizophrenic ... but he doesn't want to follow through with anything. So, he would be pending ODSP. But he's also dealing with addiction

issues. So, because of where he's at, I would not transfer him to the pending ODSP [file].… I will hang on to that file with discussion with them [ODSP] so that they know I'm still working with him because he's not ready yet to just go off and get lost. So, some of them are adamant they want to apply [to ODSP]. It's their right to do that … what will happen is if they're found not disabled, they come right back to me. So, then we work through another plan.

Only two of the people I interviewed, Clive and Pat, had been deemed eligible for ODSP. I interviewed them when they were still on OW and as they awaited the transition of their files. Interestingly, Pat made clear that she would rather have been working for pay instead of anticipating a shift from OW to ODSP for reasons of her chronic pain.

Beyond these individual barriers, other structural barriers impended the efforts of benefit recipients who saw themselves as in recovery from participating in employment, these created by the culture and organization of the Canadian labour market. Most workplaces assume an able-bodied and non–substance using worker that will perform specific tasks within a set number of hours. While flexible hours may be negotiated and work even performed at home, there are often specific outcomes to be achieved by routinized deadlines. Even people who seek to limit the harm of their alcohol or drug use cannot necessarily conform to this structural organization of paid work. Trevor said it was simply impossible for a substance user to meet their need to consume substances, "feel normal," and hold down a job.

> Because it's, it gets to a point that the person you are on drugs is you. The person you are sober isn't you anymore. So, in order to be you, you need the thing. Because it's to feel normal. Otherwise you just feel like a bag of crap. And like the body aches are ridiculous, you know. So, like trying to keep a job without having like stable drugs is like impossible. You can't get a big load of work if you don't, like, have something to take like right then.

Caseworker Gale further illustrated the disconnection between any use of substances and the organization of paid work from the perspective of a program offering employment training: "[M]any of the programs we offer have a work placement component. So, of course, those agencies don't want to send someone out with any kind of addiction because of the insurance liabilities of all of that. It makes perfect sense, and of course the employer also doesn't want to take on that liability. I understand that."

I also heard stories from benefit recipients who indicated their desire to participate in employment training to their caseworker, only to then learn that even programs designed to support people living with addiction can determine eligibility based on participants being in recovery – with recovery meaning abstinence. For example, Jules's relapse when attending a program resulted in her being told she was no longer eligible to participate.

> I didn't complete the program.... How am I supposed to gain employment in the field that I was going to school for when I wasn't able to complete the program? And I wasn't able to complete the program because they told me to leave. They should have let me come back and finish that.

That the design and organization of the program had zero accommodations for Jules further illustrates how moving forward in recovery can be inhibited by structural barriers.

Shawn also alluded to how few employers would accommodate someone on methadone and who perhaps needed to adjust their paid work performance (e.g., including hours of work) according to their management of their dose. Caseworker Gale shared Shawn's view and explained how there can even be harmful implications of employment programs that exclude OW clients on methadone. For example, methadone "use" can exclude benefit recipients from participating in programming even if they see themselves as working on recovery and have a goal of transitioning into employment.

> The XXX program, which is for youth to get into construction. So, I had a girl, a client, right age frame.... She was housed, she was on methadone. But I couldn't send her to the program because what they said was, "We will not take anybody who is on methadone or suboxone at all. They have to be totally clean. And if we [urine] test them ... and come back dirty, they will never be allowed to take it [the program] again." I couldn't set her up for the failure ... you have to say to this client who is working extremely hard, that I can't refer her to the program. So now she's sad because she can't go, so where we've now devolved to is she's now homeless, she's still doing her methadone, though, but she's all over the place.

Clive had found his experience in a job search program a poor one. Because there was a lack of fit between his needs and what the program provided, he quit the program and the result was "[N]ow she [caseworker] doesn't want to give me my cheque." When he next met his caseworker, he said he resorted to performing the role of a "broken man": "[C]rying: 'Do you really think I would be here doing this if I had any other choice?'" The caseworker, in turn, "Shoved me [sic] off to someone else instantly." This transfer of Clive to another caseworker also supports Adrienne's argument that people living with addiction need caseworkers that understand their lived realities.

People living with addiction have needs and wants related to employment that stem from their own agency; benefit recipients shared about their choices, these sometimes different from those outlined in case management as per dominant policy discourses. There are, however, not just individual, but structural barriers that impede their achievement of employment and eventual exit from the OW caseload. These structural barriers include eligibility requirements (as well as caseworkers who may not understand these) within the programs themselves. They also include the macro-level barriers within the culture and organization of paid work in Canadian society. While the latter is considerably difficult to change – though I have ideas for how to begin this cultural change that I will discuss in the last chapter of this book – some of the former barriers could be changed more quickly in the short term. Specifically, there is a need for structural change in the provision of employment activity programs. People living with addiction need employment activity programs that fit with their unique situations, including, for example, being in methadone treatment.

Resolved and Hopeful amid Systemic Poverties – and Barriers

In moving forward, in beginning something different than old patterns of substance use in some way, in doing the work of recovery – whether through abstinence or harm reduction – some people I met living with addiction were hopeful – and resolute. They had goals they believed they could achieve. Of course, other benefit recipients were not practising recovery, but even they shared stories of how they were aware of the necessity of their being unwavering, purposeful, and determined should they desire to change their substance use patterns. I conclude this chapter by considering this hope and resolve in view of the poverties benefit recipients contend with in their daily lives.

I have made clear through benefit recipients' stories that poverty is not just the experience of low income. It also includes the lack of something or more than one thing, material or intangible, that can facilitate the meeting of individual needs. The very system of OW re-produces these poverties in this sense, but in concert with systemic poverties re-produced elsewhere. Consider social services in a community at a system level: the not-for-profit services for those living with addiction, including provisions of employment programming, are lacking. The systemic poverties (re-)produced and perpetuated by OW and other related systems (e.g., addictions and mental health, the criminal justice system, and the child welfare system) then create and entrench systemic barriers. That is, where systems themselves lack, barriers are then (re-)produced within them too.

We need not accept these system-wide poverties and barriers as societally normal. Hope and resoluteness in moving forward, in living without or differently with substance use, does not lie with the individual alone. It is my contention that we can be hopeful and resolute in supporting persons living with addiction collectively too. As I will argue in the next and final chapter, we can overturn the stigmatization of addiction at a discursive, societal level, simultaneous with making change in how we offer programming and support for people living with addiction at the practical level of OW policy and administration, through a collective praxis of hope.

PART THREE

De-stigmatization, Hope, and
Potential for Change

9 Supporting Substance Users on Welfare: Of Hope among Us

Right now, I have hope and belief. But I had hope before I had belief. Franco

Franco's words represent the promise of how things may be different for persons working through substance use challenges: through hope and the potential it brings. In this final chapter, I substantiate my overall argument of this book. Specifically, I argue for the de-stigmatization of addiction by dwelling on hope. I extrapolate hope as a point of transition, a feeling and practice to pursue, from the main findings of my study. I unearth the sociology of hope and then explore what hope can be and do when we are all part of hope for people living with addiction. I revisit policy implications of my findings and conclude with attention to near "tipping points" that suggest that this is the time for a collective praxis of hope.

Lives Lived, De-stigmatized

Throughout this book, I have been telling a big story about the experiences of low-income people living with addiction, engaging in recovery, or still using drugs or alcohol, and accessing Ontario Works (OW). I set out to tell this story through qualitative research, and specifically the application of discourse and narrative theory, methods, and analytical strategies. I contextualized my study in the wider literature that I saw to link to what we know and do not know about the relationships among poverty, substance use, and income support. I also situated this study in broad theorizing on social change as productive of both greater individual choice and social inequality. I observed the processes of individualization as linking to and shaping the contemporary Canadian welfare state too, with the state itself further transformed through the parallel ideology and discourse of neoliberalism and its affinity with responsibilization and the curtailment of social rights of citizenship.

I presented a big story of living with addiction and accessing OW as a narrative arc: of becoming, being, and beginning anew. I began with sharing benefit recipients' stories of how their becoming a substance user was somehow connected to the meanings they gave and the experiences they had of their social environments (e.g., their households, their peer group; of violence) and relationships with those within them (e.g., family members, friends). I discussed women's and men's agentic decisions and corresponding actions and behaviours amid moments of their life course, and the relationships they had with institutions. In essence, I showed that the use of substances became part of individuals' personal biographies (or "reflexive project of the self") fully intentionally, or not. The becoming of a substance user was shaped by processes of socialization, self-development, survival, and aging over the life course. Some of the same actions, interactions, and processes that benefit recipients saw as somehow connected to their substance use contributed to their accessing OW even if at times the connections were more ethereal than causal.

Once on OW, I found benefit recipients' lives were shaped by interlocking and shifting discourses underscored by neoliberalism, such that being on OW was not as simple as receiving a benefit cheque each month. There was an implicit subject and certain normative ways of being assumed when accessing OW, these constituted by policy discourse and caseworker practice. Benefit recipients were to meet some expectations regarding their substance use, most often demonstrating their choice of treatment and/or recovery. Their adoption of the discursively constituted subject position of "the recovering addict" conditioned their receipt of income support. Caseworkers could rigidly conform to the standardized rules of their work *or* show small acts of kindness towards benefit recipients in exercising their discretion. Benefit recipients themselves could perceive this regulation of their benefit receipt and potential limiting of their lives but were clearly still agentic in many aspects of their daily lives.

Other facets of benefit recipients' daily lives continued parallel to and overlapping with their experience of policy constructions and regulation. Each day of living with addiction while on OW was filled with variable, limitless, and often simultaneous experiences: trying to fill the time in a long day when sober and with little to no money for leisure, getting the next fix of one's substance of choice, going to a day treatment program, working on recovery, providing self-care and care to others, and navigating health care systems to pursue relief from mental or physical pain. For mothers or fathers in particular, a typical day could include caring for children directly, such as making sure children arrived at school on time, or indirectly through relationships with children's guardians. These were but a few everyday experiences and though not all were shared by all participants, any of these experiences were universally situated in the normative frames of family and gender relations (including paid and unpaid work), the wider neoliberal social policy context, and shaped by poverties: the poverty that is the reality of receiving OW and the poverty associated with lack of specific resources and social supports that would make a difference in efforts to manage addiction or overcome it.

Some people I interviewed were hopeful and resolute in their efforts to live a life not dependent on substances and amid these poverties. They worked on themselves and often with others to imagine different ways of living or new beginnings, in ways that resisted the "recovering addict" subjectivity constituted by OW policy and discourse. They moved forward through introspection and subsequent determination because they were tired of living the life they did while using, and/or because of life-changing events. Men and women who worked on recovery seemed to see this work as possible through a re-conceptualization of their self – their "project" and therefore biography and life course trajectory began to transform, but also largely through their social support relationships with others such as counsellors, caseworkers, family members, and friends. Once committed to recovery, their emotional, mental, and physical work was constant and sometimes had to be pursued in the face of other challenges. These challenges could be deeply personal and psychological and yet often also included the lack of structural support of their recovery efforts. An example of a structural barrier included the labour market assuming able-bodied, sober, and reliable employees versus employees engaged in methadone treatment that limits the time of day in which they are physically able to work. Again, I note that the work of recovery for the relevant participants I interviewed included abstinence *or* harm reduction. It bears repeating this because as an outsider looking in, it seemed to me that the definition of the self in recovery – however defined by each unique individual – was the key to living differently.

As I have said at the outset of this book, I am keenly aware of how dependence on or addiction to alcohol or drugs has and continues to be pathologized, and in scholarly literature too. Individuals' substance use that seems uncontrollable may still be perceived as "deviant," a marker of something morally wrong or abnormal with the individual user and resounding in the harms experienced by the user and those with whom they are close or with whom they interact. Again, I do not deny the individual and social harms associated with participants' use of alcohol or drugs, these ranging from individual mental and physical discomfort, family and intimate relations unravelling in tandem with a user's behaviour, to organized crime around drug trafficking within neighbourhoods. And neither would the women and men I met. Each person I met, even if they were still using substances and even if ambivalent about their use, was transparent in sharing how they hurt themselves or others, mentally, emotionally, and perhaps even physically. A few participants told stories of how they felt self-revulsion for some of their behaviour while using, or the awfulness of their social conditions while impoverished. They could well understand why others would feel repulsed too. Their courage in sharing these stories with me was incredibly powerful in their impact. I will never forget a story Franco told me to try to get me to understand why stability of social environment, particularly safer and more affordable housing, is crucial to his work of recovery.

> I've been living in bed bug–infested places for ten years. I've woken up with a rat on my belly, pooping on me.... It was a mouse, not a rat. But when a mouse is pooping on you, or when they're leaning up against you for warmth.... When a mouse isn't afraid of you, you're at a low.

In knowing the individual and societal harms of substance use, I am nonetheless convinced that there is a need to move away from the limits on social inclusion that I see created for people who use drugs and alcohol when addiction is stigmatized. Through stories I heard firsthand: people are not their addiction. The people I interviewed were family members, sometimes mothers or fathers themselves, and friends to others in their communities. They were students, musicians, caregivers, computer nerds, crocheters, bakers, craftspeople, and labourers. They were contributing members of their communities, whether in paid work, through participation in their children's schools, or sources of support in a group treatment program. The women and men I interviewed could not be reduced to only the identity of "addict" or "recovering addict." They were people with multifaceted selves made up of many identities – who happened to also experience suffering associated with their use of alcohol or drugs, perhaps characterized by lack of control and impeded social functioning. Of course, herein lies the rub I laboured to reveal much earlier in this book: participants' relationships with OW policy and even caseworkers were such that the subject position constituted was that of "the recovering addict" in order that they continue to receive income support. OW receipt may have been just one part of their lives too. And it certainly staved off their absolute poverty. But OW receipt also involved elements of social control and regulation. While this could be tempered through novel and empathetic decisions by some caseworkers, benefit recipients shared how they worked to surpass "addict" as their only identity and to present to caseworkers and others, or even re-claim, other facets of their self, for example, as mothers, as students. They had to be hopeful, agentic, and resolute to change or subvert the meaning of "recovering addict" in their relationships with themselves, but especially with OW caseworkers and policy discourse.

In total, people's lives as lived inspired me to reach a specific place of argumentation: if addiction is but one part of a complex life lived through social relations, it is therefore incomprehensible to stigmatize – to label/stereotype/separate/degrade/discriminate in the words of Link and Phelan (2001) – those working through a substance use challenge. Indeed, Goffman (1963) saw stigma as an attribute in a person that defines them as tainted and to be discounted. When addiction is instead understood as but part of an everyday life for *any one* person, not their defining attribute or "master status" (Hughes, 1949), we disturb this one-to-one association.

Returning to a point I made earlier in this book, I want to make clear once again that I am not arguing for the normalization of substance use because I think to do so would be to obscure the individual and societal harms associated with substance use dependency. I am seeking a middle ground. I contend that addiction should not be seen as "normal" (Fraser et al., 2017); but, nor should it be seen as "other" and a means by which to socially exclude. I am desiring that living with addiction be seen as *what may be* as part of any individual's life course *writ large*, and from the perspective of a shared, collective consciousness. If addiction to alcohol or drugs is not a part of our own individual, everyday lives now, this does not mean that we ourselves may not one day experience an addiction at some time. Moving beyond ourselves, substance use dependency may already be something persons dear to each of us and who make up our circles of intimate and extended family relations and friends are working through. I therefore take my argument one step further. If addiction is a part of our communities and society itself – *which it is* – then stigmatization of addiction does little but hinder the potential of us all as people sharing in the experience of humanity.

I conclude this section with a caveat. I admit that to argue for "the destigmatization of *addiction*" might seem incongruous. That is, I still am using the morally charged language of addiction itself. This is a point I have wrestled with several times in this book and know it is an ongoing debate echoed in scholarly literature and in media of the broader lay public. However, after completing this study and reaching these points of extrapolation in this book, I remain certain that I am not yet keen on abandoning addiction entirely. I have noted that there exists perhaps lesser stigmatizing concepts available, such as that of "substance use dependency" or referring to "people who use drugs," and I have used some of these throughout this book. In my view, however, it is imperative to retain the language of addiction when it is meaningfully useful. Let me provide just one example. From the stories I heard, some participants' new beginning only emerged out of their deep identification with addiction, associating it with harm to their self and others, and then wrestling with its continued relevance for their lives to imagine a way forward. As well, I do think we can maintain the understanding that a person's substance use is constitutive of harm to themselves and others by the signification that occurs when applying the concept of addiction while simultaneously we can avoid limiting the present and future lives of persons on OW to that of ever and always being an "addict" or "recovering addict." In the remainder of this final chapter, I further argue that we can collectively achieve the de-stigmatization of addiction and the implications this brings through a collective praxis of hope.

On Pursuing Hope – A *Collective Praxis* of Hope

Generally speaking, praxis refers to the translation of an idea into action (Spronk, 2011), or the coupling of theory with practice. In *Critique and Praxis*, Harcourt (2020) reviews the scholarship of critical scholars (e.g., Karl Marx, Max Horkheimer, Judith Butler) and shows how they pursued and then retreated from praxis in answer to the question "What is to be done?" He observes how Michel Foucault, too, made different forays in answering this question. It is Harcourt's contention that there has been a turn away from praxis in philosophy and a shift towards critical interpretation. Having no ambition to delve further into the historical debates he covers so well, I refer to Harcourt's text mainly because I find his central argument inspiring: that we need to reinvigorate critical praxis during these unprecedented critical times in which we live. For Harcourt (2020, p. 17), we no longer ask "What is to be done?" and instead must start asking "What more shall I do, and what work is my praxis doing?"

I am uncomfortable with ending this book in a way that implies or has the potential to be read as another miserabilist interpretation of the lives of people living with addiction. I refuse to end with a *hopeless* tone characterizing my conclusions, something Back (2015) also recognizes as common to sociological research. Thus, in this section I outline a collective praxis of hope in theory, tentative application, and implication. In my use of praxis, I define it further as pushing thought towards human liberation (Harcourt, 2020), a use that echoes the social change assumed and imagined in the critical realist paradigm and pursued through critical discourse studies. I ask that readers read my call for a collective praxis of hope, perhaps rife with contradictions that philosophers can see, as my initial musings on what *could be* an avenue for social change, as a pursuit and way forward. Indeed, how through a different lens we may better conceptualize, respond to, and work with people living with addiction and on social assistance, in policies like OW and even through our shared human experience. I begin to sketch this collective praxis of hope by returning to the promise implied in Franco's words at the onset of this chapter: first hope, then belief. And to this I will add specifically the potential for actionable hope.

Before I get ahead of myself, let me be clear that the collective praxis of hope that I conceptualize assumes a particular way of understanding hope linked to what others have written about. According to Zygmunt Bauman (2004), hope is integral to the human condition. In our very ways of speaking, such as in our use of "no" as refusal and rejection, or even our use of the future tense, Bauman writes:

> [W]e, the humans, can't stop imagining things as different from what they are now. We can't just settle for what "is" because we cannot grasp what "is" without reaching beyond it…. We expect things to change – and we resolve to change them. Small things and big things alike…. As inevitably as the meeting of oxygen and hydrogen results in water, hope is conceived whenever imagination and moral sense meet. (2004, p. 64)

However, while clear that hope is part of our humanity and it is something we do and can do as sociologists too – as he himself did in much of his work (Lyon, 2017) – Bauman is nonetheless evasive on what specifically defines the meaning of hope. Other scholars have taken on this challenge. It seems that, like addiction, it is difficult to reach consensus on the meaning of hope, especially across academic disciplines and differing social-historical contexts (Back, 2015; Folkman, 2010; Petersen & Wilkinson, 2015).

In *The Sociology of Hope*, Desroche (1976) defined hope as analogous to the Fakir's rope that a shaman throws into the air and it holds; the rope continues to hold as humans pull themselves up with it. Back (2015) perceives Desroche to define hope as "constitutive imagination" and having properties of the future, often utopian in design. In Fallding's (1981) review of the text, wherein they underscore the analysis of religion, they further explain Desroche's theorizing of hope: in envisioning an ideal society, one can generate personal motivation. And yet, since this text was published, Petersen and Wilkinson (2015, p. 114) convincingly argue: "one cannot point to a substantial body of literature in the sociology of hope as one can for, say, the sociology of risk or the sociology of the body." For them, hope is a blind spot in sociology.

Meanwhile, Petersen and Wilkinson (2015) observe how health medicine and health care are replete with discourses of hope (p. 113). There has been considerable growth in research on hope in these and other disciplines. For example, one only has to look to psychology to observe the increasing development of standardized constructs and tests of hope (Martin & Stermac, 2009; Petersen & Wilkinson, 2015), such as Pentti et al.'s (2019) twelve-item Adult Trait Hope Scale derived from Snyder's (1989) cognitive model of hope. As I have observed earlier, specific to psychiatric research, recovery itself can be conceptualized to include learning to hope or being "full of hope for the future" (Roberts & Boardman, 2013; Heyes, 2005). On balance, Petersen and Wilkinson (2015) find that across these disciplines hope seems to be: articulated in the context of individual despair, pain, and suffering; an attitude desirable for "good health" that can be instilled in others; an orientation, attribute, or value that provides the basis of resilience and will for healing; and a means to appeal for funding for new drugs and treatments. In their own, earlier meta-analysis of research on hope in nursing, Kylmä and Vehviläinen-Julkunen (1997) found that hope can be described as an emotion, an experience, or a need.

Many interdisciplinary scholars seem to side with Desroche (1976), that hope ultimately encapsulates individuals' future aspirations, such as those I heard articulated by people I interviewed and shared in the preceding chapter. Around the time in which I began thinking more carefully about hope and its meaning for this study, I received an alumni magazine from my alma mater, the University of Alberta. The spring 2020 edition devoted an entire article to hope that reviewed related research of university faculty in education, nursing, and psychology. Education researcher Denise Larsen echoed the linking of hope to the future: "hope is the ability to envision a future in which we want to participate." Larsen's career has involved the development of programs to teach teachers and students how to strive for hope in their lives (Filkow, 2020, p. 30). Larsen viewed hope as motivating. Colleague and nursing researcher Wendy Duggleby oriented to hope in the same way but placed greater emphasis on hope as possibilities for a different future, not just expectations, with this future subject to change. She observed that for someone who is dying, hope can range from being directed at simply breathing better for a few minutes or seeing family members in the next hour. Augustine Parattakudi, a registered psychotherapist who teaches counselling psychotherapy, maintained that hope is something you awaken through relationships with others: "cultivating hope is cultivating human connection" (Filkow, 2020, p. 32).

Sociologist Les Back (2015) theorizes on hope in the present with an emphasis on emotion, feeling, and desire. Back points to how Ernst Bloch wrote *The Principle of Hope* and, in contrasting hope with the rise of fascism in the 1930s, saw it as an emotion that could be learned and one that required work, the result of which would be "people who throw themselves actively in what is *becoming*, to which they themselves belong" (Bloch, 1954, cited in Back, 2015, np, italics mine). Back (2015) also cites Jonathon Lear's *Radical Hope* (2006) and his argument about how Plenty Coups, the last Chief of the Crow Nation, and his people negotiated their experience of impending colonial and cultural devastation of the Crow Nation's way of life through the complex affect of hope (see also Farley, 2009 for a far more nuanced interpretation of this story and Lear's contribution). Thus, for Back (2015), hope can involve attention to the present, and then an expectation that *something* will happen and opportunities will be created.

Hope as possibility, however, has not yet a decided conclusion. Indeed, as Back (2015) sees it, hope is not a destination but more an improvisation with a future not yet realized. This understanding connects with what Kylmä and Vehviläinen-Julkunen (1997, p. 367) call generalized hope. For these researchers, generalized hope is different from particularized hope, the latter when hope can be connected to a specific time or matter or with an identifiable object. Hope creates promise and possibilities, with a far reach beyond what we may think is possible for the context of our lives (Back, 2015; Duggleby as cited in Filkow, 2020).

Mulling over these conceptualizations of hope, I arrive at my own that I entrench in a collective praxis of hope. My sense of hope is that it is emotional and social and, for some, spiritually infused. Hope is an orientation to that which might be in the future. Hope is a feeling of opening, orienting to something different, a perceived space of potential, and created through relations with others. The hope that I invite others to join in, individually, and at the level of our collective social experience and consciousness, is that which I heard implied in benefit participants' stories about new beginnings. In imagining a different way of being and becoming regarding their substance use, participants were hopeful. And, to me, the participants who seemed resolute in their work on recovery were those who had transformed hope into belief, as in Franco's words: what they hoped for could come to fruition. They then acted upon this belief, making hope actionable.

To apply this conceptualization of hope in a way that may transform how we collectively support persons using substances or in recovery, two interrelated changes must take place. We need to: (1) shift the discourse on hope and (2) cultivate and practise individual and collective hope.

Seeking a Collective *Discourse*

Though they focus on health studies, Petersen and Wilkinson (2015) write of discourses of hope and of the power–knowledge relations constitutive of these. It is worth reviewing how they and others see discourses of hope to have shifted with modernization such that I would now argue for a *collective* discourse on hope.

The case can be made that the dominant discourse on hope is that it resides within the scope and agency of the individual. In health studies, for example, individuals are encouraged to manage their own health, including their hope (Petersen & Wilkinson, 2015). Hope is often articulated through narratives of choice, personal control, and empowerment and therefore individualized, a linking on par with O'Malley's (2009) observation of the increasing "individual responsibilization" characteristic of contemporary politics, power, and social policy. Moreover, the processes of individualization, reflexive modernization, and de-traditionalization that are assumed in the theoretical framing of this study have bearing on this moment's discursive construction of hope. Individuals are free to construct their own less scripted and more flexible personal biographies. They are assumed to have relationships with the state, but these contingent on their demonstration of self-sufficiency, risk taking, and responsibility. To be clear, the individual responsibilization of hope does seem to fit lockstep with the idea of the neoliberal subject in late modernity.

Indeed, hope is privatized and commodified. For example, hope is to be created through individual consumption of therapies that promise to alleviate suffering or facilitate new selves (Petersen & Wilkinson, 2015). Any notion of actionable hope seems most about individuals making themselves more resilient or better able to face challenges; collective actions are less obviously part of the discourse of hope today. Bauman (2004) maintains that even the pursuit of happiness is privatized.

People are to succeed or fail in today's economy or in their social existence through their own volition. They are then held responsible and accountable for the results of their efforts, even in view of interactional and structural adversities not of their own making. The neoliberal discourse of welfare dependency can be read as assuming this same view of the individual, with the implication that the happy person is one who is not relying on the state for their economic livelihood.

Individualized hope starkly contrasts with earlier conceptions of hope that were prevalent in the middle of the twentieth century and were more social and emancipatory (Petersen & Wilkinson, 2015). The works on hope by scholars like Bloch and Desroche were written during or after world wars, at a time when the harms of technologies of mass destruction were starkly present and inviting of debate about humanity and progress. Scholars observe how utopian alternatives created through collective action and change were therefore part of the public imaginary (Bauman, 2004; Peter & Wilkinson, 2015), though Bauman is careful to also observe the harm of taking too seriously the goal of a perfect society, for example, what he calls the "enlightened" despotism of Adolf Hitler. Since then, there has been a waxing of utopian visions amid sharp criticism of them as misguided. Still the idea of some collective solidarity in the then social climate persisted, as evidenced in the growth of the post-war welfare state premised on public responsibility for survival and welfare (albeit with its histories of exclusions too). It is the idea of collective solidarity and responsibility that has now been reversed, says Bauman (2004), and indeed the post-1980s general trend of neoliberal reform in Canada suggests this.

Bauman (2004) maintains that there is one idea endemic to all utopias worth saving:

> [T]hat everyone's happiness depends on the happiness of all, that anybody's happiness can be secure only in the company of secure people, and that pursuit of happiness worthy of that name needs to be aimed at the ways and means of human togetherness. That, in other words, *pursuit of individual happiness is a collective affair*. (p. 65, italics mine)

For Bauman, we are far too close to forgetting a core idea of the "ancients," that goodness can only be attained in a good *society* (p. 65, italics in original).

What I am seeking is for us to think anew about a collective orientation towards hope that is actionable. Reframing hope and reclaiming it as praxis may make a difference in the lives of citizens, centring the experiences of those living with addiction and on welfare especially.

Just as hope is integral to humans, so too is our performativity of it. We have the capacity in language and symbols of hope to (re-)shape individuals' thinking, actions, entities, and identities (see also Petersen & Wilkinson, 2015).

Actioning Hope, Individually and Collectively

It would be remiss to overlook the sheer work involved by individuals imagining something different when their life as lived may seem characterized by lack of control, chaos, and trauma surrounding substance use, or so narrowly focused on avoiding homelessness and food insecurity that recovery is the least of individuals' worries (see also Bryant & Ellard, 2015; Sælør et al., 2015). Some benefit recipients even shared stories that were suggestive that entertaining a different way of being was not their concern. Thus, it bears repeating that my pursuit of a collective praxis of hope is inspired by participants who were in a place of new beginnings concerning their substance use, often specifically working on recovery. And in their cognitive resoluteness to do and be something different, they suggested their hope. In their actions, their actionable hope.

To *collectively* enact hope for persons living with ongoing use of alcohol or drugs, attempting to reduce harms of their use, or practising abstinence in their recovery, is to do many interrelated things at the individual and collective level:

- to have space, or make room for hope;
- to recognize individuals' own hope and their belief and knowing that their lives could be something different and of their own agentic design; and to recognize that this something different can be brought into being;
- to seek and create hope, and to want and to have hope for others; and
- to support others and ourselves in actionable hope.

Let me begin with the individual because in the enactment of hope through a collective praxis of hope, the individual does not disappear. Hope may be instilled in them by others and learned. Hope can also be a choice. And hope is certainly shaped and realized through social relations. Maholmes's research (2014), for example, shows how hope can make a profound difference in the lives of children who grow up poor, leading them to overcome adversity. Sælør et al. (2015) explored firsthand accounts of hope experienced by persons with co-occurring mental health and substance use problems. For the participants in their study, hope was inextricably tied to hoping for change and having trust as a foundation of hope. They found that when an individual had been marginalized and stigmatized or when recovery seemed difficult to pursue amids the challenge of securing food and shelter, they can face hopelessness. Thus, their participants overwhelmingly demonstrated that they had to have hope in order to have the courage to transform their life (Sælør et al., 2015).

I keep circling back to Franco's words when I think of the enactment of hope because I really do think he was on to something in linking hope with belief. Kylmä and Vehviläinen-Julkunen (1997) observe how some define hope as a belief in one's tomorrow. Groopman (2005), who wrote the book *The Anatomy of Hope: How People Prevail in the Face of Illness*, argued:

> Hope can flourish only when you believe that what you do can make a difference, that your actions can bring a future different from the present. To have hope, then, is to acquire a belief in your ability to have some control over your circumstances. You are no longer entirely at the mercy of forces outside yourself. (p. 26)

To believe in possibilities can also create the ability for people to endure, as in Groopman's analysis, harmful side effects in the pursuit of a cure for an illness.

I further propose that in the collective praxis of hope, hope is that which is giving rise to potentialities. My use of "potential" is deliberate, as it captures the capacity to achieve and become something that is different, and it is awareness of potential or capacity that I think some benefit recipients were speaking about in their conceptualization of new beginnings if not describing their actual actions undertaken per se. I am not alone in my thinking. I am indebted to Bryant and Ellard's (2015) work for how it enabled me to flesh out my initial imagining of potentialities through hope. Bryant and Ellard (2015) observe that hope is not limited to present situations or future aspirations and can include the capacity to take action. In their study of marginalized Australian youth, for example, they found youths' future thinking, and specifically planning and choice-making, was inhibited by the uncertainty of their lives. They saw this as a side effect of individualization: the demand placed upon youth to construct a reflexive project of the self. Despite youths' perception of "minimal opportunity structures," however, they still had agency in their future thinking because they had hope for something better, for example, to live happily (Bryant &

192 Part Three: Potential for Change

Ellard, 2015). And I owe much to Kylmä and Vehviläinen-Julkunen's (1997) argument that there is a functional dimension of hope, the linking of hope with potential and action. They note that hope is a mental, social, physical, and spiritual activity. Citing still other scholars, Kylmä and Vehviläinen-Julkunen observe that hope both requires activity on the part of the individual (Dufault & Martocchio, 1995) and that it is a necessary condition for activity (Farran & Popovich, 1990).

In my thinking, it is the potentialities inherent in hope that may spur on belief as per Franco and Groopman's perspective. I further contend that belief in the potentialities brought about by hope can then translate into actionable hope. If readers are seeking me to name what individual actions may stem from potentialities and what may be achieved, however, they will be disappointed. I digress to note that I struggled with the decision between wanting to think and write about benefit recipients' potentialities through hope, or about their capabilities through hope. As I made clear at the beginning of this book, I find Amartya Sen's capabilities approach illuminating, for example, the experience of poverty as capability deprivation. I remain intrigued by his argument that capabilities, what a person is able to do or be, can be seen broadly as freedoms (Sen, 2005). Stopping myself before I engage in a completely tangential argument, I will instead briefly state that while I am not writing a study of welfare economics, the discipline in which Sen's work has had such impact (Atkinson, 1999), I think hope can cultivate the capabilities of which he writes. Nonetheless, I remain more invested in seeing benefit recipients' new beginnings as hope, of what could be different and so of potentialialities, with the specificity of these being left intentionally limitless. Besides, the cross-sectional study I undertook did not permit me to assess and uncover specific capabilities that may be achieved through hope, as in the vein of Nussbaum's (2003) ten-point list of central human capabilities.

It would be an oversight to write of a collective praxis of hope in only a positive light and to avoid any attention to the dangers hope presents, including the despotic pursuit of utopias of which Bauman (2004) writes. Individuals themselves can be misguided in their hope or have false hope and so achieve undesirable and harmful outcomes of their actions (Groopman, 2004; Petersen & Wilkinson, 2015). As well, there is danger in attempting to outline a collective praxis of hope while neoliberalism still drives social policy reforms in Canada. There is a certain risk that the desiring of hope in how we live collectively with addiction as a part of our everyday lives is too easily subverted by individualism or becomes co-opted and made complicit with the continued governance of the neoliberal subject. I am aware of these dangers but want to reiterate here that my argument for a collective praxis of hope is one grounded in the stories of the people living with addiction that I met. I am indeed assuming that some people who have lived with addiction want to live differently, that they desire sobriety and recovery and to perhaps conform in some way to normative ways of being, including earning an income to support themselves and others – because this is what I heard. The collective praxis of hope I write of here assumes individuals who have used or do use drugs and alcohol but are seeing and believing in their potential for living differently.

I now turn my attention more fully to the "collective" I impose in this praxis of hope, to those notions I sketched out at the start of this section, of wanting and having hope for persons working through substance use challenges. Earlier I indicated that to cultivate hope collectively is to reclaim what has been lost, the notion of social good that has been subject to regulation and privatization alongside the pursuit and achievement of individual security and responsibility amid neoliberalism. The reclaiming or shift towards the collective discourse on hope that I desire is a shift away from the individual alone and inclusive and outward to the collective, while still holding the population of interest in this study as its centre. Assuming a cultural shift in discourse on hope as underscoring praxis links with two key assumptions I have made in the analysis of data I undertook for this book: that discourse can and does shape social experience; that discourse analysis can produce change.

Bryant and Ellard (2015) provide additional fertile ground for how the enactment of hope can be achieved at the level of the collective. They, too, acknowledge existing scholarship on hope as prioritizing the individual and see too little attention given to the social processes that can produce or inhibit hope, or how they might engender the capacity to change a future trajectory (p. 495). Bryant and Ellard (2015, p. 496) wish to overturn this and argue that hope can be (re-)framed as a "cognitive experience or even practice" that is socially produced through normative discourse. They substantiate their argument with a nod to the work of Connell (1987), who wrote about gendered practice as transformative, as changing over time through the influence of normative discourse and individuals' agentic shapings of their lives. For example, in "doing hope" for youth, of *possessing hope* for them, they further argue that others provide youth with the necessary condition to shape their futures and engender their agency (p. 496, italics mine). The primary challenge to be taken on to achieve this doing of hope is the creation of social, structural processes that they specifically call "hope-engendering strategies" (Bryant & Ellard, 2015).

In *Ontario Works*. A collective praxis of hope that embeds this notion of Bryant and Ellard's (2015) "hope-engendering strategies" can be brought to bear on re-thinking OW policy. Of course, I am assuming this exercise at a theoretical level and on par with substantiating policy implications of my findings I have already discussed. My comfort with this exercise is strengthened by a comment Atkinson (1999) made in response to a scholar questioning the ability to actually implement (and evaluate) Sen's capability approach. To paraphrase loosely, Atkinson (1999) responded to this critique by maintaining that an idea can be operationally effective and powerful in theoretical terms even just through its effectiveness at causing people to think a different way.

On one level, a collective praxis of hope can mean a re-thinking of the OW client–caseworker relationship. This re-thinking is not to discount the supportive relationships that caseworkers have with their clients, an important finding of this study. More generally, I argue for hope to become part of the default caseworker relationship, grounding caseworkers' response to any benefit recipient who demonstrates a change in their thinking about their use patterns, shares their tiredness in using, indicates their want for relationships with others, including their children, or may even be ambivalent in how they see their substance use. Hope as a default response, however, requires time and energy on the part of caseworkers. Thus, a rather straightforward hope-engendering strategy within OW design and administration would simply be the introduction of addictions or PREP caseloads that are manageable in size so that people who desire to do so can meet more often with caseworkers. The anonymizing potential of the caseworker–client relationships and its implications for substance use may then be reduced.

Sweeping changes cannot happen immediately. The "distance from the labour market" discourse still shapes OW caseworkers' practice in Toronto and is even not without merit. And yet, I contend that the management of the benefit recipient according to this discourse and the subjectivity constituted within it may indeed change. For example, the question that the caseworker may ask is no longer what does this "recovering addict" need to become closer to the labour market, but *what does this unique human living a life mediated by complex poverties and social relations need?* Such a simple shift has the power to make room for perceiving benefit recipients' multiple identities, overturn the "one size fits all" orientation that still infiltrates current OW policy (noticed most with regard to its employability imperative), and, ultimately, contribute to the de-stigmatization of addiction.

To actionize hope as a caseworker could also mean making people's benefit receipt less conditional upon their participation in some form of recognized treatment but in seeing treatment as but one potential action, with still others possible through hope. I am not advocating for a turn away from treatment and will not propose a list of universal recommendations for how to enact hope in treatment. However, I remain optimistic about how a collective praxis of hope can create space for treatment to occur differently too. I see considerable promise in the work of psychologist Paul Wong. Wong (2013) worried that overcoming addiction may be circumvented by individuals' false hope. Based on his analysis of the existence and response to patterns of addiction in the downtown east end of Vancouver, he advocates for a meaning-centred approach (MCA) to treatment. This approach provides a sense of optimism based on faith and meaning and is an alternative to mainstream approaches to addiction (e.g., the disease model). MCA assumes the benefits of a healing community, which translates into addressing people's needs for psychosocial integration and continued social support. The approach treats people holistically, and while recognizing that an individual's reality may seem bleak, pushes an orientation that there is hope for every person who identifies with living with addiction. Treatment must instill hope and provide hope in recovery (Wong, 2013).

Time spent in the beginnings of recovery, time that some participants defined as limitless or characterized by nothing to do, may be transformed through a collective praxis of hope. To have space for hope can be as simple as having something to do during the day that is fulfilling of the spirit. This is not to discount existing programming in this vein, such as programs offered through Toronto Employment and Social Services (TESS) that are about building life skills to support individuals' journeys towards paid work, or the offerings of art-based therapy programs through organizations like the Centre for Addiction and Mental Health (CAMH). The programming I am imagining, though, is simply about creating space with the smaller purpose of learning about or doing an activity, and perhaps a larger result of social inclusion and facilitation of hope. This activity program would create opportunity for (peer) support but would not be centered around recovery, life skills, or employment activities. My thoughts are inspired by Jesse, who had the insightful idea that learning something new can make a difference to people overwhelmed by the work of recovery. He believed in the importance of "getting people knowing how to cook, or something like that" when I asked him what recommendations he would make to change programming for persons living with addiction. Jesse also believed in the importance of education: "No matter how old you are you can still learn." When I think of Jesse's suggestions and then remember how crotcheting became such a passion for Bianca, I think there is room for "pre-employment" programming that differently "fills the day."

On yet another level, hope-engendering strategies are those that involve changes in other structural conditions that interact with OW policy. A collective praxis of hope invites public spending and growth in available and accessible treatment, better mental and physical health care, improved benefit incomes, and accessible and affordable housing. It forces discussion about improving the employment activity programming contracted by the City of Toronto to provide benefit recipients with paid work skills and experience. That is, hope-engendering strategies would include the invitation of service providers to create programs to work with persons who want to engage in paid work but are in methadone treatment. As well, hope-engendering strategies would include more plentiful spaces for detoxing when wanted, resources and programs that are consistently offered even when relapse occurs, and improved harm-reduction initiatives. Indeed, more accessible, safe injection sites that save lives are needed *right now* in the province of Ontario, instead of even their potential introduction becoming mired in political and moral judgments about what life is worth saving. Ontario still does not have a stand-alone harm-reduction policy and in 2017, the end point of this study, was observed to be woefully behind other provinces in Hyshka et al.'s (2017) analysis. There is boundless potential for individuals' greater self-esteem, self-worth, and self-actualization and long-lived lives through structural conditions that engender hope.

If we see people working through substance use challenges as not limited to the identity of "addict" or "recovering addict," we create space for human potential. And if we join in hope for people working through recovery or managing substance use to see this potential themselves, we do not ignore addiction but remove it as reason to stigmatize and socially exclude. To have hope for others living with addiction can change social relations of which they and we are part and creates opportunities for their belief, for their actionable hope. As revealed in especially this book, sometimes the experience of addiction for individuals is that of loss of connectivity, isolation from others, and overwhelmingly social exclusion. Should we not stigmatize addiction and instead collectively cultivate and support hope for those who experience it, this no longer need be the case.

Near Tipping Points

Back (2015) argues that a sociology of hope requires attention to the social conditions that make it possible. Throughout this book, I have endeavoured to reveal the everyday life conditions or social relations encompassing the being of a person who uses substances or is managing recovery from them, while also experiencing low income and conforming to the rules and regulations of OW. The findings I present lead me to argue that the de-stigmatization of addiction can be possible through hope and make hope possible. There are potentialities offered through hope, and actionable hope is viable for individuals and society. I see my study findings to specifically invite a collective praxis of hope in how we engage and interact with each other now and in the future, and over how we experience problems in our own or others' substance use, or in support of others who work to set aside patterns of use for something different.

As I sit and write this call for a collective praxis of hope, it is November 2020. Canadians are experiencing the eighth month of the SARS-CoV2, or COVID-19, pandemic declared to be of global proportions by the World Health Organization in March 2020. No longer in the exact same "lockdown" practices, practices of living and being have nonetheless dramatically changed, with mask wearing enforced indoors in some places, changing restrictions placed on social gatherings in many provinces, and social distancing universally mandated. Running parallel with this pandemic, social movements around anti-Black racism and anti-Indigenous racism in North America, never not present, crystallized more visually in public demonstrations in the wake of the police killings of Breonna Taylor in Louisville, Kentucky (March 2020); of George Floyd in Minneapolis, Minnesota (May 2020); and the video-recorded racist treatment of Indigenous woman Joyce Echaquan by Quebec hospital staff as she was dying (September 2020). I write while I, too, await the results of the 2020 American election, the lead-up to which has been characterized by unprecedented behaviour of an American president and politicians. And I write as one of the headlines in CBC News is "Canada's opioid crisis kills 13 people a day in 2018, prevention report shows" (Zafar, 2020).

In straying somewhat off topic in the preceding paragraph and only scratching the surface in so many ways, my intent was as a reminder of the broader and challenging social conditions and relations in which living with addiction occurs. We are, as Harcourt (2020, p. 10) made so powerfully clear, living at a critical moment:

> the looming cataclysm of global climate change, the hegemonic rise of neoliberalism and growing inequalities within nations, the surge of a

fascist New Right at the international dimension, the emerging threat of pandemics, nuclear proliferation, and conflict between rogue nations. We are living through one of the most critical periods, if not the most critical, in human history – with critical taken in its most formative etymological sense. Our politics, our world, our very Earth are in critical condition and are situated at turning points from which we may never recover.

To be clear, Harcourt's (2020) entire text is devoted to outlining critical praxis as a response to these social conditions and relations. Drawing from Harcourt, it is my contention that there are other near "tipping points" pushing the arguments I make in this final chapter. I do not employ this concept as per Grodzins (1957) and prefer instead Gladwell's (2002) usage, to refer to when social behaviour crosses a threshold, its effect unstoppable. In what follows, I outline near tipping points that deserve further mention and are suggestive of the need for broad changes in how we co-exist as it pertains to human suffering associated with substance use. This necessitates a confrontation with human mortality and a still deeper introspection about the broader policy implications of this study. It requires the slightly awkward strategy of discussing "before" COVID-19, when this study was undertaken, and "during" COVID-19; indeed, with the goal to further extrapolate the significance of this study to this moment and beyond.

Canada has been facing an opioid crisis since at least 2016. In this year, the rate of opioid-related deaths was 7.9 per 100,000 people, with British Columbia (BC) and Alberta the provinces with the highest rate of deaths (20.7 per 100,000 versus 14.4, respectively). Men and people aged 30–9 were dying most. Indigenous populations on reserve unfairly devastated by these deaths and nations put out calls for recognition of a crisis emerging in southern Alberta as early as 2014. Deaths were attributed to increasing use of prescription opioids and the toxicity of drugs sold illegally (e.g., laced with fentanyl) (Belzak & Halverson, 2018). In 2018, about thirteen people died opioid-related deaths each day (Zafar, 2020). Nearly half of these deaths were among those aged 30–49 and still primarily among men. Now, during the COVID-19 pandemic, the numbers climb. CBC News reported that between April and September 2020, over one hundred Torontonians died opioid-related deaths; this was double the number in the same period in 2018 and 2019. Thus, the opioid crisis persists and is changing given the constraints on behaviour and interaction in view of the pandemic. In general, drug users faced the closure of safe injection sites across Canada early on and now in 2020 grapple with concerns over their deepening social isolation and how to access safe drugs during mandated social distancing practices, as well as reduced access to treatment and harm-reduction services (Canadian Centre on Substance Use and Addiction, 2020).

The state of formal supports for persons living with addiction during the pandemic are made to seem direr still by recalling much earlier struggles to achieve social inclusion voiced by participants in this study. I remember listening to "The Current" on CBC News Toronto in April 2017 during my data collection. Anna Maria Tremonte was interviewing long-time activist Donald MacPherson. MacPherson (2001) wrote the "four pillars approach" (treatment, prevention, policing, and harm reduction) in response to drug-related problems he witnessed in Vancouver just under two decades ago. Reflecting on his years of work, he said: "And unfortunately, my experience is that many people have to die before something comes along," in this case, safe injection sites. Listening to this interview and then researching his work after, I was struck by his simple argument: if not for the ability to reduce harm, folks using drugs risk death. During the remainder of the interview with Tremonte, MacPherson argued not for de-criminalization of drugs or legalization but controlling and regulating drug use for persons through a public health perspective. Adopting such a perspective would mean users no longer needlessly suffer non-fatal overdoses, supporting their stability informs their mental health and well-being, and they can maintain their housing, etc. This approach, however, is not in favour even today. Instead the legal and criminal war on drugs, or criminalization of drug use, persists. And, so, people continue to die. For MacPherson, this is "One of the unspoken about and largest social injustices of our time" (CBC Radio, 2017). While the conclusion of this book is not an argument for or against decriminalization or legalization, MacPherson's thoughts still resonate with me and prompt me to imagine how broader and sweeping legal and policy change could very well be part of a collective praxis of hope concerning individuals' experiences of addiction and low income.

Before COVID-19, there were still other tipping points suggestive of this being the time to pursue a collective praxis of hope. They were told in the stories of caseworkers and benefit recipients alike. Too often people felt restricted to the identity of "recovering addict" in their relationships with OW caseworkers. Of course, as I have shown, some participations were working on recovery to surpass this identity and begin anew. But they, too, felt the weight of being perceived as only ever an "addict." If this constitution of the subject in discourse and practice within casework persists, there does seem to be little choice but to continue to think of persons living with addiction as "other" and "different than." Related problems include exclusionary employment programs and workplaces at the very time a person perceives they are ready for something different. Another near tipping point includes custody disputes over children, such as when mothers' desires to parent children while working on their recovery are not or cannot be supported by others. Current structural conditions, whether OW policy, the labour market, or child welfare policy, seem to only work best for the sober, neoliberal subject. These near tipping points are exacerbated and transformed during the COVID-19 pandemic. Indeed, anti-poverty advocates remain concerned about how receipt of OW benefits is contingent on the report of employability efforts when, meanwhile, some benefit recipients have health problems that make them immune-compromised and/or are unable to report because they cannot access computers given public library closures (Durrani, 2020). OW caseworkers as one source of intimate face-to-face support for benefit recipients living with addiction is no longer possible, with several offices now closed in Toronto and casework performed by phone.

I argue that a collective praxis of hope is the now thinkable shift in view of these near tipping points. Something has to give. To be sure, the people I met were living with addiction in 2016 and 2017. But before and since then, too many people have lost loved ones to drug or alcohol addiction, whether because of splintered relationships or death by overdose. Risk of death should not be the final tipping point for a collective praxis of hope for persons working through substance use challenges. But just possibly, awareness of the risk *now* may spur on a change in our individual and societal, collective conscience. A collective praxis of hope means hope *for life*. We need to think differently and, for example, no longer continue to focus only on how to heal "the addict" so that they are ready to engage in paid work. Collective hope means we can think about fixing paid work opportunities too, so that persons in recovery, and even if they are in methadone treatment, can thrive. For parents, the identity of addict will no longer replace the identity of mother or father. The former may have to be reconciled to pursue new beginnings, and it seems nigh impossible to remove the necessary oversight of child welfare professionals if children are deemed at risk. But the latter identity will never be lost in a collective praxis of hope. A collective praxis of hope is receptive to, and inclusive of, potentialities alongside challenges, in many ways receptive to the contradictions that seem characteristic of the process of individualization in late modernity.

Perhaps there is movement along these lines already in Ontario. For example, at the same time sweeping changes and challenges were brought to Canadian culture by COVID-19, in March 2020 the Ontario government released the *Roadmap to Wellness: A Plan to Build Ontario's Mental Health and Addictions System*. Over $3 million is be invested into creating a "comprehensive" and "connected" mental health and addictions system based on four pillars: improving quality, expanding existing services, implementing innovative solutions, and improving access. In its infancy, this plan nonetheless may even already be one step towards a collective praxis of hope.

Moreover, there is considerable room for still other steps forward in a collective praxis of hope, these steps taking the form of future research. Assuming the limitations of this study, these discussed at length in Appendix C (e.g., including the non-generalizability of my findings), I suggest only a few directions for future research here. First, opportunity exists to move beyond Ontario and engage in comparative research of social assistance programs across Canada and the experiences of people living with addiction with the intention of mobilizing a collective praxis of hope – from a place of collective cross-Canada knowledge. Second, taking this study as inspiration to begin from a different starting place, shedding the language of addiction entirely and centring the subjectivity of people who use drugs while accessing welfare, would certainly yield, I think, greater experientially based argumentation for involving all of us in hope-engendering strategies. Finally, future research on people experiencing substance use challenges while accessing welfare could better integrate health-related research. This research could bridge the intersections between sociology and health studies by understanding and working against the dovetailing processes of, say, criminalization and medicalization, in overturning stigma and the pursuit of hope.

Conclusion

"We are in the realm of hope – and not mere wishing – when we make meaning in relation to a world without the illusions we use to protect ourselves from what is difficult" (Farley, 2009, p. 547). I heed Farley's caution. We cannot only romanticize and must see risk in what I have outlined as a collective praxis of hope. And yet I contend that, collectively, we face an opportunity as humans to change our attitudes, behaviours, practices, norms, and values about living with an addiction to drugs or alcohol and on low income. We can de-stigmatize and see the person and a life lived richly, not *just* the addiction. We can experience the emotion of hope for others. We can practise hope through social relations with others, in our discourses and actions, in our creation of opportunities for actionable hope, and in our adoption of hope-engendering strategies structurally and institutionally. To me, there is a simple way we can all begin anew: when people living with addiction seek something different in their relationship with a substance than what was, we need to *all* be ready – without stigma, with hope.

Appendix A: Public Use Policy Documents

City of Toronto. (2012). *Working as one: A workforce development strategy for Toronto.*

City of Toronto. (2015). *Operating budget overview.* Toronto Employment and Social Services.City of Toronto. (2016a). *Toronto poverty reduction strategy: Year 1 report to community.* City of Toronto.

City of Toronto. (2016b). *Workforce development annual report.* Toronto Employment and Social Services.

City of Toronto. (2017). *Meeting many needs: Advancing Toronto's workforce development and poverty reduction strategies annual report.* Toronto Employment and Social Services.

City of Toronto. (2018). *Making a difference by making connections annual report.* Toronto Employment and Social Services.

Government of Ontario. (2014). *Ontario's poverty reduction strategy annual report. Archived.*

Lankin, F., & Sheikh, M. A. (2012). *Brighter prospects: Transforming social assistance in Ontario.* A Report to the Minister of Community and Social Services. Commission for the Review of Social Assistance in Ontario.

Legislative Assembly of Ontario. (2009). *Bill 152 (Chapter10, Statutes of Ontario, 2009): An act respecting a long-term strategy to reduce poverty in Ontario.*

Legislative Assembly of Ontario. (7 May 2012). *40th parliament, official report of debates (Hansard).* Standing Committee on the Legislative Assembly.

Ministry of Children, Community and Social Services. (2016b). *6.10: Persons in residential programs for the treatment of substance abuse.* Ontario Works Policy Directives.

Ministry of Children, Community and Social Services. (2018). *6.10: Persons in residential programs for the treatment of substance abuse.* Ontario Works Policy Directives.

Ministry of Children and Youth Services. (2009). *Breaking the cycle: The first year.* Ontario's Poverty Reduction Strategy Annual Report.

Ministry of Community and Social Services. (2006). *McGuinty government helping people break free of substance and welfare dependencies.* Archived, Ontario News Room.

Ministry of Community and Social Services. (2009). *8.4 addiction services initiative (ASI)* Ontario Works Policy Directives.

Ministry of Community and Social Services. (2011). *Results-based plan briefing book 2010–2011.* Ministry of Community and Social Services.

Ministry of Community and Social Services. (2012). *Results-based plan briefing book 2011–2012.* Ministry of Community and Social Services.

Ministry of Community and Social Services. (2013). *Results-based plan briefing book 2012–2013.* Ministry of Community and Social Services.

Ministry of Community and Social Services. (2014). *Results-based plan briefing book 2013–2014.* Ministry of Community and Social Services.

Ministry of Community and Social Services. (2015). *Results-based plan briefing book 2014–2015.* Ministry of Community and Social Services.

Ministry of Community and Social Services. (2016a). *Estimates briefing book 2015–2016.* Ministry of Community and Social Services.

Ministry of Community and Social Services. (2016b). *Ontario Establishing Income Security Reform Working Group.* Toronto, Ontario.

Ministry of Community and Social Services. (2017). *Estimates briefing book 2016–2017.* Toronto, Ontario.

Ministry of Community and Social Services. (2018). *Estimates briefing book 2017–2018.* Toronto, Ontario.

The Ontario Social Assistance Review Advisory Council. (2010). *Recommendations for an Ontario income security review: Report of the Ontario Social Assistance Review Advisory Council.* Ministry of Community & Social Services.

Appendix B: Interview Guides

Interview Guide for *OW Caseworkers*

I. Managing Clients on OW

To begin, I am interested in discussing addiction in general.

ADDICTION
- How do you think OW defines addiction?
- How do you define addiction?
- *Now let's talk about your relationships with clients living with addiction.*
- How do you learn they have an addiction? (probes: How do you learn that their substance use impacts their employability? What do you do to make clients comfortable in disclosing they have an addiction?)
- What treatment expectations do you have for clients? (probes: Do you refer clients to treatment programs? Do they receive help fast enough? Do you have expectations of their participation in treatment?)
- What is your role as a caseworker in helping someone seek treatment?
- What kinds of treatment programs do your clients participate in?
- What are the situations that make it difficult for clients to participate in treatment programs?
- Do you feel you are able to support clients enough in their management of their addiction?
- How do you feel OW could do a better job in supporting clients with an addiction?

PAID WORK
- *I'd like to now discuss the paid work expectations you have for clients.*
- Do you have paid work expectations for your clients? (probes: When do you discuss how your clients should seek paid work? When they are sober? What do you talk about?)

- What kinds of employment assistance activities do your clients participate in?
- What things make it difficult/easy for your clients to do employment activities?
- *The next questions are about how prepared or motivated you think your clients are about paid work.*
- What are your paid work goals for clients?
- Do you feel your clients have enough education and skills to get the job they want? (probe: What job do they want? How hopeful are they about getting a job?)
- *Let's conclude this section with a general discussion of people's relationships with OW. Not everyone's experience on OW is the same.*
- How do you think your client's experiences on OW are different than the experiences of other people on OW who are NOT using substances?

II. Imagining a Different OW for People Living with Addiction

- *We are reaching the end of the interview. I understand that OW does not expect you to be an addictions counsellor, but I am interested in your thoughts about how you think OW might change to better respond to clients who are ready to stop using and become closer to the labour market.*
- *I've heard it's sometimes difficult to access treatment in Toronto. Would it be helpful if OW referred clients to one treatment counsellor who could:*

  • Complete assessments of their overall health and well-being so they can better understand their substance use? (probe: Your psychological, mental, physical, spiritual health and well-being?)
  • Provided ongoing case management of their efforts to recover?
  • Made it easier for them to learn about and receive supports needed to address their substance use?

- What are some other ways that OW could help clients in their efforts to manage recovery/stay sober? (probe: For example, ensure access to affordable/available childcare so program can be attended?)
- *It's also difficult to find a good paying job in today's labour market.*
- Would it be helpful if OW completed assessments to help clients discover a job that best suits them?
- What are some other things that OW could do to help clients find work? (probe: Training?)
- Finally, if clients were to work again, what supports would they need to stay working and manage their recovery? (probes: Would

it be helpful to have someone to check in with each month? Should OW be a source of this kind of support, e.g., a Job Retention Support Worker, or not?)

Interview Guide for *OW Clients*

I. *Typical Day/Week*

- *We begin the interview with a series of questions designed to get a sense of your daily life. Your answers will help direct my questioning in the remainder of the interview.*
- What does a typical day look like for you? (probe: What sort of activities, e.g., paid work, school, treatment, volunteering, do you do during the day/week?)
- Can you tell me about the people you live with and your relationships with them (probe: children/grandchildren, partner, parents, parents-in-law, friends/others?)
- Who do you spend time with during the week? About how many people, e.g., family, friends, counsellors, do you see each week?
- What is the biggest challenge you face each day?
- How has addiction impacted your daily life? (probe: For how long?)
  Applicable to participants with children or other dependents:
  Who does the household chores in your house?
  Who does the caring work (or childcare) in your house?

II. *History of Use, OW Receipt*

- *We now turn to some questions that explore the history of your use and access to OW.*
- *Existing research shows that children who grew up in families in which they experienced trauma are more likely to experience substance use in adulthood. I'd like to begin by asking you some questions about your upbringing and if you see it as linked to your substance use.*
- What was your childhood like? And your teenage years? (probes: Did you feel happy? Sad?)
- How would you describe your family growing up? (probe: As stable or prone to conflict/violence?)
- Was your family connected to any government systems? (probes: Was your parent on welfare [OW]? Was child welfare [Children's Aid Society] involved in your life?)
- Is there a history of addiction in your family? (probe: Were drugs or alcohol readily used in your house?)

- Can you tell me about your experiences in school? (probes: What was your experience learning? Was school easy?)

    - Applicable to participants who did not finish high school:
    - Why did you not finish high school?
    - When did you move out of your family home? (probe: Why?)
- *Let's focus more on the history of your substance use.*
- Can you recall your first experience with substance use? (probe: Was there anything about that time in your life that you see as connected to your trying drugs/alcohol?)
- Can you tell me about how your use became a problem? (probe: What do you think you needed at that time?)
- It costs money to use drugs/alcohol. How did you do afford it? (probes: Were you working? Can you tell me, roughly, about how much you were spending a week?)
- *And now I'd like to discuss the reasons for your being on OW.*
- How did you come to be on OW? (probes: Did you come to be on OW because of your substance use? Did you lose your job?)

III. Managing Addiction

- *Let's now talk about your current situation, about your living with substance use challenges and being on OW.*
- What is the substance you have trouble with? Alcohol and/or drugs?
- Are you currently using? (probes: Approximately how long have you been using? How long have you been clean?)
- Are there other substances that you use that are not a problem for you?
- Have you ever received help for managing your addiction? (probes: What kind of treatment are you in? Day or evening program? AA?)

    - Applicable to participants not in treatment:
    - Why are you not in treatment?
    - Applicable to participants in treatment:
    - How did you learn about and access your treatment?
    - Is your treatment readily available? And close by?
    - Does your treatment conflict with the other activities you do each day/week?
    - What are you learning about yourself in treatment?

- What do you like about your treatment? What do you not like? (probe: Do you feel more hopeful?)
- Do you have any other mental or physical health conditions that make it difficult to recover from your addiction? (Probes: Are you smoking? Experience chronic pain? Anxiety or depression?)
- *I am also interested in what you think about addiction. Many people use substances, but some find it becomes a problem for them.*
- How do you define addiction? (probe: What does having an addiction mean to you?)

IV. Receiving OW

Now, my questions are more about your relationship with OW.

ADDICTION
- *Let's start with some questions focused on addiction.*
- How do you think OW understands addiction?
- How do you think your specific caseworker understands addiction?
- Your caseworker knows you use substances. How did s/he find out about this? (probe: Are you on a caseload with a worker who specializes in addiction?)
- Do you feel supported by your interaction with your caseworker? (probe: Would you find it helpful if your worker followed up more with you?)
- What could caseworkers do to make it more comfortable for you to discuss your substance use and any challenges you face because of it? (probes: What have your relationships been like with caseworkers?)
- If you need more help with your addiction, would you feel like your OW caseworker would be someone you can go to? (probes: How often do you see your caseworker? Would it be helpful to see her/him more often?)

  - Applicable to participants in treatment:
  - Did your OW caseworker refer you to your current treatment program? Did you receive help fast enough?

PAID WORK
- *I would like to now discuss your experiences working for pay now or in the past and your thoughts about how OW supports your paid work efforts.*

- Are you currently working for pay? (probe: Or volunteering?)
- When was the last time you worked for pay? (probe: Why did this job end?)
- Does your caseworker have any expectations of you to participate in paid work? (probes: Have you discussed when you should seek paid work? What do you talk about?)
- Are the expectations of your OW caseworker reasonable? (probe: What expectations should OW have for people recovering from addiction?)
- Are you participating in any employment assistance activities? (probes: Are you completing your GED? Training, ESL, OASIS; Have you participated in one in the past?)
- What things make it difficult/easy for you to do employment activities?
- *The next questions are about how prepared or motivated you feel about paid work.*
- I understand everyone develops a personal employment plan in consultation with their caseworker at some point. Can you tell me about yours?
- What is your personal goal concerning paid work?
- Do you feel you have enough education and skills to get the job you want? (probe: What
- job do you want? How hopeful are you about getting a job?)
- How do you feel about going back to work? (probe: Are you nervous?)

  - Applicable to participants working for pay or participating in employment activities:
  - How has your participation in this activity helped with your recovery?

- *Let's conclude this section of the interview with a general discussion of people's relationships with OW. Not everyone's experience on OW is the same.*
- How do you think your experiences on OW are different than the experiences of other people who are using substances? (probes: Provide comparison category for participant, e.g., How are your experiences different from a single parent?)
- How do you think your experiences on OW are different than the experiences of other people on OW who are NOT using substances?

IV. Supports Given, Received, and Needed[1]

- *This section of the interview focuses on the supports you need while living with an addiction.*
- Do your family and friends know you use substances?
- Do relationships with family members, both younger and older, encourage or support your recovery? (probes: How? Help with monthly bills? Emotional support? etc.)
- Do relationships with friends, both younger and older, encourage or support your recovery? (probes: How? Help with monthly bills? Emotional support? etc. Has this changed?)
- *Sometimes people have friends that feel more like family than their actual mothers, fathers, siblings, etc.*
- Can you tell me if you have friends like this and if they encourage or support your recovery?
- *Let's talk about supports you receive beyond family and friends.*
- Do you receive any support from community organizations that aid in your recovery? (probe: e.g., parenting programs, childcare, job training, food bank, other programs such as counselling or nutrition, seniors programs, etc.)
- Finally, are you receiving any other financial support from the government?
  (probe: e.g., besides OW, do you receive child benefits? etc.)
- *And now let's talk about the quality and quantity of support you receive.*
- Do you find this support helpful? (probe: Does it help with your overall health, mental/physical, and well-being?)
- Do you receive enough support for managing your addiction? (probes: Do you feel alone in managing your addiction? Would you like more emotional, financial, material, spiritual, etc. support?)

---

1 The following definitions of support will be assumed:
   Physical/practical support (instrumental) to friends and family: home maintenance (e.g., snow shovelling, spring cleaning, repairs), grocery shopping, and providing transportation.
   Caregiving support: household chores, preparing meals, minding children, and even assisting with personal care.
   Emotional (expressive) support: a shoulder to lean on when needed, give advice to adult family members or children, or give the help that talking with someone provides. Spirituality can also play an important role in their giving and receiving of emotional support.
   Material support: clothes, food, etc., you may give or loan to family members or friends.

– How does the support you receive help you manage everything
 else in your daily life? (probe: Your addiction, caring for others [e.g.,
 children, dependents], and meeting the expectations of OW?)

Applicable to clients not in treatment:

- You're not in treatment. Do you want to change the way you use
 substances?
- What do you think treatment is? (probe: Did you know you can
 get help in managing your use?)
- What supports do you need to consider sobriety?

– *My next questions are about the support you give to others.*
– What support do you give to family members, both younger and
 older? (probes: Help with monthly bills? Emotional support? etc.
 Why?)
– What support do you give to friends, both younger and older?
 (probe: Help with monthly bills? Emotional support? etc. Why?)
– Do you engage with community organizations in any way? (probe:
 e.g., volunteering)
– Does your helping others have an impact on your substance use
 and/or recovery? (probes: Make it difficult to engage in treatment
 and/or participate in employment activities?)

V. Imagining a Different OW for People Living with Addiction

– *We are reaching the end of the interview. This last section focuses on what
 you think might be changed in how OW responds to your addiction and
 employment potential.*
– *I've heard that it's sometimes difficult to access treatment in Toronto.
 Would it be helpful if OW referred you to one treatment counsellor who
 could:*

- Complete assessments of your overall health and well-being
 so you can better understand your substance use? (probe: Your
 psychological, mental, physical, spiritual health and well-being?)
- Provided ongoing case management of your efforts to recover?
- Made it easier for you to learn about and receive supports
 needed to address your substance use?

– What are some other ways that OW could help you in your efforts
 to manage recovery/stay sober? (probe: For example, ensure access
 to affordable/available childcare so program can be attended?)
– *It's also difficult to find a good paying job in today's labour market.*

– Would it be helpful if OW completed assessments so that you can discover a job that best suits you?
– What are some other things that OW could do to help you find work? (probe: Training?)
– Finally, if you were to work again, what supports would you need to stay working and manage your recovery? (probes: Would it be helpful to have someone to check in with each month? Should OW be a source of this kind of support, e.g., a Job Retention Support Worker, or not?)

Appendix C: Methods

Ontological and Epistemological Assumptions

My approach to what can be known and how it is known about the experience of living with addiction while also accessing Ontario Works (OW) maps onto an approach that my dear friend and colleague, Katherine Bischoping, and I wrote about in our book about some qualitative methods and one that is decidedly post-positivist: this approach can be thought of as rooted in a critical realist paradigm tempered by a dose of social constructionism (Bischoping & Gazso, 2016) and straying towards the comparable relativism and sensitivity to social and historical context invited by post-structuralism. That is, in the design of my study and its completion, I maintained a healthy tension between understanding reality as something that exists independent of people's representations of it (Cruickshank, 2003), or critical realism; reality as a construct of persons and groups (Berger & Luckman, 1966), or social constructionism; and reality as unstable, contested, and contextual, or post-structuralism (Agger, 1991).

To clarify, I set out to do this study with an interest in exploring what is the experience of accessing OW while also managing substance use, and what are the consequences of making choices about substance use while also living lives rich in other experiences. I also, however, wanted to understand how individuals' experiences as persons living with substance use dependency and accessing OW were constituted by larger meaning-making systems, in my case OW policy discourse itself. I was curious how policy language was used to conceptualize and construct benefit recipients who identify as struggling with substance use and how any one way of constructing them becomes dominant over others and may change over time. I was therefore keen to unpack the power–knowledge relations constitutive of, and ideologies constructed in, OW discourse. This led me, like many orienting to social constructionism in this way, to draw on the work of Michel Foucault (Baert et al., 2011; Raskin, 2002). However, I also oriented to the work of Norman Fairclough to engage in the exercise of critique with the goal of social change; this is clearest in the final chapter of this book. Finally, I sought out people's narratives about their experiences in accessing OW and working through addiction and through their own subjective reconstructions of "knowing" and "being" (Berger & Luckman, 1966). In seeking this information, I remained sensitive to Foucault's view of epistemology and ontology: the knower may seem to know a reality, but it is already and always a construction (Bischoping & Gazso, 2016). I understood the stories told by participants as discursively constituted.

Two additional caveats are warranted to position my approach to the reality I sought to study. By no means do I purport to offer a phenomenology of the experience of living with addiction while on low income, but I do appreciate how lived experience is approached from this perspective. As linked to the work of Edmond Husserl and Alfred Schütz, the emphasis in phenomenology is on how humans experience a lifeworld. As Wagner (2002) explains further in drawing on these two theorists, "all we know and do in the social world is anchored in individual consciousness and experienced subjectively." Said differently, all reality is thought to consist of objects and events, but as they are perceived and understood by humans, and so taken for granted. What we take to be reality, then, is imbued with intersubjective meaning (Bischoping & Gazso, 2016). I was aware of this understanding when interviewing persons about their everyday lives and trying to understand how they experienced their selves and things outside of the self, for example, rules and regulations in OW discourse (see also Wagner, 2002). Finally, I am not aligning myself with an interpretivist paradigm narrowly defined as an interest in interpreting people's meanings and behaviours as only according to their subjective frame of reference (Williams, 2000). Given my invocation of social constructionism and post-structuralism, I understand even the meanings people give in their stories to be mediated by discourse.

My anchoring of paradigmatic insights together in order to meet my research objectives is not unique. Since paradigms themselves are theoretical constructs and not containing of indisputable logic, there is a growing argument among researchers that the use of multiple paradigms and methods might very well yield a better understanding of the topic of focus (see Denzin & Lincoln, 2012). The use of more than one paradigm and/or one method can facilitate the interdependent analysis of data and extrapolation of meaning and knowledge beyond that which would be achieved with only one approach (Bogna et al., 2020). Moreover, building on points I made in the introductory chapter of this book, here I note that the eclecticism of my ontological and epistemological assumptions also suits the broader theoretical situation of my research within the social change brought about by the process of individualization. In turn, my methods suit my understanding of individualization itself as a discursive field replete with discourses and concepts and contestations within.

Questions, Data, and Methods

Situated this way ontologically and epistemologically, I originally began this research with what I thought were two clear research questions: (1) What policy discourses shape eligibility for OW for persons recovering from addiction? and (2) What are the welfare-to-work experiences of persons recovering from addiction? Once I began answering these questions through an analysis of OW policy documents and governmental reports, and soon after I interviewed my first three caseworkers, these questions metamorphosed. While I could retain question one with confidence, question two required a revision to: *What are the experiences* of persons living with addiction while on OW? Chapter 6 especially shows why this revision had to occur. Two sources of qualitative data were required to answer these newly revised questions: policy discourse and personal stories or narratives.

Policy as Discourse

What is "discourse" can often seem abstract or illusive to define and made more complex because of different disciplinary views. I see discourse as the texts of social life, these being verbal, written, visual, and behavioural, and which we experience in everyday common-place settings (e.g., our households, in our communities) and in institutional settings (e.g., the university). Discourse is the "web of meanings, ideas, interactions and practices that are expressed or represented" in these same texts (Bischoping & Gazso, 2016, p. 129). Policy is one such text.

The *policy discourse* on addiction and OW that I include as data in this study is limited to "public-use" discourse from the period 2009–17 that I purposefully sampled for its informational richness; my focus on this time period is made clear in chapter 6. Public-use discourse was of two types: written and verbal. I collected documents that could be retrieved through online searches of the Internet or from university or legislature libraries. These included OW policy itself (e.g., the *Ontario*

Works Act, including Directives), annual reports and other documents produced by the ministry concerned with OW (the Ministry of Children and Community Services), or the municipal government department responsible for administering OW in the City of Toronto (Toronto Employment and Social Services, TESS). I did not retrieve any internal documentation through a Freedom of Information and Protection of Privacy Request. In imposing a limit to "public-use" policy discourse, the study in this book therefore remains silent about information that is not made known to the public. This is a limitation and a strength. I wanted to work with what is made known about living with addiction while accessing OW. The verbal text to which I refer is the Legislative Assembly of Ontario discussions documented in the House Hansard Index, between 2009 and 2017. Over this period, transcriptions of these meetings were searched and purposively sampled for any reference to addiction and OW.

Interviewing and Storying

In-depth interviews with caseworkers and benefit recipients were my method of data collection to answer my second research question. In in-depth or intensive interviewing, the researcher and participant are engaged in a search for meaning, for answers that are sometimes difficult to articulate. My style of interviewing as a feminist scholar is infused with sensitivity to researcher and participant standpoint and social location. I endeavoured to create space for participants and me to discuss experiences as conversationally as possible. Indeed, as DeVault (2004) observes, it is the way the researcher conveys their concerns and the way questions are asked that can further recruit participants in the search for meaning.

I approached interviews as a means by which we (myself and participants) would tell stories. Of course, as a researcher, I played a more directive role in seeking these stories. While I desired stories primarily about the caseworker experience from OW caseworkers, I wanted to hear stories of a life lived from OW benefit recipients (see also below). In narrative inquiry in general, stories are understood as used by individuals to describe human actions (Polkinghorne, 1995). Narratives – or stories – are simply recountings of experiences that have taken place over time (Bischoping & Gazso, 2016) or can be seen as emplotted accounts with a beginning, middle, and end (e.g., the Labov model) (Polkinghorne, 1995). From a life-course perspective, narratives are also seen to reveal individual choices, chances, events, and transitions as they unfolded in socio-historical and family context (Brettell, 2002; Dewilde, 2003; Elder,

1994; Webb & Gazso, 2017). To recall again my theoretical situation of this project, I note that Zinn (2002) understands the life course perspective's emphasis on biography and narrative to be especially suitable for capturing the process and experience of individualization.

Bamberg and Georgakopoulou (2008, p. 378) observe that it is common for researchers to listen to stories and then engage in what they call "autobiographical models" or "big story research." The analytic focus tends to be on peoples' telling of "nonshared experiences, past events" as representing their subjectivities and reflecting their identities, and an assumption that in the telling of the story, the narrator is making sense of the self. As Mishler (1986) observes, stories with some sense of chronology (beginning, middle, end) are a common response to interview questions about everyday life experiences. These big stories are different from "small stories" (Bamberg & Georgakopoulou, 2008). Small stories are those that tend to materialize in everyday talk (e.g., future projections, breaking news, references to shared experience) (Georgakopoulou, 2007) and excluded from the formal research interview. Unlike big stories, small stories are not told in monologic form, in chronological order, nor contain individually centred search for the meaning of the past. This distinction is important to note at length because this is indeed a book of big story research. The very organization of the second part of this book adopts a chronological, narrative arc.

The Participants

I used purposive and convenience sampling to recruit both OW caseworkers and OW benefit recipients because I was keen to answer my research questions from two different perspectives. My two-stage process of recruitment was facilitated by a relationship I developed with City of Toronto (specifically Toronto Employment and Social Services, TESS) managers who shared my research interests in how persons engaging in or managing substance use concurrently experienced OW receipt. While my larger interests were academic and oriented towards unearthing the experience of living with addiction on welfare from stigmatizing rhetoric, we shared interests that were also practical and applied, for example, what would we find that would provide them with information they could use, perhaps to support policy change? I deliberately use "we" here because my qualitative interview guides were designed to fit both of our interests and the findings understood to be disseminated academically (e.g., journal articles, this book) and internally within TESS; in fact, many of the findings discussed in this book have already been presented at two different research meetings with caseworkers, managers, and directors.

The interpretation of study findings and my extrapolation from them are mine alone. Any mistakes in interpretation of policy change are therefore mine as well. To be clear, I am not writing on behalf of the City of Toronto or TESS. As well, my study was not a study of TESS or its administration of OW. Some of my findings are revealing of the challenging work of casework and, of course, some of my interpretations critical of the unfair or unequal experiences of people accessing OW. And yet, in my analysis I remained acutely aware that people I interviewed would have been worse off financially if not for their OW receipt; I write at length about the social support benefit recipients received from caseworkers in this book. I am also confident that some of the findings I share are not new to scholars of poverty and the welfare state. Some of my findings are also not new to TESS itself. There are numerous City of Toronto and TESS reports and publications, some I include as my public-use policy discourse, that document the everyday struggles that people on OW face. What is new in this book is my sociological attention to the experiences of people living with addiction while accessing OW and amid multiple other poverties. What I am most critical about – and in the academic sense as a sociologist – is the limitations, consequences, and broader policy implications of how individuals living with addiction are constructed in OW policy. Moreover, it is in the concluding chapter of this book that I then present my case for how my findings lead me to argue for the de-stigmatization of addiction and to transform how we see the potential of people living with addiction and accessing OW – through hope.

I met caseworkers by processes of referral from managers. Caseworkers representing and working in OW offices in the main regions of the Greater Toronto Area received an email invitation to consider participating in the study; the letter explained my research objectives and that the findings would be useful to TESS as well. Once interested caseworkers responded positively to the invite, I followed up with each of them and explained that their participation in the study would in no way jeopardize their employment. I shared that I would preserve confidentiality by using pseudonyms and also by making no connections between their experiences and their office location. I interviewed seven caseworkers in total and at their office locations, each different in physical design but with a security presence. While security measures such as the employment of security guards could undoubtedly ensure the safe interaction among individuals in these locations, I admit I found the requirement that I, too, had to interact with security guards in order to have a meeting in a place of social welfare support to be somewhat disconcerting. I was reminded of how physical space can create the experience of social control, regulation, and marginalization too.

Turning my focus to OW benefit recipients, I set out to interview people who self-defined as living with addiction to substances, specifically drugs or alcohol. I began my research assuming these drugs would include criminalized and illicit drugs such as cocaine, crack cocaine, heroin, and crystal methamphetamine. I also assumed that some people I interviewed may prefer yet another illegal substance of choice that I would learn about, or that some people would name prescription drugs (e.g., opioids) as their preference. I understood alcohol use to include hard liquor and spirits, beer, and wine. I had the thought that some people would be using methadone. I admit that this hunch stemmed not from a great familiarity with substance use literature but from my past employment as a corrections officer for Corrections Canada. I have had firsthand experience "supervising" individuals' ingestion of the drug in prison in lieu of opioids and as they sought recovery. While caseworkers speak of their relationships with their clients, in line with how welfare claimants are largely framed as consumers of services (Baker Collins, 2016; Broad & Antony, 1999), I choose to use the language of benefit recipient or participant instead. I make clear when I am writing about caseworkers versus those they work with, benefit recipients.

Telephoning people who had conveyed interest in participating in the study to their caseworker and consented to sharing their contact information with me was the easiest part of recruitment, that is, the act of picking up my phone and dialing a number. To clarify, in the days and weeks following my interview with each caseworker, they then shared about the opportunity to complete a research interview with eight to ten prospective participants on my behalf. I assumed that since caseworkers had already been interviewed, they would be knowledgeable in describing the study to individuals on their caseload. I shared with caseworkers that I was seeking a diverse sample in terms of individuals' marital status, race, ethnicity, Indigeneity, sexual orientation, and gender and was hoping to meet people who were caring for children. Caseworkers shared that their involvement in the process of recruitment went fairly smoothly. They told potential participants about the study in face-to-face or telephone meetings and that it was quickly clear whether they were interested in participating or not. One caseworker told me that one prospective participant was not pleased at the invite to consider taking part in the project. They told the caseworker that their life experience was their own, their knowledge their own, and of value – and not to be shared with some outsider doing research. I saw this response as an illuminative example of exactly why reflexivity is needed in research. I was indeed an outsider doing research and affiliated with an institution for which research could be perceived to not always benefit those with whom the researcher meets.

There was no good time of day to reach people. I tried the telemarketer tactic of phoning between 5:00 p.m. and 7:00 p.m. (and felt some guilt doing it), but that was of little use. If I left a voice mail, I could not count on being called back. On average, I left three voice mails, about three days apart, before giving up and turning to the next name and number on my list. Once I was able to connect with someone on the phone, I would explain the project as quickly and simply as possible and remind them that their caseworker had already told them about it. I asked if they had any questions about the project and would entertain being interviewed. I explained that if we met, they would be given the opportunity to formally consent to participate in an interview. I also confirmed that they would receive a $25 gift card to Shoppers Drug Mart or a grocery store and Toronto Transit Commission travel tokens in thanks for their participation. If possible, I scheduled the interview then and there and within the next week.

After our initial verbal contact, many people wanted to communicate via text message. Since I primarily text with my family and friends, I found it entirely odd to text someone I did not know to confirm a meeting time. However, the act of texting seemed to work for connecting with many prospective participants. Perhaps it was the lesser intimacy permitted by texting that some people found appealing. Of the interviews I did complete, I often felt they happened because of sheer luck. For example, three times I drove to meet a person at an agreed upon location and they were not there. When this happened a second time with another prospective participant, I soon learned to text before I left the house – and to pull my car over at a rest stop and text on the way. This tactic of constantly checking in by text became particularly important when I was driving on wintry highways in February in southwestern Ontario.

I conducted interviews at homes, coffee shops (e.g., Tim Hortons), and fast food restaurants (e.g., McDonalds); three interviews were completed by telephone at the request of the participant. I audio-recorded all interviews. For people I met in person, I became incredibly adept at using the Internet and Google maps to suggest a location to meet near their home address. Most participants did not want to be interviewed at home. I believe this reflected their concerns for their privacy but also their housing situation. Many people I interviewed lived with a roommate, some lived in rooming houses, and four were temporarily housed at a friend's house but otherwise homeless. Since I lived north of Toronto, I spent a lot of time in my car driving to the interview location and hoping that my maps app was not leading me astray. I felt excited and nervous to meet people and hear their stories as I drove, which often meant that the car journey felt like it took forever when in fact it was the usual 1–1½ hour drive.

Once I reached a location, the next challenge was to meet the correct person. When I was to meet Jesse, the very first benefit recipient I would meet, he said, "look for the man wearing a beanie hat." So, I did look for him at the time we agreed upon at a coffee shop. I was feeling like he had stood me up only to then realize that he was the man in the line-up for coffee wearing what I would call a pom-pom toque. I noticed him because he was doing what I was doing: glancing around as if he were looking for someone. A "beanie" in my mind was a tight-fitting unadorned knit hat. Following this misunderstanding, I became proactive and told participants to "look for the woman with black glasses and a gigantic blue shoulder bag, maybe with papers in front of her at a table."

The main challenges while interviewing in coffee shops or restaurants were the noise and curiosity of others. I did my best to make it seem I was not interviewing by covering my recorder with a piece of paper and placing my questionnaire and interview guide out of view. Whenever I could, I made sure I purchased refreshments and food for myself and participants. I missed this opportunity only if the person I was to meet arrived long before I did. The setting of the interview likely shaped how participants told their stories in two ways. Some participants may not have been as forthcoming in sharing their stories in a public setting. In contrast, some participants may have perceived a greater anonymity in sharing their stories in this less intimate environment than a face-to-face interview in a closed office.

It took me a long time to interview twenty-eight people living with addiction: from November 2016 to September 2017. This was partially because it was so difficult to reach people by phone, gain their agreement to meet for an interview, and then meet in person to have the interview. But it was also because there were so many reasons that a person figuring out how to manage their substance use or working on recovery would have to not make an interview, even if scheduled and even if they knew I was en route to our chosen location. Finally, the lengthier period of data collection was also my decision. It was after only my third interview that I realized I needed to take time to sit with stories shared and engage in an emotional detox of sorts. I soon conducted only one interview a week at best. This was not because I became depressed while interviewing, but rather because I found the interviews heavy, characterized by a mix of stories of fear, pain, hope, and pursuing new beginnings in a life to live.

The total sample size of participants in this study was thirty-five, including seven caseworker participants and twenty-eight benefit participants. This study was not funded by an outside agency and was completed with the support of small grants of internal funding from my home university. This lack of grant funding was intentional; I did not apply for any. For the first time since the completion of my PhD program (over ten years ago), I wanted to do research informed by my own experiences, interests, and efforts. I desired a slower and very exploratory way of working rather than the imposition of a tight timeline and strict organizational framework that I have found to be conditioned by the receipt of external grant funding. Though I collaborated with TESS to meet participants, I wanted to, and did, interview each person of whom I speak or share stories. I used my small amount of internal university funding to pay for invaluable research assistance with transcribing interviews, an interdisciplinary literature review, collection and organization of policy discourse, and reviewing early drafts of this book. I note that I transcribed half of the interviews myself based, I believe, in the importance of remembering how my intimate conversations with people unfolded, a practice that I found served me well in then coding the talk data, which I discuss below. I have worked this study from start to finish, the finish being this very book – and *enjoyed* it. Having lost the feeling of joy in doing research for several years, this study has reminded me that it exists and can be mine.

The majority of the seven OW caseworkers I interviewed were white and had one or more years of experience in case management. They included five women and two men. Each of my caseworker interviews were about 1–1½ hours in length. My interest was in how caseworkers thought OW defined addiction and how they defined addiction; their case management relationships, including their paid work expectations for benefit recipients; and how OW could better respond to people living with addiction (see Appendix B).

I sought more detailed demographic information from the twenty-eight people who self-defined as living with addiction while accessing OW using a short questionnaire. I have found such questionnaires beneficial when doing in-depth interviews because they permit the establishment of a loose backstory that then helps me contextualize how I ask further questions about participants' life courses. I asked participants about their gender, education, age, marital status, parental status (e.g., children in their care or others), household size, accommodation, years in receipt of OW, and past employment. I also asked people to self-define their cultural heritage and/or race and/or ethnicity. There was a level of awkwardness in asking such a complex question (see also Gazso & Bischoping, 2018). Sometimes this awkwardness materialized because I am a white researcher seeking information about people's race and ethnicity when, given our earlier phone conversations, this did not seem to be the focus of our interview. I persisted in asking this question for three reasons. First, the history of the construction of Canada as a nation – and that which we know as law, policy, etc. – is that of colonialism and systemic racism that continues to produce inequalities that shape the lives of Black, Indigenous, and people of colour (BIPOC). Second and relatedly, I ask this question because people's experiences of their social realities, including receipt of OW and substance use, differ depending on their social positions, with their race/ethnicity being one of many anchors of their positionality. Finally, I ask this because I find that while awkward moments may arise, people are quite reflective in their answers. Cultural heritage, race, and ethnicity mean something to people's identities as they ponder them in an interview moment, even if their answers are divergent from others' answers, confusing, or wandering, and even when we as researchers cannot always agree on what they mean. I found this to be the case with many of the twenty-eight benefit recipients I interviewed: they often tried to offer a deeper clarification of their answer. Twenty-two participants defined themselves as "white" but desired to make it known that they were "Canadian," "Italian," "French-Canadian," or "Irish," for example. Of the remaining participants, six people identified as "Black," "Caribbean," "mixed race," or "Middle Eastern."

The people that I interviewed ranged in age from sixteen to sixty-seven. I interviewed more women than men (sixteen versus twelve), and in my presentation of findings I adopt the gender pronoun that participants identified with. I did not seek information about sexual orientation directly but gathered that all but one participant saw themselves as heterosexual persons in their stories of their past or current marital or co-habitating relations. Only through her stories of her marriage and child did I learn that Theresa self-defined as a white, lesbian woman who had raised her daughter with her partner until she passed away. Six women identified as lone mothers with children in their care. Most participants (twenty-two) defined as single and had previous common-law or marital relationships. Of these single persons, eighteen were parents and in some way engaged in co-parenting children in the care of guardians or ex-partners. The highest level of completed education for most participants was high school, although eleven recipients also had some post-secondary education and had attended college or university. Not all participants completed high school; nine did not. As made clear in chapter 5, some participants found spending time with friends and using substances during high school hours and later to be a more enjoyable use of their time. Clive, a self-proclaimed alcoholic, explained how high school attendance can gradually wane over time: "So, once I had money and got my own place ... [y]ou're up drinking all night, well, you don't get up and go to school in the morning." All twenty-eight benefit recipients had past paid work experience. Several people (eleven) had been involved with the criminal justice system. At the time of the interview, all recipients had been on OW for one year or more and resided in rental housing.

The twenty-eight people who consented to be interviewed by me seemed comfortable self-defining as living with addiction, the language I used in our initial conversations. In total, participants had experienced addiction to opioids (prescription or illicit) (seventeen participants); alcohol (seven participants); and cocaine, including crack cocaine (four participants). Some people indicated their poly-substance use but pinpointed the substance they had the most difficulty managing or overcoming. Twenty-three participants shared their pursuit of recovery and engaged in various forms of treatment, including Alcoholics or Narcotics Anonymous and day programming. Eight participants specifically participated in methadone treatment, and two participants participated in suboxone treatment. Five people independently pursued sobriety and abstinence. Being in recovery or using substances, however, were not necessarily mutually exclusive for some participants; some of those engaged in methadone treatment were also still randomly using. Five participants did not report being in recovery or any form of treatment. These five engaged in random substance use.

Analysis

The strategies undertaken to analyse interview talk and discourse were those that map onto the theoretical framework outlined in my introductory chapter and the ontological and epistemological assumptions I outline above. I used two strategies, discourse and narrative analysis, and worked both inductively and deductively, resulting in my production of data-driven and theory-driven findings (see also Gazso, 2019).

Discourse Strategies

My analysis of policy discourse falls in line with "critical discourse studies," what Wodak and Meyer (2016) define as projects in which the goal is to deconstruct ideologies and power in text. In critical discourse studies, no one theorist or approach is favoured, and rather it is incumbent upon the scholar to make clear their critical goals and methods that produce their scholarly contribution (van Dijk, 2013).

I analysed policy discourse for the discourses it represented, but also the ideologies and power relations it reflected, the subjectivities it constituted, and the feeling rules it contained. I sought to deconstruct and define the discourses represented and their ideological work, drawing on this insight from Critical Discourse Analysis (or CDA) (Fairclough & Wodak, 1997). I explored whether these discourses (re-)produced ideology or organized systems of meaning-making (e.g., ideas and values) and prescriptions for a collective (see Hall, 1996; van Dijk, 1998). I maintained the distinction between ideology and discourse for analytical reasons. For example, familiar with the existing scholarship on welfare reform in Canada, I was attentive to whether the discourse of welfare dependency and its linkage with neoliberal ideology would be replicated in the policy discourse I sampled.

In *Discourse and Social Change* (1992), Fairclough observed that one can study discourse for how it is produced and shared but also how it is changed, and through motives of power, oppression, and resistance. I queried whether new discourses seemed apparent and for what apparent reasons, leaning heavily on the definition of discourse as webs of meaning and resounding in implication I shared earlier. I also drew upon Fairclough and Wodak's (1997) understanding of discourse as constitutive of society and culture. I explored whether and how meaning assigned to addiction and low income was filtered through policy discourse, culminating in definitions of eligibility over time and crafted by those with power (e.g., social actors, politicians, experts, etc.).

Indeed, in critical discourse studies, language is understood as imbued with power (Bischoping & Gazso, 2016). Power, however, is not simply in the Weberian sense, of exercising one's will over others (Weber, 1964), as in the case of social actors involved in the design and administration of OW. Power is also relational, an assumption shared by both CDA scholars and theorist Michel Foucault (with the former drawing heavily from the latter in explaining this assumption). According to Foucault, power changes, power is productive, and power is constraining. Power is "not an institution, and not a structure; neither is it a certain strength we are endowed with; it is the name one attributes to a complex strategical situation in a particular society" (Foucault, 1978, p. 93).

Assuming Foucault's more nuanced understanding of power, the subject positions constituted by power-knowledge relations inherent in discourse were a third interest of mine. I specifically draw on Foucault's notion of disciplinary power as including the regulation and normalization of human experience, or the socialization of people to rules of behaviour via discourse (Brodie, 2008; Foucault, 1977). Subjectification, or how individuals may self-discipline or "work on themselves" to conform to a discourse, is linked to disciplinary power (Rabinow & Rose, 2006). As is made clear in chapter 6, I worked to uncover the subject positions made available to persons living with addiction *through* discourses in OW and related policy documents and the talk of participants about OW policy and practice, a point I will return to again below.

In undertaking analysis of the talk of benefit recipients, I soon came to see that people's work on themselves also involved their emotions or feelings, an observation made by Arlie Hochschild (1983) and originally from a symbolic interactionist vantage point. Hochschild understands social relations to shape individuals' emotions (e.g., of anger) and how they manage them – how they consciously try to feel – in the form of "feeling rules." In situations in which individuals experience a conflict between these feeling rules and their experiences, individuals engage in mental (e.g., change their thinking) and physical (e.g., breathing deeply) emotion work. Hochschild (2013) more recently and fully observed these "feeling rules" are interactionally produced *and* ideologically and discursively constituted and constrained. I drew on this understanding to explore how especially parents engaged in emotion and identity work in relation to discourses about family relations, addiction, and poverty and their feeling rules. Finally, I undertook discourse analysis with the broader objective of putting the product of my analysis to the ends of social justice or to endeavour to bring about social change. This is a goal I share with many critical discourse scholars (Bischoping & Gazso, 2016) and obvious in my argumentation for the de-stigmatization of addiction and the call for a collective praxis of hope in how we understand and support low-income people living with addiction.

Narrative Strategies

I read caseworker interviews as containing their stories of their experiences interpreting OW policy rules and regulations and applying them in their casework. My analysis of benefit recipients' stories went deeper and focused on the meaning they gave to events and transitions in their lives and how they saw these to shape how their lives unfolded following them. Like in my other research with Jason Webb, I was also interested in how people living with addiction while on OW might discuss turning points or fateful moments that resulted in their altering the course of their lives (see Berger, 2008; Giddens, 1991; Webb & Gazso, 2017). In knowing that participants have many subjective interpretations of and meanings for life course events they have experienced (Bischoping & Gazso, 2016), I assumed that I was exposed to but one or a few in the moments of our interview.

Alongside my desire to present a big story of living with addiction and accessing OW, I was especially interested in how benefit recipients made sense of their identities in their storytelling (Webb & Gazso, 2017). In their stories in response to my questions, I assumed people were talking about their identities of the past, in the present, and those they aspire to in the future. People experience multiple identities over time and any one moment lived is not limited to one identity alone (Raskin, 2006). Different facets of identities are more salient in some contexts than others (Widdicombe, 1998). Further, as assumed in the process of individualization, the broad theoretical frame of my study introduced in chapter 1, identity is unlimited and to be ongoingly crafted by each individual. I therefore paid attention to how people seemed to decide, change, and create their identities over time, including that of substance user or "addict" and in relation to their experiences with others (see also Mead, 1984 [1934]). To return to Hochschild's conceptualization of emotional labour, I looked for instances in interview transcripts where it seemed that benefit recipients were: (1) performing emotional labour in response to "feeling rules" at the time of their sharing a story with me; and/or (2) telling me a story about emotional labour they performed in the past in response to "feeling rules" (Hochschild, 1983). I also explored whether benefit recipients were engaging in identity work simultaneous to this emotional labour (Gazso, 2021). Chapter 7 of this book is especially revealing of how I use narrative and discourse analysis to explore how benefit recipients engage in emotion and identity work in relation to discursively constituted "feeling rules" to move past only ever being seen and known as an "addict."

Discourse/Story/Discourse. I saw my use of two analytic strategies to complement each other and to enable the answering of my research questions. I approached and understood policy documents to reflect discourse. I also saw the talk of participants, their narratives told during our interview, to reflect or represent discourse(s). I made several analytical assumptions in drawing this connection between story and discourse. Individuals' stories were understood to reveal changing identities over their life courses, with these changes brought about through interactions with others as well as with discourse(s). Besides analysing interview talk for what I thought stories revealed, I also set out to uncover participants' explicit (re-)production of policy discourse or other discourses on family, addiction, and poverty, as well as the unspoken, implicit ideologies and taken-for-granted assumptions (or hegemony as per Gramsci, 1971) that underpinned these (see also Gazso, 2019). One example of a connection I explored in this vein goes as follows: I sought to discover benefit recipients' storied experiences of living with addiction while on OW and how they were discursively shaped by policy regulations and caseworkers' constructions of *what they should be*.

Coding Specifics

I adopted a process of coding interview transcripts largely informed by some of the coding principles of grounded theory, specifically open and axial coding (Strauss & Corbin, 1998). In open coding, the experiences of interview participants are given conceptual labels. In this first attempt at grouping data, attention is given to patterns and shared dimensions of experiences in participants' responses. In axial coding, the goal is higher-level development of categories, the careful grouping and interpreting of several "open code" categories into broad themes. I applied this coding strategy to participants' stories in my use of NVivo, a qualitative software, and worked with the two groups of interview data, caseworker interviews and benefit recipient interviews, separately. The coding schema for each group was maintained as separate, as I wanted to compare the themes for the caseworker and benefit recipient talk (see, for example, chapter 6). In presenting interview themes throughout the remainder of the book, I share what I believe to be exemplary quotes from caseworker or benefit recipient interviews.

I applied similar coding principles in my discourse analysis. I first read and coded my public-use policy documents separately. For example, I coded each ministry annual report for key words, ideas, or phrases. I then re-read these in total (e.g., all ministry annual reports from 2009 to 2017), to determine if some of these words and ideas could be grouped categorically (what I saw as themes), or if there seemed to be language used to conceptualize benefit recipients or direct policy change (what I saw as discourses). I then queried whether these seemed to change over time, for example, one discourse replacing another. My confidence in seeing a discourse was supported if I read across the policy discourse writ large and saw any one discourse reproduced or changing in multiple documents at the level of the provincial ministry (e.g., annual reports, reports of the Social Assistance Advisory Council) and the City of Toronto municipal government.

Ethical and Editorial Decisions

The study completed was approved by the ethics board at the university where I am employed. As mentioned, voluntary consent of participants was integral to the entire recruitment process. In the chapters of the book, I preserve anonymity and confidentiality by adopting pseudonyms for caseworkers and benefit recipients. Though caseworkers referred people to me, I deliberately do not attend to the one-to-one caseworker/benefit recipient relationship, though it would have been possible to do so. This is done to protect the identity and experience of all participants.

I offer edited interview transcripts in this book. While I preserve the style of talk, including pauses, repetition of words, and change of direction in my presentation of quoted excerpts, I sometimes remove my participation in the talk. For example, I remove my side of the conversation in cases when a participant was telling a lengthier story and my contribution was primarily a sign of my active listening, for example, my use of "Hmmhmm," "I see what you mean," "Right," "Okay." I made some other choices for reasons of presentation and organization of quotes. I use ellipses "…" deliberately, to signal that conversation continues and yet I have chosen to break the flow of it for analytical purposes. There is always a risk of making such a decision, but I did my best to not lose context. My use of ellipses was mainly to remove redundant or "off topic" information. I used square brackets "[]" to add wording to clarify a sentence. Some readers may find it awkward how I sketch out the demographic backstory of benefit recipients the first time I introduce them and present quoted excerpts from their stories. I am aware that this could come across as, for example, reifying the social constructs of gender, race, and ethnicity. I had different intentions. It is important to me to name (via pseudonym) and share some backstory for each benefit recipient because I want to honour their standpoints and/or social positions and aspects of the self that they made known to me.

The editorial decisions I made culminate in the structure of this book. I chose to organize and present the experiences and stories of people accessing OW and using substances or in recovery from use as phases of a persons' total life course – up until I met them. I organized and wrote interview questions from a life course perspective, with its emphasis on individuals' experiences and perceptions of events, transitions, and trajectories. So, it is not surprising that I heard stories of becoming a substance user, of being a substance user, and of new beginnings of transcending use and mightily endeavouring to subvert the identity and stigma of "addict" and do something different or become someone else. I organize my presentation of findings according to these phases in the second part of this book, and yet spend the most time writing about the phase of being an active or recovering substance user on OW. I devote three chapters to this because, given my analysis strategies, I see an important analytical moment to compare discursive constructions of being, as through OW policy and procedure and caseworkers' application of it, as opposed to or in allegiance with individuals' actual living of everyday lives.

Inherent Biases and Limitations

The final sample of participants does suffer from bias. I met caseworkers who were invited by a program manager to consider their involvement in the study. It is possible that the caseworkers who agreed to participate were either keen on showing support for their superior or fearful of negative repercussions should they not. It is entirely reasonable to assume that caseworkers decided on which people to refer to me. I suspect that this was the case with at least two caseworkers I interviewed mainly because of how they spoke in ways that implied they had mutual trust and good rapport with some and not other benefit recipients.

My final sample of benefit recipient participants suffers from heteronormative bias. By chance, most benefit recipients I interviewed did present themselves as heterosexual through the stories they told. I also wonder if caseworkers' whiteness (with the exception of one caseworker) and the relationships they had with benefit recipients is at least partially linked to how the sample of benefit recipients I obtained over-represents the experiences of white women and men. I can only speculate whether caseworkers had caseloads that included disproportionality white individuals since "race"-based data for OW caseloads are not publicly available. I also cannot know the quality of relationships between Black, Indigenous, and people of colour (BIPOC) accessing OW and living with addiction and their caseworkers. Given the ongoing harm and violence they are exposed to in their relationships with colonial, surveying, and regulatory systems, it may be the case that some BIPOC benefit recipients do not desire a close relationship with white caseworkers. It is also possible that not all eligible BIPOC benefit recipients were asked to consider participating in the study and referred to me. In my purposive sampling, I phoned people who conveyed interest to their caseworker, knowing nothing about them except that the caseworker felt they fit my recruitment criteria. My final sample of benefit recipients is also one of convenience. Since I telephoned over twenty-five more people than my final sample size of twenty-eight, I tend to think that some caseworkers did quite forthrightly ask any eligible client to entertain participating and collected the names of those who agreed to discuss the project with me by phone. Although my sample does not lend itself to a deep critical engagement, I endeavour to attend to how I see social constructions of race to dovetail with the experiences of racialized participants living with addiction and accessing OW where possible.

Living with addiction, as I soon learned from people I interviewed, may require the deception of others with whom one is close, such as by keeping substance use secret and hidden. It can also be isolating in that a person may choose (sometimes unconsciously it seems) to avoid interactions with others, simply not have enough economic resources to enable their interactions with others, or experience mental health challenges that inhibit their interactions with others. Any of these reasons for isolation need not be mutually exclusive. Mulling over this at one point during my interviews with benefit recipients, I made an entry in my field notes under the question: "So why share with me?" Beneath I jotted my musings, which are suggestive of other potential biases in my sample. It initially seemed to me that people appeared to agree to meet for one of four different reasons. First, in seeming to believe me when I said I was not interviewing them to pass judgment on their lives, some participants approached the interview with an attitude of: "This is me. Take it or leave it." Second, some participants seemed to thrive on being a teacher. Having heard me when I shared that I do not have my own backstory of living with addiction, some participants seemed to adopt the attitude of "Ah, I will teach you what it's like" in the interview. Third, some participants seemed to genuinely have the attitude of "I will share a story that could bring about others' hope and make things different for someone else." Fourth, some participants seemed to approach the interview for therapeutic reasons. This purpose became clearest when participants shared, to roughly paraphrase, "I am still working on this/I am learning this about myself/I see now" in the interview itself. As I wrote in my fieldnotes, especially these participants seemed to use the interview as a means of "coming to terms with the self."

As time has passed and I have engaged in further reflection, I am also confident that the benefit recipients I interviewed felt a mix of being ambivalent about participating, trusting their caseworker's recommendation to participate, wanting to please their caseworker by participating, or fearing retribution from their caseworker if they did not participate (e.g., heightened surveillance or sanctioning). I also believe that I interviewed people who wanted something to do. As is made clear in chapter 6, a typical day when working on recovery and on OW, for example, can be a day with a lot of time to fill. I am also fairly sure I interviewed some people who were incentivized by the promise of a gift card and tokens. In my fieldnotes about my interview with Dante, I note how he made a joke that he could "sell the gift card to go get high." And how he laughed when I replied: "Well, yes. You can do whatever you want with the card." Dante was not alone in his thoughts. Charise further explained how drug dealers will accept gift cards but usually not at their full dollar amount; a $25 gift card given to a dealer may only get the purchaser a $20 amount of their substance of choice. It is impossible to know if Dante or Charise were incentivized to participate in the interview for these reasons. Their insights, however, shed light on the ins and outs of buying and selling in the "black market" economy of drugs on the street. During data collection and now, I recognize too, that the people I interviewed could be contacted. They owned or shared cell phones or had a land line that they had paid to access. While I have not interviewed each person I was referred to by a caseworker, there was always the possibility that I could. Potential participants, unlike others living with addiction and in low income in Toronto, had some kind of residence, even if temporary, and a consistent means of affordable communication.

Remembering the training I have received as a methodologist I can identify another final limitation of this study: the total sample is small. A non-random sample of seven caseworkers and twenty-eight client participants is not the stuff upon which generalizations can be made. The number of people I interviewed is small by comparison to larger-scale randomized quantitative study samples, and even the scope of some qualitative research. As a qualitative researcher I am familiar with how the value of sociology for policy change has been, in some circles, associated with "evidence-based" decision-making thought to be only achievable by survey results and subsequent statistics gleaned from a random sample of 1,000 people or more. On more than one occasion, I have even come to learn how in some inner academic circles there is little space for sociological research that offers the deep interpretation and intimate familiarity with a small number of participants' lives that narrative analysis can permit. By contrast, I align myself as a researcher with the more nuanced argument that a smaller sample of participants is desirable for the richness of and closeness to the data it affords, and the size of the sample understood to be largely informed by the nature of the research topic and resources (Crouch & McKenzie, 2006; Gaskell, 2000). Moreover, in narrative analysis, the assumption is that the analysis of even one story told by one person or just a few stories is methodologically worthy given the transparency of the researcher's objectives and how they achieved them (see, for example, Ahmed, 2013; Berger, 2008). It is my hope that in outlining how I approached the data here, and then presenting my findings throughout this book, the adequacy of my interview sample will be confirmed for readers. By the time I had interviewed my twenty-eighth client participant, I felt I was hearing a story with patterns that echoed the stories of many of the others I heard, though of course still reflective of the unique participant too. I assessed that further data collection would not yield any new information such as surprising behaviours or new patterns (O'Reilly & Parker, 2013). Finally, one last comment is useful, this being that critical discourse studies and narrative analysis are not meant to be used to generalize to a larger population, but rather have the purposes that I outlined earlier.

One Last Note

As I stated in the introduction of this book, I have a place of privilege in this study. I set out to hear and collect the stories some people volunteered to share with me. It is worth repeating that it is I – not the participants themselves – that have chosen to showcase their voices, to highlight their experiences and perceptions of these, in a book. Thus, I wish to make it crystal clear once again that I am telling a story too. I am telling the big story of what it is like to live with addiction while on OW as I interpret and understand it given my theoretical and methodological assumptions. Essentially, I am narrating participants' narratives. Especially benefit recipients' words about their actions, feelings, and pinnacle events or transitions in their lives are words I have audio recorded, then ordered – organized by my interpretation – and put on the page. I have tried to do so with utmost care and responsibility, to share all participants' stories in their original intent and meaning. But it goes without saying that in my analysis and in view of my own research objectives, I have made decisions. And I may have made mistakes. For example, I did not return to my participants after I analysed their transcripts to ask them to confirm the validity of my interpretations of their stories. I took the approach, as did participants who agreed to talk with me, that ours was a "one-off" meeting. Of course, for some, this will invite some valid methodological criticism. I ask readers to nonetheless hear the stories shared, especially by benefit recipients – holding and musing over them alongside what is clearly my own sense of them – as inestimable in value. No matter how presented, the stories of people living with addiction and accessing OW reveal a too-long untold part of our collective, daily lives, stories too often and too easily silenced and marginalized.

Appendix D: Benefit Recipients' Backstories and Profiles

1 = JESSE
Age 28, single man; sometimes lives with girlfriend
Caucasian (Scottish, Irish, German, English)

"Look for the man wearing the beanie hat."

Jesse was my first benefit recipient participant. He was the man in the line-up for coffee at the coffee shop where we met, wearing what I would call a pom-pom toque. I perceived him as living a hard life. He was thin, very pale (he was white) and very tall. He was patient and had a relaxed demeanour. Jesse was introduced to different drugs and experienced an escalation of his use through a new peer group. He explained that the new peer group he was exposed to was *in treatment*. At the time of the interview, Jesse was participating in Drug Treatment Court in lieu of jail time for offences associated with his drug use.

2 = SMITRI
Age 43, mother of three children in care of guardian; common law, lives with boyfriend
Mixed-race (Jamaican or Black; Caucasian)

Smitri shared "little flashbacks" – her words – to sketch out her history of use.

I met Smitri at an OW office location. She had a warm presence about her; at the time, she was finishing up her participation in Drug Treatment Court in lieu of jail time. Despite the questions I asked her, Smitri approached the interview through telling me the stories she wanted to tell most. Smitri went to the School of the Arts in Mississauga for visual arts, where she started "getting into" cannabis and doing a lot of LSD.

When she was fourteen, she was introduced to crack by a random man in the school yard. Through our interview, I learned that her beginnings of use and participation in drug trafficking began in adolescence and there were some (but not clear) articulations about the connection between her use, her experience of multiple-perpetrator sexual assault, and the related trauma.

3 = JULES
Age 28, lone mother of three children <12, two in care of others; sometimes lives with boyfriend
Caucasian (Italian, Polish)

We ended up sitting in my car to chat for the hour-long interview.

At the time of our interview together, Jules was a lone mother of three children, one who was in guardianship of her own mother; another child lived with his father, her ex-partner. She understood her past use of OxyContin to be somewhat problematic. On suboxone treatment when I met her, she did not identify as having a substance use addiction. Through her view, her use of substances was tied to her own experience of gendered trauma, specifically a miscarriage. Jules was not receiving her full income support payment from OW for reasons of alleged welfare fraud. She was in the process of appealing the charge of fraud and in extreme poverty, relying heavily on the financial support provided by her boyfriend at the time. We drove to a Shoppers Drug Mart after our interview so she could purchase some cold medication.

4 = DARLENE
Age 37, lone mother of two children <12; shares an apartment with her children; separated
Caucasian (Scottish)

I met Darlene at a downtown coffee shop on a wintry day.

Darlene was a lone mother raising a daughter and son under the age of twelve. She defined herself as in recovery and told me that her drug of choice in the past was OxyContin. She connected her escalating use of the prescription drug use to her experiences of chronic pain associated with her having been diagnosed with fibromyalgia and car accidents. She found it difficult to raise her children on her monthly income and that strategies of making ends meet were integral to their survival. CAS became involved in her mothering of her children through the behaviour of her ex-husband, and not because of her use of opioids.

5 = ARASH
Age 36, single man; has accommodation through participation in a treatment program
Middle Eastern (Iranian)

After we concluded our interview, we set off walking together towards the subway, on our way to our next and separate adventures.

Arash immigrated to Canada from Iran when he was a child with his mother, father, and sister. We met for our interview in a cafeteria on a University of Toronto campus. He identified himself as in recovery from an addiction to alcohol and cocaine. I remember Arash had a calm demeanour and mindful presence about him. I also found Arash to be deeply introspective, philosophical, and well-read in his answers. Arash looked back on his adolescence as the time in which using substances was fun and more fun than attending school. Arash had completed a prison sentence in a federal correctional centre for the crime of armed robbery. It was Arash's parole officer that referred him to OW because he had no immediate means to support himself upon release from prison.

6 = FRANCO
Age 29, single man; has accommodation through participation in a treatment program
Caucasian (Italian)

Undoubtedly, the most gracious man I interviewed.

Franco recalled events in his childhood, adolescence, and young adulthood as harrowing and productive of his suffering. After our interview, he walked me to the bus stop and waited with me for the bus, as he knew I was navigating a part of Toronto that I was less familiar with. Franco was of medium-build and about 5'7" in height. I remember his shoes, black lace-up loafers that were well worn and scuffed at the toes. I remember them because he made a point of drawing my attention to them and telling me that he had these shoes for years; purchasing new shoes was not a luxury he could easily afford on his single-person income on OW. Franco lived in a rooming house for men in treatment for substance use. He was attending a trauma counselling group when I met him for our interview. Franco was sober and defined as "in recovery" for about one year prior to the time of our meeting. Franco was certain in his drawing of a connection between his experiences of traumatic events over his life course thus far and his descent into repeated use of alcohol and crack cocaine no matter the consequences.

7 = CARIE
Age 37, single woman; shares an apartment with her good friend
Caucasian (Scottish, Irish)

She seemed to enjoy her role as "teacher" of all things related to the topic of the interview.

Carie was a gregarious single white woman. She was in methadone treatment and defined as in recovery. She lived with a roommate and did not have children, though she shared that she saw children as a future possibility at some point in her life. My interview with Carie included stories about herself and her life experiences, but she also used the interview as a way to teach me information about drug use subculture that she thought I should know, some of it disturbing in detail. Her own experiences of pain were associated with her use of prescription drugs. Carie worked for years with a moving company and so would suffer from back pain. She told about how she would not take medication for it. Once she broke her foot, however, she did eventually agree to take what she was prescribed for pain: OxyContin. She traced her addiction to OxyContin to this experience, once even living on the street when her use escalated.

8 = CLIVE
Age 55, single man; father of child <18 in care of mother; divorced; has an apartment
Caucasian (Scottish)

Clive expressed himself with candour and tongue-in-cheek humour.

Clive was a self-proclaimed alcoholic. His one daughter from a previous relationship lived with her mother after the two divorced. Even though Clive said he did not see or speak to his daughter often, his view was that they were close. Clive felt that his daughter provided him opportunities to be a father even if his fathering just meant being available to visit, to talk and listen, when she came to town. Clive seemed comfortable with his decisions and behaviours of use; he mentioned drinking a lot, especially after his divorce, but this was just one facet of his self; he was still a father too. He would drink in high school, and his school attendance gradually waned over time as a result of staying up all night to drink with friends. By the time I met Clive, he perceived that he was mainly unemployed because of pain. He had a favorite "local" (pub) in his neighbourhood.

9 = CODY
Age 36, single man; father of two children <15 in care of others; separated; lives with his father in his childhood home
Caucasian (Scottish; mixed-race ancestry)

Cody had an infectious smile.

Cody's immersion into a lifestyle where he used substances for their recreational effects (e.g., he had fun), often with peers or friends, began early. Cody seemed to embrace this way of living and began throwing raves before he was of the legal age to consume alcohol. His parents were fairly laid back about his experimentation with drugs at a young age (e.g., even making cannabis cigarettes available) as long as his use was limited to softer drugs. When we met, Cody was one year sober and defined as in recovery. It seemed the sheer youthful excitement involving a life of partying had passed by the time he was in his twenties, and following a series of events, including a break-up and loss of his child, he transitioned into using heroin. Cody was eventually sentenced to federal prison for crimes of break-and-entry theft that he committed while he perceived he was most addicted to drugs. Cody had been on and off OW over the ten years before we met. When Cody reflected more deeply on his entrance into criminal behaviour and his later federal incarceration, he saw his heroin use to be spurred on by his immense anger and frustration over losing custody of his eldest daughter to her mother.

10 = ALEXEI
Age 47, single man; father of child <18 in care of ex-wife; divorced; has an apartment
Caucasian (Russian)

Alexei had startling blue eyes and short greying hair.

Alexei wore a jogging or "leisure" suit and a gold chain around his neck. He was fit and single; he had been divorced from the mother of his children for over ten years. I learned that Alexei had immigrated to Canada from the then Soviet Union (now Russia) in his early twenties and in the early 1990s. Alexei was open and honest about his patterns of using heroin and his being in and out of treatment or pursuing sobriety at different moments in his life. As we neared the end of our interview and were discussing how his father seems to continue to support him emotionally and financially regardless of his use, I asked about his mother. He responded that she died in the Soviet Union. With discomfort, he told me that he was in the process of coming to terms with seeing the loss of his mother and the way it happened when he was an adolescent as somehow linked to his escalating use of drugs as he entered adulthood.

11 = THERESA
Age 53, single woman; mother of child >19 living alone; widowed;
has an apartment
Caucasian (British)

We met at a Tim Hortons in her neighbourhood and she was dozing off in her wheelchair when I walked in; this was a space where Theresa was known.

Theresa was the mother of a twenty-four-year-old daughter. Theresa had lost the use of her legs through her prolonged drug use in earlier years and was confined to a wheelchair. She was transparent about her daily use of alcohol. In fact, Theresa was brutally honest and blunt and used deadpan humour to tell stories about her experiences. Theresa acknowledged that her main source of physical pain each day stemmed from years of using heroin in the past. Theresa found that her attendance in group programs was not effective in her determination to change her use habits. She explained the growing appeal of her practice of harm reduction. It enabled her to develop a slow, evolving approach to managing her alcohol and cocaine use.

12 = SEASON
Age 38, lone mother of five children <19; shares an apartment with
her children
Mixed-race (Caucasian; Indigenous)

Our code word for talking about OW was "work." Season was the mother of Justice.

Season was a lone mother of six children in her care, worried about how she could pinpoint her triggers but could not seem to overcome them, observing her triggers as excuses that were harmful to herself and others. Season grappled with her mental health (she was diagnosed with PTSD) and with household poverty as a daily challenge. Season observed that even including the child support payment she received from two of her children's father, there was not enough money to help her afford shoes, clothing, or recreational activities for all six of her children. Besides caring for her kids and trying to continue to focus on recovery while sometimes randomly using, Season grappled with her experience of the child welfare foster system as an adolescent. Season had been incarcerated for two years, which became a challenge to achieving gainful employment due to having a criminal record.

13 = JUSTICE
Age 18, lone mother of infant son; shares an apartment with her mother and siblings
Mixed-race (Jamaican; Caucasian; Indigenous)

Ours was the shortest interview. Justice was the eighteen-year-old daughter of Season.

Justice was the only lone mother I interviewed who could rely on her own mother to support her caring for her infant son; her son's father was not financially supportive of her and the baby. I interviewed Justice by phone. This was the shortest interview I had and characterized by Justice's lack of talk and my perception of her as guarded. She randomly used cannabis and drank but did not define as living with addiction. Justice shared that she had already been asked to leave the family home and had been in foster care a time before being allowed to return. Despite their troubles and her mother's addiction, Season was a large source of support in her life and, by association, the life of her son.

14 = DANNI
Age 35, single woman; mother of two children <12 in care of father; has an apartment
Caucasian (Irish, Dutch, Italian)

She lived alone in an apartment on the outskirts of Toronto. She lived steps away from a beautiful walk beside Lake Ontario.

Danni was an attractive white woman but almost painfully thin. She had been on OW for two years when we met. She self-defined as clean and in recovery from a heroin and fentanyl addiction. In recovery, she smoked marijuana as needed to curb her anxiety and dampen the appetite suppressant side effect of her methadone treatment. Danni was also the mother of two young children – unfortunately she lost custody and visitation rights. The children were being raised by her ex-partner and their biological father. Danni saw her substance use to have changed her perception of her reality and was harmful to her sense of self to the extent that she was institutionalized a few times in her life. Danni's eventual escalation of use took place throughout her twenties into her thirties; she said her experiences of trauma shaped this escalation.

15 = PAT
Age 64, single woman; mother of three children >25; divorced; shares an apartment with a roommate
Caucasian (French, Ukrainian)

Pat did the quitting herself. Pat had powerful stories of strong relationships with her children, especially her one daughter.

Pat was an attractive single woman and mother of three adult children. She was in recovery and had been on methadone about twenty years. She started using street drugs and alcohol in her teenage years when she left home. She primarily left home to escape the physical abuse she received at the hands of her mother. She traced her escalating misuse of drugs to physical pain she experienced. By the time she was in her forties, she understood her use of Percocet as an addiction. Her exposure to Percocet occurred while she was incarcerated in a provincial correctional institution.

16 = JIM
Age 54, single man; has an apartment
Caucasian (English, Irish, Welsh)

At times, our interview was characterized by confrontation, Jim letting me know when I was doing a poor job of listening.

Jim had a university degree in the Sciences. His story of accessing OW was textured by what he saw as an incredibly scary time in young adulthood. Soon after convocation from university, he suffered a bout of plantar fasciitis. While he did remember his alcoholism during this time too, he applied for OW primarily because of his inability to move about and maintain employment because of pain, and how it seemed to affect his overall mental health and well-being. Jim worked hard to make me understand that I was misguided in seeing his caseworker as aware of his alcoholism and supportive of his recovery.

17 = TREVOR
Age 25, single man; has an apartment
Caucasian

Trevor had been going to college, had a girlfriend, and had an entrepreneurial spirit. And then, "all of them, boom! Dead."

For Trevor, addiction equates with loss. Trevor experienced multiple deaths in the family before I met him. At the time of our interview, he identified as being in recovery, on methadone, and on and off OW for about six years. His parents were not wealthy. He shared memories of his own suffering over the processing of these deaths and connected them to his escalating substance use. The pressure to have enough money to afford drugs was related to his shift from using OxyContin to heroin.

C18 = BIANCA
Age 43, single woman; mother of four children <19 in the care of others; separated; lives in a suite in her childhood home
Caucasian (Italian)

Bianca overcame a crack cocaine addiction to try to maintain a relationship with her children. And then used heroin. She laughed at what she saw as the absurdity of this.

Bianca defined herself as a proud Italian woman and seemingly implied her experience of addiction as a supernatural force. She was on house arrest in her parents' home as she awaited her court date when we met; she was charged with trafficking drugs with her ex-partner. Bianca had four children with her ex-partner, whom she lived with as common-law for many years. They ranged in age from thirteen to nineteen. Her nineteen-year-old son lived nearby in his own apartment. Her youngest children lived nearby, in the custody of her brothers and sisters-in-law. Bianca had been clean for over one year when we sat down to chat. She had been on OW for over twenty years. In the course of our interview, I learned that she partially traced her drug use to how being with her friends and using drugs or alcohol became more fun than going to school.

19 = DANTE
Age 44, single man; has an apartment
Black (Caribbean)

He moved agilely, talked with his hands, and "performed" others he spoke about. Dante genuinely seemed to like to laugh.

Dante was about 5′8″ in height and average in build. Dante explained that he began using substances as a young man in high school. He was a good student and often impressed his peers by getting good grades and still being able to really "party it up." Dante felt his use made him stick out in the crowd of his predominately white classmates. By the time I met him, he had spent several years using a combination of drugs, stealing to support his habit (and moving in and out of provincial jail), and engaging in paid work, mostly construction. For Dante, the self in its entirety is consumed by addiction such that the mind–body binary dissolves. It seemed a surprise to Dante that once he moved out of his parents' home and no longer had his mother's support, he could no longer maintain a balance between his substance use and the semblance of a scheduled day.

20 = ADAM
Age 27, single man; has an apartment
Caucasian

As a musician, Adam had lived a party lifestyle. We shared a good laugh about the Snoop Dogg (featuring Dr. Dre) song, "Smoke Weed Everyday," as it pertained to his past.

Adam defined as a recovering alcoholic. He had been accessing OW for one year when we met. He first used cannabis in his adolescence; he thinks likely as a coping strategy for his depression. At the time I met him, he still used but now practised harm reduction. While in his late teens and early twenties, he experimented with mushrooms, acid, and cocaine and cited MDMA as a problem for him. During this time, his use was tied to his band's performances at festivals. Adam defined primarily as a recovering alcoholic because he felt he easily gave up the drugs, like acid, but could not control his alcohol use.

21 = STEVE
Age 53, single man; has accommodation through participation in a treatment program
Caucasian

Steve liked to talk. He seemed as pleased to be ending his day of work to chat on the phone as I was to talk to him.

Steve was the only person I interviewed who had the unique experience of participating in a residential program run by the Salvation Army for persons committed to recovery. Steve worked in a laundry; taking part in the program involved his working to build employment skills and contribute to the community. Steve had led a rich life in the past, of working for pay as a high-rise window washer and living in a rented apartment. Eventually, his drinking and substance use patterns culminated in his inability to continue his work and he lost his apartment and became homeless for some time before he participated in the residential treatment program. He saw that one challenge of his participation was to continue to live in the residence for some time in order to save enough money to afford an apartment of his own.

22 = CHARISE
Age 54, single woman; mother of child >19 living with ex-husband; divorced; shares an apartment with a roommate
Caucasian (French, Hungarian)

After two failed attempts, I finally met Charise. Charise refused to cancel our interview even though I wondered if we should.

Charise lived with a friend in his apartment. She saw her addiction to crack cocaine as somehow supernaturally out of her control. Charise had applied for OW while she was in a relationship with an abusive partner. When we met, she observed that her participation in a program each week was linked to her ongoing receipt of benefits. She was in the process of working on recovery but still randomly used crack cocaine. Her adult son lived with her ex-partner, his father.

23 = TYNESHA
Age 27, single woman; mother of three children <8 in care of ex-partner; separated; has an apartment
Mixed-race (Caucasian; Trinidadian)

On a very rainy fall day, I drove to midtown Toronto to meet Tynesha at a McDonald's restaurant near to where she was living.

Tynesha had mothered three children who were currently in the custody of, and living with, their biological father and her ex-partner. Her children were removed from her care by the Children's Aid Society. Tynesha saw this as the consequence of her alcohol use but did not share the same understanding of her use as that which seemed to be shared by her ex-husband and child welfare caseworkers. She did not define her use of alcohol as an addiction but saw it as a coping strategy she used at times, such as in response to a tumultuous childhood and sexual abuse at the hands of her father as a child, and later the abuse she suffered at the hands of her ex-partner as an adult.

24 = SHAWN
Age 53, single man; father of child >19 living with his ex-wife; divorced; temporarily living in a house he is renovating
Caucasian (Scottish, English)

He wore a ball cap over his sandy brown hair, long in the back. Shawn's clothing choices especially made me think of the shared dress code of my father and his friends.

Of all participants, Shawn was perhaps the clearest in articulating a perspective on his addiction that resonated with a biomedical explanation. He was a white man with a slim build. When we discussed his first memories of substance use, we also talked about his experiences growing up in his middle-class family of origin. Shawn was still randomly using heroin when I interviewed him. He recognized that others, specifically his caseworker for OW, saw his use as problematic. Shawn, however, seemed ambivalent about it and fairly satisfied with his ability to make ends meet through his receipt of OW and his casual employment as a handyperson.

25 = ANAIS
Age 28, single woman; shares an apartment with roommates
Mixed-race (Indigenous; Caucasian, Scottish)

Anais had straight brown hair to her waist and big brown eyes. I drove her home when our interview was over.

Anais quit her use of prescription opioids on her own "cold turkey." She defined as in recovery and had participated in a methadone treatment program for a short period of time before I met her. She had moved to Toronto in the last year and applied for OW because she was unemployed. Anais was in the process of taking next steps towards pursuing post-secondary education and had an OW caseworker who encouraged her to think about possible funding opportunities if she also pursued an application for a Status Card given her Indigenous heritage.

26 = ADRIENNE
Age 33, lone mother with partial custody of 17-year-old; shares an apartment with her son, her partner and son's father living elsewhere
Caucasian

Her apartment was spacious and had an incredibly comfortable couch that we both sank into as we chatted. Her son and partner were in and out of the room during our interview.

Adrienne saw addiction as all consuming. She was a lone mother with a seventeen-year-old son and was sober nine months when I met her at her home. She was actively pursuing recovery from an opioid addiction with a suboxone treatment program and one-on-one counselling. When we spoke about her adolescence, she shared about an earlier experience of miscarriage as a profoundly frightening time. She connected this event with her subsequent substance use.

27 = MARNIE
Age 33, lone mother of child <5; lives with her child and her parents in her childhood home
Caucasian (Irish, Scottish)

Marnie had just finished working out at a local gym and had already even bought a coffee by the time I met her in the coffee shop.

Marnie was a lone mother of a four-year-old child. She was a recovering cocaine user and was in a suboxone treatment program. She had been clean in the last year and a bit that she had been on OW. Marnie had been admitted into an institutional detox program and while housed there, a caseworker doing outreach referred her to OW. Marie was raising her young daughter with the support of her parents and even lived in their home. Marnie's perception of herself as defined by more than her past addiction was not always shared by caseworkers.

28 = TARA
Age 53, single woman; mother of three children; two < 19 in care of ex-husband; divorced; has an apartment
Caucasian (Irish)

In talking with Tara, I felt like I was talking to an intimate and much older family member.

Tara was the mother of twin daughters who were in the care of her ex-partner. Her eldest daughter lived on her own. Tara had revisited changing her patterns of crack cocaine use several times and was sober by the time of our interview. Tara, however, was clear that she engaged in harm reduction as part of a process of recovery. Tara was pursuing further change in her life by attending a bridging program at a local college. Tara understood addiction as producing a loss of the self, a hollowing out that inhibits some identities beyond that of addict.

References

Adjei, P. B., Mullings, D., Baffoe, M., Quaicoe, L., Latif, A. Shears, V., & Fitzgerald, S. (2017). The "fragility of goodness": Black parents' perspectives about raising children in Toronto, Winnipeg, and St. John's of Canada. *Journal of Public Child Welfare, 12*(4), 461–91. https://doi.org/10.1080/15548 732.2017.1401575

Adrian, M., & Barry, S. (2003). Physical and mental health problems associated with the use of alcohol and drugs. *Substance Use & Misuse, 38*(11–13), 1575–1614. https://doi.org/10.1081/ja-120024230.

Agger, B. (1991). Critical theory, poststructuralism, postmodernism: Their sociological relevance. *Annual Review of Sociology, 17*(1), 105–31. https://doi .org/10.1146/annurev.so.17.080191.000541

Ahmed, A. (2013). Structural narrative analysis: Understanding experiences of lifestyle migration through two plot typologies. *Qualitative Inquiry, 19*(30), 232–42. https://doi.org/10.1177/1077800412466050

Aldridge, H. (2017). *What does the data tell us about rising income inequality in Canada?* Maytree. https://maytree.com/wp-content/uploads/What-does -the-data-tell-us-about-rising-poverty-in-Canada.pdf

American Addiction Centres. (2019). History of American substance abuse treatment centres. *American Addiction Centres.* https://americanaddictioncenters .org/learn/us-trends-addiction-treatment/

American Psychiatric Association. (2013). *Diagnostic and statistical manual of mental disorders.* American Psychiatric Association.

Anderssen, E. (2017, December 11). Most mental health patients don't get timely psychiatric care in Ontario, study finds. *The Globe and Mail.* https:// www.theglobeandmail.com/news/national/most-mental-health-patients -dont-get-timely-psychiatric-care-in-ontario-study-finds/article37285740/

Anthony, W. (1993). Recovery from mental illness: The guiding vision of the mental health service system in the 1990's. *Psychosocial Rehabilitation Journal, 16*, 11–23. https://doi.org/10.1037/h0095655

Atkinson, A.B. (1999). The contributions of Amartya Sen to welfare economics. *Scandinavian Journal of Economics, 101*(2), 173–90. https://doi.org/10.1111/1467-9442.00151

Augsberger, A., & Swenson, E. (2015). "My worker was there when it really mattered": Foster care youths' perceptions and experiences of their relationships with child welfare workers. *Families in Society: The Journal of Contemporary Social Services, 96*(4), 234–40. https://doi.org/10.1606/1044-3894.2015.96.34

Back, L. (2015). Blind pessimism and the sociology of hope. *Discover Society* (27). https://discoversociety.org/2015/12/01/blind-pessimism-and-the-sociology-of-hope/

Baert, P., Weinberg, D., & Mottier, V. (2011). Social Constructionism, postmodernism and deconstructionism. In I. C. Jarvie & B. J. P. Zamora (Eds.), *The SAGE handbook of the philosophy of social sciences* (pp. 475–86). Sage.

Baker, M., & Tippin, D. (1999). *Poverty, social assistance, and the employability of mothers: Restructuring welfare states.* University of Toronto Press.

Baker Collins, S. (2016). Value discretion in a people-changing environment: Taking the long view. *Journal of Sociology & Social Welfare, 43*(2), Article 5. https://scholarworks.wmich.edu/jssw/vol43/iss2/5

Baker Collins, S., Smith-Carrier, T., Gazso, A., & Smith, C. (2020). Resisting the culture of poverty narrative: Perspectives of social assistance recipients. *Journal of Poverty, 24*(1), 72–93. https://doi.org/10.1080/10875549.2019.1678551.(on-line 2019).

Bamberg, M. (2013). Identity and narration. In P. Hühn (Ed.), *The living handbook of narratology.* Hamburg University.

Bamberg, M., & Georgakopoulou, A. (2008). Small stories as a new perspective in narrative and identity analysis. *Text & Talk, 28*, 377–96. https://doi.org/10.1515/TEXT.2008.018

Barret, B.J., & St. Pierre, M. (2011). Variations in women's help-seeking behaviours in response to intimate partner violence: Findings from a Canadian-based population study. *Violence Against Women, 17*(1), 47–70. https://doi.org/10.1177/1077801210394273

Bartram, M. (2021). 'It's really about wellbeing': A Canadian investigation of harm reduction as a bridge between mental health and addiction recovery. *International Journal of Mental Health and Addiction, 19*, 1497–1510. https://doi.org/10.1007/s11469-020-00239-7

Battle, K., & Torjman, S. (1989). *How finance re-formed social policy.* The Caledon Institute of Social Policy. https://maytree.com/wp-content/uploads/474ENG.pdf.

Battle, K., & Torjman, S. (1995). How finance re-formed social policy. In D. Drache & A. Ranachan. (Eds.), *Warm heart, cold country: Fiscal and social policy reform in Canada* (pp. 407–41). Caledon Institute of Social Policy.

Bauld, L., McKell, J., Carroll, C., Hay, G., & Smith, K. (2012). Benefits and employment: How problem drug users experience welfare and routes into work. *Journal of Social Policy, 41*(4), 751–68. https://doi.org/10.1017/S004727941200030X

Bauman, Z. (2004). *Work, consumerism and the new poor.* Open University Press.

Bauman, Z. (2007). *Liquid times.* Polity Press.

Beck, U. (2007). Beyond class and nation: Reframing social inequalities in a globalizing world. *The British Journal of Sociology, 58*(4), 679–705. https://doi.org/10.1111/j.1468-4446.2007.00171.x

Beck, U., & Beck-Gernsheim, E. (1995). *The normal chaos of love.* Polity Press.

Beck, U., Giddens, A., & Lash, S. (1994). *Reflexive modernization: Politics, tradition and aesthetics in the modern social order.* Stanford University Press.

Becker, H.S. (1953). Becoming a marihuana user. *American Journal of Sociology, 59,* 235–42. https://doi.org/10.1086/221326

Becker, H.S. (1955). Marihuana use and social control. In A. M. Rose (Ed.,) *Human behavior and social processes: An interactionist approach.* (pp. 589–607). Houghton Mifflin.

Becker, H.S. (1963). *Outsider: Studies in the sociology of deviance.* The Free Press of Glencoe.

Béland, D., & Daigneault, P-M. Eds. (2015). *Welfare reform in Canada: Provincial social assistance in comparative perspective.* University of Toronto Press.

Belzak, L., & Halverson, J. (2018). Evidence synthesis–The opioid crisis in Canada: A national perspective. *Health Promotion and Chronic Disease Prevention in Canada, 38*(6), 224–33. https://doi.org/10.24095/hpcdp.38.6.02

Benbow, S., Gorlick, C., Forchuk, C., Ward-Griffin, C., & Berman, H. (2016). Ontario's poverty reduction strategy: A critical discourse analysis. *Canadian Journal of Nursing Research, 48,* 100–9. https://doi.org/10.1177/0844562116684729

Bendle, M.F. (1999). The death of the sociology of deviance? *Journal of Sociology, 35*(1), 42–59. https://doi.org/10.1177/144078339903500103

Benoit, C., Carroll, D., & Chaudhry, M. (2003). In search of a healing place: Aboriginal women in Vancouver's downtown eastside. *Social Science & Medicine, 56*(4), 821–33. https://doi.org/10.1016/S0277-9536(02)00081-3

Benoit, C., & Magnus, S. (2017). "Depends on the father": Defining problematic paternal substance use during pregnancy and early parenthood. *Canadian Journal of Sociology, 42*(4), 379–402. https://doi.org/10.1186/s12939-015-0206-7

Benoit, C., Magnus, S., Phillips, R., Marcellus, L., & Charbonneau, S. (2015). Complicating the dominant morality discourse: Mothers and fathers' constructions of substance use during pregnancy and early parenthood.

International Journal for Equity in Health, 14, 72. https://doi.org/10.1186 /s12939-015-0206-7

Berger, P.L., & Luckmann, T. (1966). *The social construction of reality: A treatise in the sociology of knowledge.* Doubleday.

Berger, R.J. (2008). Agency, structure, and the transition to disability: A case study with implications for life history research. *The Sociological Quarterly, 49*(2), 309–33. https://doi.org/10.1111/j.1533-8525.2008.00117.x

Bezanson, K. (2006). *Gender, the state, and social reproduction: Household insecurity in neo- liberal times.* University of Toronto Press.

Bischoping, K., & Gazso, A. (2016). *Analyzing talk in the social sciences: Narrative, conversation & discourse strategies.* Sage.

Bloch, E. (1954). *The principle of hope: Volume 1.* MIT Press.

Bogna, F., Raineri, A., & Dell, G. (2020). Critical realism and constructivism: Merging research paradigms for a deeper qualitative study. *Qualitative Research in Organizations and Management: An International Journal, 15*(4), 461–84. https://doi.org/10.1108/QROM-06-2019-1778

Bolhaar, J., Ketel, N., & van, der Klaauw, B. (2020). Caseworker's discretion and the effectiveness of welfare-to-work programs. *Journal of Public Economics, 183,* 14080. https://doi.org/10.1016/j.jpubeco.2019.104080

Boucher, A. (2013). Familialism and migrant welfare policy: Restrictions on social security provision for newly-arrived immigrants. *Policy and Politics, 42*(3), 367–84. https://doi.org/10.1332/030557312X655602

Bourgois, P. (2000). Disciplining addictions: The bio-politics of methadone and heroin in the United States. *Culture, Medicine, and Psychiatry, 24*(2),165–95. https://doi.org/10.1023/A:1005574918294

Boychuk, G. (1998). *Patchworks of purpose: The development of provincial social assistance regimes in Canada.* McGill-Queen's University Press.

Boychuk, G.W. (2015). Federal policies, national trends, and provincial systems: A comparative analysis of recent developments in social assistance in Canada 1999-2013. In D. Béland and P. M. Daigneault. (Eds.), *Welfare reform in Canada: Provincial social assistance in comparative perspective.* (pp. 35–52). University of Toronto Press.

Boyd, S. (1999). *Mothers and illicit drugs: Transcending the myths.* University of Toronto Press.

Boyd, S., & MacPherson, D. (2018/19). Community engagement – The harms of drug prohibition: Ongoing resistance in Vancouver's downtown eastside. *BC Studies* 200, 87–96. https://doi.org/10.14288/bcs.v0i200 .191462

Bradburn, J. (2015, June 8). Electing Mike Harris: Twenty years ago today, Ontario voted in one of its most controversial governments. *The Torontoist.* http://torontoist.com/2015/06/electing-mike-harris/

Breitkreuz, R., Williamson, D., & Raine, K. (2010). Dis-integrated policy: Welfare-to-work participants' experiences of integrating paid work and unpaid family work. *Community, Work & Family, 13*(1), 43–69. https://doi.org/10.1080/13668800902923753

Brettell, C.B. (2002). Gendered lives: Transitions and turning points in personal, family, and historical time. *Current Anthropology (Chicago), 43,* S45–S61. https://doi.org/10.1086/339565

Broad, D., & Antony, W. (1999). *Citizens or consumers? Social policy in a market society.* Fernwood Publishing.

Broadbent Institute. (2012). Towards a more equal Canada: A report on Canada's economic and social security. https://assets.nationbuilder.com/broadbent/pages/7723/attachments/original/1592496641/towards_a_more_equal_canada.pdf?1592496641

Brodie, J. (1997). Meso-discourses, state forms and the gendering of liberal-democratic citizenship. *Citizenship Studies, 1*(2), 223–42. https://doi.org/10.1080/13621029708420656

Brodie, J. (2002). Citizenship and solidarity: Reflections on the Canadian way. *Citizenship Studies, 6*(4), 377–94. https://doi.org/10.1080/1362102022000041231

Brodie, J. (2008). The social in social citizenship. In E. F. Isin (Ed.), *Recasting the social in citizenship* (pp. 20–43). University of Toronto Press.

Brodie, Janine. (2007). The new social "isms": Individualization and social policy reform in canada. In C. Howard (Ed.), *Contested individualization: Debates about contemporary personhood* (pp. 153–69). Pagrave Macmillan.

Brooks, D. (2019). Winning the war on poverty: The Canadians are doing it: We're not. *The New York Times.* https://www.nytimes.com/2019/04/04/opinion/canada-poverty-record.html

Bryant, J., & Ellard, J. (2015). Hope as a form of agency in the future thinking of disenfranchised young people. *Journal of Youth Studies, 18*(4), 485–99. https://doi.org/10.1080/13676261.2014.992310

Buchman, D. Z., Reiner, P. B., & Illes, J. (2011). The paradox of addiction neuroscience. *Neuroethics, 4*(2), 65–77. https://doi.org/10.1007/s12152-010-9079-z

Buchman, D. Z., Skinner, W., & Illes, J. (2010). Negotiating the relationship between addiction, ethics, and brain science. *AJOB Neuroscience, 1*(1), 36–45. https://doi.org/10.1080/21507740903508609

Bungay, V., Johnson, J.L., Varcoe, C., & Boyd, S. (2010). Women's health and use of crack cocaine in context: Structural and 'everyday' violence. *International Journal of Drug Policy, 21*(4), 321–9. https://doi.org/10.1016/j.drugpo.2009.12.008

Bush, I.R., & Kraft, K.M. (2001). Self-sufficiency and sobriety. Substance-abusing women and welfare reform. *Journal of Social Work Practice in the Addictions, 1*(1), 41–64. https://doi.org/10.1300/J160v01n01_05

Calnitsky, D. (2016). "More normal than welfare": The Mincome experiment, stigma, and community experience. *Canadian Review of Sociology/Revue Canadienne De Sociologie, 53*(1), 26–71. https://doi.org/10.1111/cars.12091

CAMH (2020). *Addiction.* https://www.camh.ca/en/health-info/mental-illness-and-addiction-index/addiction

Campbell, N.D. (2010). Toward a critical neuroscience of 'addiction'. *Biosocieties, 5*(1), 89–104. https://doi.org/10.1057/biosoc.2009.2

Canada. (1994a). *The context of reform: A supplementary paper.* Ministry of Supply and Services. Government of Canada.

Canadian Mental Health Association. (2021). *Substance use and addiction.* Canadian Mental Health Association. https://ontario.cmha.ca/addiction-and-substance-use-and-addiction/

Canadian Centre on Substance Use and Addiction. (2020). Impacts of the COVID-19 pandemic on people who use substances: What we heard. https://ccsa.ca/impacts-covid-19-pandemic-people-who-use-substances-what-we-heard

CBC News (2020, January 8). Cancellation of basic income pilot 'devastating': Lakehead researcher says. *CBC News.* https://www.cbc.ca/news/canada/thunder-bay/basic-income-research-1.5418728

CBC News. (2017, August 30). Young Canadians struggling to access mental health services: study. https://www.ctvnews.ca/health/young-canadians-struggling-to-access-mental-health-services-study-1.3568988

CBC Radio. (25 April 2017). *The Current.* https://www.cbc.ca/radio/thecurrent/the-current-for-april-25-2017-1.4083138/april-25-2017-full-episode-transcript-1.4085470

Centre for Addiction and Mental Health (CAMH). 2023. Fundamentals of addiction: Key concepts in addiction. https://www.camh.ca/en/professionals/treating-conditions-and-disorders/fundamentals-of-addiction/f--of--addiction---key-concepts-in-addiction

Chapple, A., Ziebland, S., & Hawton, K. (2015). Taboo and the different death? Perceptions of those bereaved by suicide or other traumatic death. *Sociology of Health & Illness, 37*(4), 610–25. https://doi.org/10.1111/1467-9566.12224

Cheetham, A., Allen, N.B., Yücel, M., & Lubman, D. I. (2010). The role of affective dysregulation in drug addiction. *Clinical Psychology Review, 30*(6), 621–34. https://doi.org/10.1016/j.cpr.2010.04.005

Choo, H. Y., & Myra Max Ferree, M.M. (2010). Practicing intersectionality in sociological research: A critical analysis of inclusions, interactions, and institutions in the study of inequalities. *Sociological Theory*, *28*(2), 129–49. https://doi.org/10.1111/j.1467-9558.2010.01370.x

Christopher, K. (2012). Extensive mothering: Employed mothers' constructions of the good mother. *Gender & Society*, *26*(1), 73–96. https://doi.org/10.1177/0891243211427700

Citizens for Public Justice. (2018). *Poverty trends 2018*. https://cpj.ca/wp-content/uploads/Poverty-Trends-Report-2018.pdf

City of Toronto. (2023). *Monthly Ontario Works amounts*. https://www.toronto.ca/community-people/employment-social-support/employment-support/employment-seekers-in-financial-need/ontario-works-rates/

City of Toronto. (2012). *Working as one: A workforce development strategy for Toronto*. Economic Development Committee. https://www.toronto.ca/legdocs/mmis/2012/ed/bgrd/backgroundfile-45320.pdf

City of Toronto. (2015). *Operating budget overview*. Toronto Employment and Social Services. https://www.toronto.ca/legdocs/mmis/2015/ex/bgrd/backgroundfile-77441.pdf

City of Toronto. (2016a). *Toronto poverty reduction strategy: Year 1 report to community*. https://www.toronto.ca/wp-content/uploads/2017/11/97da-Toronto-Poverty-Reduction-Strategy-Year-One-Report-backgroundfile-98562.pdf

City of Toronto. (2016b). *Workforce development annual report*. Toronto Employment and Social Services. https://www.toronto.ca/legdocs/mmis/2017/ed/bgrd/backgroundfile-102726.pdf

City of Toronto. (2017a). *16- & 17-year old's*. https://www.toronto.ca/community-people/employment-social-support/support-for-people-in-financial-need/assistance-through-ontario-works/policies-and-procedures/16–17-year-olds/

City of Toronto. (2017b). *Meeting many needs: Advancing Toronto's workforce development and poverty reduction strategies annual report*. Toronto Employment and Social Services. https://www.toronto.ca/legdocs/mmis/2018/ed/bgrd/backgroundfile-114676.pdf

City of Toronto. (2018). *Annual report: Making a difference by making connections annual report*. Toronto Employment and Social Services. https://www.toronto.ca/wp-content/uploads/2019/07/99a9-tess-annual-report-2018.pdf

City of Toronto. (2020). *Monthly Ontario Works amounts*. https://www.toronto.ca/community-people/employment-social-support/employment-support/employment-seekers-in-financial-need/ontario-works-rates/

Clarke, J. (2011). The challenges of child welfare involvement for Afro-Caribbean families in Toronto. *Children and Youth Services Review*, *33*(2), 274–83. https://doi.org/10.1016/j.childyouth.2010.09.010

Cleck, J.N., & Blendy, J.A. (2008). Making a bad thing worse: Adverse effects of stress on addiction. *The Journal of Clinical Investigation, 118,* 454–61. https://doi.org/10.1172/JCI33946

Collins, A.B., Strike, C., Guta, A., Turje, R.B., McDougall, P., Parashar, S., McNeil, R. (2017). "We're giving you something so we get something in return": Perspectives on research participation and compensation among people living with HIV who use drugs. *International Journal of Drug Policy, 39,* 92–8. https://doi.org/10.1016/j.drugpo.2016.09.004

Comas-Diaz, L., Hall, G.N., & Neville, H.A. (2019). Racial trauma: Theory, research, and healing. Introduction to the special issue. *American Psychologist, 74*(1), 1–5. https://doi.org/10.1037/amp0000442

Community Development Halton. (1998). *The social assistance reform act: An information package.* https://cdhalton.ca/1998/12/05/social-assistance-reform-act-an-information-package/

Connell, R. (1987). *Gender and power: Society, the person, and sexual politics.* Stanford University Press.

Connidis, I. A. (2001). *Family ties and aging.* Sage.

Coulter, K. (2009). Women, poverty policy, and the production of neoliberal politics in Ontario, Canada. *Journal of Women, Politics and Policy, 30*(1), 23–45. https://doi.org/10.1080/15544770802367788

Crawley, M. (2018). Welfare reform is the Ford government's next big project. CBC News. https://www.cbc.ca/news/canada/toronto/doug-ford-welfare-social-assistance-ontario-works-odsp-1.4885584

Crouch, M., & McKenzie, H. (2006). The logic of small samples in interview-based qualitative research. *Social Science Information, 45*(4), 483–99. https://doi.org/10.1177/0539018406069584

Cruickshank, J. (2003). *Critical realism: The difference it makes.* Routledge.

Culhane, D. (2003). Their spirits live within us: Aboriginal women in downtown eastside vancouver emerging into visibility. *American Indian Quarterly, 27*(3/4), 593–606. https://doi.org/10.1353/aiq.2004.0073

Curcio, G., & Pattavina, A. (2018). Still paying for the past: Examining gender differences in employment among individuals with a criminal record, *Women & Criminal Justice, 28*(5), 375–96. https://doi.org/10.1080/08974454.2018.1441773

Daily Bread Food Bank. (2017). *Who's hungry? 2017 profile of hunger in Toronto.* Daily Bread Food Bank. https://www.homelesshub.ca/sites/default/files/attachments/Whos-Hungry-2017.pdf

Danziger, S.K., Corcoran, M., Danziger, S., & Heflin, C. (2000). Work, income, and material hardship after welfare reform. *The Journal of Consumer Affairs, 34*(3), 6–30. https://doi.org/10.1111/j.1745-6606.2000.tb00081.x

Daoud, N., Matheson, F., Pedersen, C., Hamilton-Wright, S., Minh, A., Zhang, J., & O'Campo, P. (2016). Pathways and trajectories linking housing instability and poor health among low-income women experiencing intimate partner violence (IPV): Toward a conceptual framework. *Women & Health, 56*(2), 208–25. https://doi.org/10.1080/0363 0242.2015.1086465

Dassieu, L., Kaboré, J.-L., Choinière, M., Arruda, N., & Roy, E. (2020). Painful lives: Chronic pain experience among people who use illicit drugs in Montreal (Canada). *Social Science & Medicine, 246*, 112734, 1–8. https://doi.org/10.1016/j.socscimed.2019.112734

Dawson, M. (2012). Reviewing the critique of individualization: The disembedded and embedded theses. *Acta Sociologica, 55*(4), 305–19. https://doi.org/10.1177/0001699312447634

Deegan, P. (1996). Recovery as a journey of the heart. *Psychiatric Rehabilitation Journal, 19*. https://doi.org/10.1037/h0101301

deGroot-Magetti, G., & Blackstock, S. (2009). Activists strengthen anti-poverty legislation. *Toronto Star, Opinion.* https://www.thestar.com/opinion/2009/05/07/activists_strengthen_antipoverty_legislation.html

DeKeseredy, W.S., Schwartz, M.D., Alvi, S., & Tomaszewski, E.A. (2003a). Crime victimization, alcohol consumption, and drug use in Canadian public housing. *Journal of Criminal Justice, 31*(4), 383–96. https://doi.org/10.1016/S0047-2352(03)00031-X

DeKeseredy, W.S., Schwartz, M.D., Alvi, S., & Tomaszewski, E. A. (2003b). *Under siege: Crime in a public housing community.* Lexington Books.

Dennis, F. (2016). Encountering triggers: Drug-body-world entanglements of injecting drug use. *Contemporary Drug Problems, 43*(3), 126–41. https://doi.org/10.1177/0091450916636379

Dennis, F. (2017). The injecting 'event': Harm reduction beyond the human. *Critical Public Health, 27*(3), 337–49. https://doi.org/10.1080/09581596.2017.1294245

Dennis, F. (2019). *Injecting bodies in more-than-human worlds.* Routledge.

Denzin, N. K., & Lincoln, Y. S. (2012). *The landscape of qualitative research* (4th ed.). Sage.

Desroche, H. (1979). *The sociology of hope.* Routledge and Kegan Paul.

Devault, M.L. (2004). Talking and listening from women's standpoint: Feminist strategies for interviewing and analysis. In S. N. Hesse-Biber, P. Leavy, & M.L. Yaiser (Eds.), *Feminist perspectives on social research* (pp. 227–50). Oxford University Press.

Dewilde, C. (2003). A life-course perspective on social exclusion and poverty. *The British Journal of Sociology, 54*(1), 109–28. https://doi.org/10.1080/0007131032000045923

Dobrowolsky, A., & Jenson, J. (2004). Shifting representations of citizenship: Canadian politics of "women" and "children". *Social Politics, 11*(2), 154–80. https://doi.org/10.1093/sp/jxh031

Dodge, R., Daly, A., Huyton, J., & Sanders, L. (2012). The challenge of defining wellbeing. *International Journal of Wellbeing*, 2(3), 222–35. https://doi.org/10.5502/ijw.v2i3.4

Dohan, D., Schmidt, L., & Henderson, S. (2005). From enabling to bootstrapping: Welfare workers' views of substance abuse and welfare reform. *Contemporary Drug Problems*, 32(3), 429–56. https://doi.org/10.1177/009145090503200306

Doucet, A., & Mauthner, N. (2002). Knowing responsibly: Ethics, feminist epistemologies and methodologies. In M. Mauthner, M. Birch, J. Jessop and T. Miller. (Eds.), *Ethics in qualitative research.* (pp. 123–45). Sage.

D'Sylva, F., Graffam, J., Hardcastle, L., & Shinkfield, A.J. (2012). Analysis of the stages of change model of drug and alcohol treatment readiness among prisoners. *International Journal of Offender Therapy and Comparative Criminology*, 56(2), 265–80. https://doi.org/10.1177/0306624X10392531

Duclos, Y.-J., Tiberti, L., & Araar, A. (2018). Multidimensional poverty targeting. *Economic Development and Cultural Change*, 66(3), 519–54. https://doi.org/10.1086/696105

Dufault, K.J., & Marocchio, B. (1995). Hope: It's spheres and dimensions. *The Nursing Clinics of North American*, 20(2), 379–91. https://doi.org/10.1016/S0029-6465(22)00328-0

Duff, C. (2008). The pleasure in context. *The International Journal on Drug Policy*, 19(5), 384–92. https://doi.org/10.1016/j.drugpo.2007.07.003

Duff, C., Asbridge, M., Brochu, S., Cousineau, M.M., Hathaway, A.D., Marsh, D., & Erickson, P. G. (2012). A Canadian perspective on cannabis normalization among adults. *Addiction Research and Theory*, 20(4), 271–83. https://doi.org/10.3109/16066359.2011.618957

Durrani, T. (2020). Low-income Ontarians facing partial claw back of federal assistance during COVID-19. *Healthy Debate*. https://healthydebate.ca/2020/04/topic/ontario-low-income-cerb-covid

Dwyer, P. (2002). Making sense of social citizenship: Some user views on welfare rights and responsibilities. *Critical Social Policy*, 22(2), 273–99. https://doi.org/10.1177/02610183020220020601

Eichler, M. (1997). *Family shifts: Families, policies, and gender equality.* Oxford University Press.

Elder, G. H. (1994). Time, human agency, and social change: Perspectives on the life course. *Social Psychology Quarterly*, 57(1), 4–15. https://doi.org/10.2307/2786971

Employment and Social Development Canada. (2021). *Understanding systems: The 2021 report of the national advisory council on poverty.* https://www.canada.ca/content/dam/esdc-edsc/documents/programs/poverty-reduction/national-advisory-council/reports/2021-annual/advisory-council-poverty-2021-annual(new).pdf

Erickson, P.G., & Callaghan, R.C. (2005). The probable impacts of the removal of the addiction disability benefit in Ontario. *Canadian Journal of Community Mental Health = Revue Canadienne De Santé Mentale Communautaire, 24*(2), 99–108. https://doi.org/10.7870/cjcmh-2005-0017

Fairclough, N. (1992). *Discourse and social change.* Polity.

Fairclough, N., & Wodak, R. (1997). Critical discourse analysis. In T. A. van Dijk (Ed.), *Discourse studies: A multidisciplinary introduction, Vol. 2, Discourse as social interaction* (pp. 258–84). Sage.

Fallding, H. (1981). The sociology of hope [Review of *The Sociology of Hope* by H. Desroche]. *The Canadian Journal of Sociology, 6*(2), 209–11. https://doi.org/10.2307/3340090

Farley, L. (2009). Radical hope: Or, the problem of uncertainty in history education. *Curriculum Inquiry, 39*(4), 537–54. https://doi.org/10.1111/j.1467-873X.2009.00456.x

Farran, C.J., & Popovich, J. (1990). Hope: A relevant concept for geriatric psychiatry. *Archives of Pyschiatric Nursing, 4*(2), 124–30. https://doi.org/10.1016/0883-9417(90)90019-H

Faupel, C.E., Horowitz, A.M., Weaver, G., & Corzine, J. (2013). *The sociology of American drug use* (3rd ed.). Oxford University Press.

Fernández-González Liria, Esther, C., & Erika, B. (2019). Women victims of intimate partner violence in shelters: Correlates of length of stay and subsequent re-entries. *Violence Against Women, 25*(12), 1433–49. https://doi.org/10.1177/1077801218821445

Figley, C.R. (Ed.). (1985). *Trauma and its wake, volume 1: The study and treatment of post-traumatic stress disorder.* Brunner/Mazel.

Filkow, A. (2020, Spring). Seeking hope. *New Trail, University of Alberta Alumni Magazine,* 29–38.

Folkman, S. (2010). Stress, coping, and hope. *Psycho-oncology, 19*(9), 901–8. https://doi.org/10.1002/pon.1836

Foucault, M. (1973/1994). *The birth of the clinic: An archaeology of medical perception.* Tavistock.

Foucault, M. (1977). *Discipline and punish: The birth of the prison.* Pantheon.

Foucault, M. (1978). *The history of sexuality. Vol. 1: An introduction* (R. Hurley, Trans.). Vintage Books.

Fraser, S., Pienaar, K., Dilkes-Frayne, E., Moore, D., Kokanovic, R., Treloar, C., & Dunlop, A. (2017). Addiction stigma and the biopolitics of liberal modernity: A qualitative analysis. *International Journal of Drug Policy, 44,* 192–201. https://doi.org/10.1016/j.drugpo.2017.02.005

Frings, D., Wood, K. V., Lionetti, N., & Albery, I. P. (2019). Tales of hope: Social identity and learning lessons from others in Alcoholics Anonymous: A test of the social identity model of cessation maintenance. *Addictive Behaviors, 93,* 204–11. https://doi.org/10.1016/j.addbeh.2019.02.004

Funk, L., & Kobayashi, K. (2016). From motivations to accounts: An interpretive analysis of "living apart together" relationships in mid-to later-life couples. *Journal of Family Issues, 37*(8), 1101–22. https://doi.org/10.1177/0192513X14529432

Garrett, P.M. (2018). *Welfare words: Critical social work & social policy.* Sage.

Gaskell, G. (2000). Individual and group interviewing. In M. Bauer & G. Gaskell (Eds). *Qualitative researching with text, image and sound* (pp. 38–56). Sage.

Gazso, A. (2006). *Gendering the responsible risk taker: Social assistance reform and parents' citizenship, market and family care relations in three western provinces* [Unpublished PhD dissertation].

Gazso, A. (2007a). Staying afloat on social assistance: Parents' strategies of balancing work and family. *Socialist Studies, 3*(2), 31–63. https://doi.org/10.18740/S4F018

Gazso, A. (2007b). Balancing expectations for employability and family responsibilities while on social assistance: Low income mothers' experiences in three Canadian provinces. *Family Relations, 56*(5), 454–66. https://doi.org/10.1111/j.1741-3729.2007.00473.x

Gazso, A. (2009). Gendering the 'responsible risk taker': Citizenship relationships with gender-neutral social assistance policy. *Citizenship Studies, 13*(1), 45–63. https://doi.org/10.1080/13621020802586743

Gazso, A. (2012). Moral codes of mothering and the introduction of welfare-to-work in Ontario. *Canadian Review of Sociology, 49*(1), 26–49. https://doi.org/ DOI: 10.1111/j.1755-618x.2011.01279.x

Gazso, A. (2019). Dueling discourses, power, and the construction of the recovering addict: When social assistance confronts addiction in Toronto, Canada. *Critical Social Policy, 40*(1), 130–50. https://doi.org/10.1177/0261018319839158

Gazso, A. (2023). Managing more than poverty when living with addiction: Parents' emotion and identity work. *Journal of Family Issues, 44*(1) . https://doi.org/10.1177/0192513X211041981

Gazso, A., Baker, C. S., Smith-Carrier, T., & Smith, C. (2019). The generationing of social assistance receipt and "welfare dependency" in Ontario, Canada. *Social Problems, 67*(3), 585–601. https://doi.org/10.1093/socpro/spz032

Gazso, A., & Bischoping, K. (2018). Feminist reflections on the relation of emotions to ethics: A case study of two awkward interviewing moments." *Forum Qualitative Social Research* 19(3). https://dx.doi.org/10.17169/fqs-19.3.3118

Gazso, A., & McDaniel, S. (2010/2011). The great west 'experiment': Neo-liberal convergence and transformations in citizenship in Canada. *Canadian Review of Social Policy, 63/64*, 15–35.

Gazso, A., McDaniel, S., & Waldron, I. (2016). Networks of social support to manage poverty: More changeable than durable. *Journal of Poverty, 20*(4), 441–63. https://doi.org/10.1080/10875549.2015.1112869

Gazso, A. & McDaniel, S. (2015). Families by choice and the management of low income through social supports. *Journal of Family Issues, 36*(3), 371–95. https://doi.org/10.1177/0192513X13506002

Georgakopoulou, A. (2007). *Small stories, interaction and identities.* John Benjamins Pub. Co.

Gibson, K., & Hutton, F. (2021). Women who inject drugs (WWID): Stigma, gender and barriers to needle exchange programmes (NEPs). *Contemporary Drug Problems, 48*(3), 276–96. https://doi.org/10.1177/00914509211035242

Giddens, A. (1991). *Modernity and self-identity: Self and society in the late modern age.* Polity Press.

Giddens, A. (1998). *The third way: The renewal of social democracy.* Polity Press.

Gilhula, A. (2006). Lawyer went out of way to help Kimberly Rogers. *Sudbury. com.* https://www.sudbury.com/police/lawyer-went-out-of-way-to-help -kimberly-rogers-209668

Gingrich, L.G. (2008). Social exclusion and double jeopardy: The management of lone mothers in the market-state social field. *Social Policy & Administration, 42*(4), 379–95. https://doi.org/10.1111/j.1467-9515.2008.00610.x

Gladwell, M. (2002). *The tipping point: How little things can make a big difference.* Back Bay Books.

Goffman, E. (1963). *Stigma: Notes on the management of spoiled identity.* Penguin Books.

Gorlick, C.A., & Brethour, G. (1998). *Welfare-to-work programs: A national inventory.* Canadian Council on Social Development.

Government of Canada. (2018). *Opportunity for all – Canada's first poverty reduction strategy.* Government of Canada. https://www.canada.ca/en /employment-social-development/programs/poverty-reduction/reports /strategy.html

Government of Ontario. (2022, July 29). *Renewal and recovery: Ontario's vision for social assistance transformation.* https://www.ontario.ca/page/recovery -renewal-ontarios-vision-social-assistance-transformation

Government of Ontario. (10 June 2021). *Ontario introduces streamlined employment supports.* https://news.ontario.ca/en/release/1000282 /ontario-introduces-streamlined-employment-supports.

Government of Ontario. (2014). *Ontario's poverty reduction strategy annual report. Archived.* https://www.ontario.ca/page/ontarios-poverty-reduction -strategy-2014-annual-report

Graefe, P. (2015). Social assistance in Ontaro. In D. Béland and P.M. Daigneault. (Eds.), *Welfare reform in Canada: Provincial social assistance in comparative perspective.* (pp. 111–26). University of Toronto Press.

Gramsci, A. (1971). *Selections from the prison notebooks of Antonio Gramsci* (Q. Hoare & G. Nowell Smith, Eds. & Trans.). International Publishers.

Grant, T., Huggins, J., Graham, J.C., Ernst, C., Whitney, N., & Wilson, D. (2011). Maternal substance abuse and disrupted parenting: Distinguishing mothers who keep their children from those who do not. *Children and Youth Services Review, 33*(11), 2176–85. https://doi.org/10.1016/j.childyouth.2011.07.001

Grant, T., Younglai, R., & Yukselir, M. (2017). Census 2016: Income grows in resource-rich provinces, Ontario and Quebec lag behind. *The Globe and Mail.* https://www.theglobeandmail.com/report-on-business/economy/census-2016-statscan-income/article36242392/

Grodzins, M. (1957). Metropolitan segregation. *Scientific American, 197*(4), 33–41. https://doi.org/10.1038/scientificamerican1057-33

Groopman, J. (2005). *The anatomy of hope: How people prevail in the face of illness.* Random House.

Gubrium, J.F., & Jarvinen, M. (2014). Troubles, problems, and clientization. In J. F. Gubrium & M. Jarvinen (Eds.), *Turning troubles into problems: Clientization in human services* (pp. 1–13). Routledge.

Gueta, K., & Addad, M. (2013). Molding an emancipatory discourse: How mothers recovering from addiction build their own discourse. *Addiction Research and Theory, 21*(1), 33–42. https://doi.org/10.3109/16066359.2012.680080

Gutman, M.A., McKay, J., Ketterlinus, R.D., & McLellan, A.T. (2003). Potential barriers to work for substance-abusing women on welfare. Findings from the CASAWORKS for Families pilot demonstration. *Evaluation Review, 27*(6), 681–706. https://doi.org/10.1177/0193841X03259030

Hall, S. (1996). The problem of ideology: Marxism without guarantees. In D. Morley & K.-H. Chen (Eds.), *Stuart Hall: Critical dialogues in cultural studies* (pp. 24–5). Routledge.

Halpern-Meekin, S. (2019). *Social poverty: Low-income parents and the struggle for family and community ties.* New York Press.

Harcourt, B.E. (2020). *Critique & praxis: A critical philosophy of illusions, values, and action.* Columbia University Press.

Hartman, Y. (2005). In bed with the enemy: Some ideas on the connections between neoliberalism and the welfare state. *Current Sociology, 53,* 57–73. https://doi.org/10.1177/0011392105048288

Harvey, D. (2007). *A brief history of neoliberalism.* Oxford University Press.

Hasin, D., & Kilcoyne, B. (2012). Comorbidity of psychiatric and substance use disorders in the United States: Current issues and findings from the NESARC. *Current Opinion in Psychiatry, 25*(3), 165–71. https://doi.org/10.1097/YCO.0b013e3283523dcc

Hathaway, A.D., Mostaghim, A., Erickson, P.G., Kolar, K., & Osborne, G. (2018). "It's really no big deal": The role of social supply networks in normalizing use of cannabis by students at Canadian universities. *Deviant Behavior, 39*(12), 1672–80. https://doi.org/10.1080/01639625.2017.1411047

Hays, S. (1996). *The cultural contradictions of motherhood*. Yale University Press.

Health Canada. (2023). *About substance use*. Government of Canada. https://www.canada.ca/en/health-canada/services/substance-use/about-substance-use.html

Heisz, A. (2019). *An update on the market basket measure comprehensive review*. Income Research Paper Series, Statistics Canada. https://www150.statcan.gc.ca/n1/pub/75f0002m/75f0002m2019009-eng.htm

Henderson, S., Dohan, D., & Schmidt, L. (2006). Barriers to identifying substance abuse in the reformed welfare system. *Social Service Review, 80*(2), 217–38. https://doi.org/10.1086/501491

Herd, D., Carrasco, C., & Kim, Y. (2018). *Walk a mile in their shoes: Documenting the experiences and needs of singles in receipt of Ontario Works in Toronto*. Working Report # 2. Ontario Centre for Workforce Innovation. https://ocwi-coie.ca/wp-content/uploads/2018/06/Singles-Study-Report-2-Walk-A-Mile-In-Their-Shoes-FINAL.pdf

Herd, D., Lightman, E., & Mitchell, A. (2009). Searching for local solutions: Making welfare policy on the ground in Ontario. *Journal of Progressive Human Services, 20*(2), 129–51. https://doi.org/10.1080/10428230902871199

Heyes, S. (2005). *Art of recovery: A pocket guide to recovery from mental distress*. Speak Up Somerset.

Hill, J., & Leeming, D. (2014). 'Reconstructing 'the alcoholic': Recovering from alcohol addiction and the stigma this entails. *International Journal of Mental Health and Addiction, 12*, 759–71. https://doi.org/10.1007/s11469-014-9508-z

Hochschild, A.R. (1979). Emotion work, feeling rules, and social structure. *American Journal of Sociology, 85*(3), 551–75. https://doi.org/10.1086/227049

Hochschild, A.R. (1983). *The managed heart: Commercialization of human feeling*. University of California Press.

Hochschild, A.R. (2003). *The commercialization of intimate life: Notes from home and work*. University of California Press.

Hochschild A.R. (2013). Afterword: welfare reform: recognition and emotional labour. *Social Policy and Society, 12*(3), 487–9. https://doi:10.1017/S1474746413000122

Hogan, S.R., Unick, G.J., Speiglman, R., & Norris, J.C. (2011). Gender-specific barriers to self-sufficiency among former supplemental security income drug addiction and alcoholism beneficiaries: Implications for welfare-to-work programs and services. *Journal of Social Service Research, 37*(3), 320–37. https://doi.org/10.1080/01488376.2011.564071

Hogue, A., Dauber, S., Dasaro, C., & Morgenstern, J. (2010). Predictors of employment in substance-using make and female welfare recipients. *Journal*

of Substance Abuse Treatment, 38(2), 108–18. https://doi.org/10.1016
/j.jsat.2009.09.003

Hopson, L., Warner, L., Hardiman, E.R., & James, T. (2015). A qualitative study
of black women's experiences in drug abuse and mental health services.
Affilia, 30, 1, 68–82. https://doi.org/10.1177/0886109914531957

Howard, C. Ed. (2007). *Contested individualization: Debates about contemporary
personhood.* Palgrave Macmillan.

Hughes, E.C. (1945). Dilemmas and contradictions of status. *American Journal
of Sociology, 50,* 353–9. https://doi.org/10.1086/219652

Hughes, E.C. (1949). *Social change and status protest: An essay on the marginal
man.* Bobbs-Merrill, College Division.

Hughes, K. (2007). Migrating identities: The relational constitution of drug use
and addiction. *Sociology of Health & Illness, 29*(5), 673–91. https://doi.org
/10.1111/j.1467-9566.2007.01018.x

Hussong, A.M. (2002). Differentiating peer contexts and risk for adolescent
substance use. *Journal of Youth and Adolescence, 31*(3), 207–20. https://
doi.org/10.1023/A:1015085203097

Hyshka, E., Anderson-Baron, J., Karekezi, K., Belle-Isle, L., Elliott, R., Pauly,
B., & Strike, C. (2017). Harm reduction in name, but not substance: A
comparative analysis of current Canadian provincial and territorial policy
frameworks. *Harm Reduction Journal, 14,* Article No. 50. https://
doi.org/10.1186/s12954-017-0177-7

Ilcan, S. (2009). Privatizing responsibility: Public sector reform under neoliberal
government. *Canadian Review of Sociology, 46*(3), 207–34. https://doi.org
/10.1111/j.1755-618x.2009.01212.x

Income Security Advocacy Centre. (2020). *Inquest into the death of Kimberly
Rogers.* ISAC. http://incomesecurity.org/isac-cases/inquest-into-the-death
-of-kimberly-rogers/

Jacobs, K. & Gill, K. (2002). Substance abuse in an Urban Aboriginal population.
Journal of Ethnicity in Substance Abuse, 1(1), 7–25. https://doi.org/10.1300
/J233v01n01_02

Järvinen, M., & Miller, G. (2010). Methadone maintenance as last resort: A
social phenomenology of a drug policy. *Sociological Forum, 25*(4), 804–23.
https://doi.org/10.1111/j.1573-7861.2010.01213.x

Jenson, J. (2010). Diffusing ideas for after neoliberalism: The social investment
perspective in Europe and Latin America. *Global Social Policy, 10*(1), 59–84.
https://doi.org/10.1177/1468018109354813

Jenson, J., & Saint-Martin, D. (2003). New routes to social cohesion?
Citizenship and the social investment state. *Canadian Journal of Sociology,
28*(1), 77–99. https://doi.org/10.2307/3341876

Jones, A. (2016). No-one discipline for welfare-payment systems failure that
cost $52M to fix: minister. The Canadian Press. https://www.thestar.com

/news/canada/2016/05/02/no-one-disciplined-for-sams-failure-that-cost
-52m-to-fix-minister-says.html?rf

Jones, L.V., Hopson, L., Warner, L., Hardiman, E.R., & James, T. (2015). A
qualitative study of black women's experiences in drug abuse and mental
health services. *Affilia, 30*(1), 68–82. https://doi.org/10.1177/08861099
14531957

Kampen, T., Elshout, J., & Tonkens, E. (2013). The fragility of self-respect:
Emotional labour of workfare volunteering. *Social Policy and Society, 12*(3),
427–38. https://doi.org/10.1017/S1474746413000067

Kanellakos, S. (2006). *Report to health, recreation and social services committee.*
https://app06.ottawa.ca/calendar/ottawa/citycouncil/occ/2004/11-10
/hrss/ASC2004-CPS-PAR-0013.htm

Kelly, B. C. (2006). Conceptions of risk in the lives of club drug-using youth.
Substance Use and Misuse, 40(10), 1443–59. https://doi.org/10.1081
/JA-200066812

Kelly, T.M., Daley, D.C., & Douaihy, A.B. (2012). Treatment of substance
abusing patients with comorbid psychiatric disorders. *Addictive Behaviors,
37*(1), 11–24. https://doi.org/10.1016/j.addbeh.2011.09.010

Kim, Y., Carrasco, C., & Herd, D. (2018). *Improving our knowledge of and
responses to singles on Ontario Works in Toronto.* Working Report #4. Ontario
Centre for Workforce Innovation. https://ocwi-coie.ca/wp-content
/uploads/2018/06/Singles-Study-Report-4-Exits-to-Employment_FINAL
.pdf

Kimball, T.G., Shumway, S.T., Austin-Robillard, H., & Harris-Wilkes, K.S.
(2017). Hoping and coping in recovery: A phenomenology of emerging
adults in a collegiate recovery program. *Alcoholism Treatment Quarterly,
35*(1), 46–62. https://doi.org/10.1080/07347324.2016.1256714 https://
doi.org/10.1016/j.adolescence.2010.07.006

Klein, S., & Montgomery, B. (2001). *Depressing wages: Why welfare cuts hurt both
the welfare and working poor.* Canadian Centre for Policy Alternatives.

Klett-Davies, M. (2007). *Going it alone? Lone motherhood in late modernity.* Ashgate.

Klimas, J., Gorfinkel, L., Fairbairn, N., Amato, L., Ahamad, K., Nolan, S., Simel,
D.L., & Wood, E. (2019). Strategies to identify patient risks of prescription
opioid addiction when initiating opioids for pain: A systematic review.
JAMA Network Open, 2, 5. https://doi.org/10.1001/jamanetworkopen
.2019.3365

Kneebone, R., & White, K. (2015). An overview of social assistance trends in
Canada. In D. Beland & P-M. Daigneault (Eds.), *Welfare reform in Canada:
Provincial social assistance in comparative perspective* (pp. 53–92). University of
Toronto Press.

Krebs, E., Wang, L., Olding, M., DeBeck, K., Hayashi, K., Milloy, M.-J., Wood,
E., Nosyk, B., & Richardson, L. (2016). Increased drug use and the timing of

social assistance receipt among people who use illicit drugs. *Social Science & Medicine, 171*, 94–102. https://doi.org/10.1016/j.socscimed.2016.11.006

Kylmä, J., & Vehviläinen-Julkunen, K. (1997). Hope in nursing research: A meta-analysis of the ontological and epistemological foundations of research on hope. *Journal of Advanced Nursing, 25*(2), 364–71. https://doi.org/10.1046/j.1365-2648.1997.1997025364.x

Lander, L., Howsare, J., & Byrne, M. (2013). The impact of substance use disorders on families and children: From theory to practice. *Social Work in Public Health, 28*, 194–205. https://doi.org/10.1080/19371918.2013.759005

Lankin, F., & Sheikh, M. A. (2012). *Brighter prospects: Transforming social assistance in Ontario.* Commission for the Review of Social Assistance in Ontario. A Report to the Minister of Community and Social Services. https://www.mcss.gov.on.ca/documents/en/mcss/social/publications/social_assistance_review_final_report.pdf

Larner, W. (2000). Neo-liberalism: Policy, ideology, governmentality. *Studies in Political Economy, 63*(1), 5–25. https://doi.org/10.1080/19187033.2000.11675231

Lash, S. (2001). Individualization in a non-linear mode. Foreword by Scott Lash in U. Beck & E. Beck-Gernsheim, *Individualization.* Sage.

Lear, J. (2006). *Radical hope: Ethic in the face of cultural devastation.* Harvard University Press.

Lee, D., & Lee, B. (2020). The role of multilayered peer groups in adolescent depression: A distributional approach. *American Journal of Sociology, 125*(6), 1513–58. https://doi.org/10.1086/709425

Legislative Assembly of Ontario. (2009). *Bill 152 (chapter10, statutes of Ontario, 2009): An act respecting a long-term strategy to reduce poverty in Ontario.* Retrieved from: https://www.ola.org/en/legislative-business/bills/parliament-39/session-1/bill-152

Legislative Assembly of Ontario. (7 May 2012). *40th parliament, official report of debates (Hansard).* Toronto, Ontario: Standing Committee on the Legislative Assembly. Open Access Electronic Government Documents., retrieved from: https://www.ola.org/sites/default/files/node-files/hansard/document/pdf/2012/2012-05/house-document-hansard-transcript-1-EN-07-MAY-2012_L048.pdf

Leigh, J. P., Pacholok, S., Snape, T., & Gauthier, A. H. (2012). Trying to do more with less? Negotiating intensive mothering and financial strain in Canada. *Families, Relationships and Societies, 1*(3), 361–77. https://doi.org/10.1332/204674312X656284

Lightman, E., Mitchell, A., & Herd, D. (2005). One year on: Tracking the experiences of current and former welfare recipients in Toronto. *Journal of Poverty, 9*(4), 5–26. https://doi.org/10.1300/J134v09n04_02

Lindesmith, A.R. (1938). A sociological theory of drug addiction. *American Journal of Sociology, 43*, 593–609. https://doi.org/10.1086/217773

Link, B.G., & Phelan, J. C. (2001). Conceptualizing stigma. *Annual Review of Sociology, 27*, 363–85. https://doi.org/10.1146/annurev.soc.27.1.363

Lipsky, M. (1980). *Street level bureaucracy: Dilemmas of the individual in public services*. Russell Sage Foundation.

Little, M., & Marks, L. (2006). A closer look at the neo-liberal petri dish: Welfare reform in British Columbia and Ontario. *Canadian Review of Social Policy, 57*, 16–45.

Little, M.H. (1994). "Manhunts and bingo blabs": The moral regulation of Ontario single mothers. *Canadian Journal of Sociology, 19*(2), 233–47. https://doi.org/10.2307/3341346

Little, M.H., & Morrison, I. (1999). The "pecker detectors" are back: Regulation of the family form in Ontario Welfare Policy. *Journal of Canadian Studies. Revue D'études Canadiennes, 34*(2), 110–36. https://doi.org/10.3138/jcs.34.2.110

Little, M.H. (1998). *No car, no radio, no liquor permit: The moral regulation of single mothers in Ontario, 1920–1997*. Oxford University Press.

Lofland, L.H. (1973). *A world of strangers: Order and action in urban public space*. Basic Books.

Long, C., DeBeck, K., Feng, C., Montaner, J., Wood, E., & Kerr, T. (2014). Income level and drug related harm among people who use injection drugs in a Canadian setting. *International Journal of Drug Policy, 25*(3), 458–64. https://doi.org/10.1016/j.drugpo.2013.11.011

Luck, P.A., Elifson, K.W., & Sterk, C.E. (2004). Female drug users and the welfare system: A qualitative exploration. *Drugs: Education, Prevention and Policy, 11*(2), 113–28. https://doi.org/10.1080/0968763031000152504

Lussier, K., Laventure, M., & Bertrand, K. (2010). Parenting and maternal substance addiction: Factors affecting utilization of child protective services. *Substance Use & Misuse, 45*(10), 1572–88. https://doi.org/10.3109/10826081003682123

Lyon, D. (2017). Bauman's sociology of hope. *Cultural Politics, 13*(3), 296–9. https://doi.org/10.1215/17432197-4211266

Macdonald, D., & Friendly, M. (2017). *Time out: Child care fees in Canada 2017*. Canadian Centre for Policy Alternatives.

MacPherson, D. (2001). *A framework for action: A four-pillar approach to drug problems in Vancouver: Prevention, treatment, enforcement, harm reduction*. https://static1.squarespace.com/static/596f8b1ca803bb496e345ac8/t/59c97123f5e231aeec5a781d/1506373924623/A_Four-Pillar_Approach_to_Drug_Problems_in_Vancouv.pdf

Madden, E.F. (2019). Intervention stigma: How medication-assisted treatment marginalizes patients and providers. *Social Science & Medicine, 232*, 324–31. https://doi.org/10.1016/j.socscimed.2019.05.027

Maholmes, V. (2014). *Fostering resilience and well-being in children and families in poverty: Why hope still matters.* Oxford University Press.

Maki, K. (2011). Neoliberal deviants and surveillance: Welfare recipients under the watchful eye of Ontario Works. *Surveillance & Society, 9*, 47–63. https://doi.org/10.24908/ss.v9i1/2.4098

Malins, P. (2017). Desiring assemblages: A case for desire over pleasure in critical drug studies. *The International Journal on Drug Policy, 49*, 126–32. https://doi.org/10.1016/j.drugpo.2017.07.018

Mandell, D. (2002). *Deadbeat dads: Subjectivity and social construction.* University of Toronto Press.

Marshall, T.H. (1963). *Sociology at the crossroads, and other essays.* Heinemann.

Martin, F.S. (2010). Becoming vulnerable: Young women's accounts of initiation to injecting drug use. *Addiction Research and Theory, 18*(5), 511–27. https://doi.org/10.3109/16066351003611653

Martin, K., & Stermac, L. (2009). Measuring hope: Is hope related to criminal behaviour in offenders? *International Journal of Offender Therapy and Comparative Criminology, 54*(5), 693–705. https://doi.org/10.1177/0306624X09336131

Maslow, A.H. (1943). A theory of human motivation. *Psychological Review, 50*, 370–96. https://doi.org/10.1037/h0054346

Matthews, D. (8 May 2012). Oral questions: Mental health services. Ontario Legislative Assembly of Ontario. Edited *Hansard*, 40: 1 session. http://hansardindex.ontla.on.ca/hansardeissue/40-1/l049.htm

Maynard, R. (2017). *Policing black lives: Violence in Canada from slavery to the present.* Fernwood Publishing.

McDaniel, S.A. (2002). Women's changing relations to the state and citizenship: Caring and intergenerational relations in globalizing western democracies. *Canadian Review of Sociology, 39*(2), 125–50. https://doi.org/10.1111/j.1755-618X.2002.tb00614.x

McLaren, M.A. (2002). *Feminism, Foucault, and embodied subjectivity.* State University of New York Press.

McMullin, J.A., Davies, L., & Cassidy, G. (2002). Welfare reform in Ontario: Tough times in mothers' lives. *Canadian Public Policy, 28*(2), 297–314. https://doi.org/10.2307/3552330

McQuaid, R., Malik, A., Moussouni, K., Baydack, N., Stargardter, M., & Morrlsey, M. (2017). Life in recovery from addiction in Canada. *Canadian Centre on Substance Use and Addiction.* https://www.ccsa.ca/sites/default/files/2019-04/CCSA-Life-in-Recovery-from-Addiction-Report-2017-en.pdf

Mead, G.H. (1984 [1934]). *Mind, self, and society: From the standpoint of a social behaviorist.* University of Chicago Press.

Metsch, L., McCoy, C., Miller, M., McAnany, H., & Pereyra, M. (1999). Moving substance-abusing women from welfare to work. *Journal of Public Health Policy, 20*(1), 36–55. https://doi.org/10.2307/3343258

Mills, S. (2004). *Discourse.* 2nd edition. Routledge.

Ministry of Children, Community and Social Services. (2018). *6.10: Persons in residential programs for the treatment of substance abuse.* Ontario Works Policy Directives. https://news.ontario.ca/mcys/en/2016/6/ontario-establishing -income-security-reform-working-group.html

Ministry of Children, Community and Social Services. (2019). *Who to contact if you suspect fraud.* https://www.mcss.gov.on.ca/en/mcss/programs/social /fraud.aspx

Ministry of Children and Youth Services. (2009). *Breaking the cycle: The first year.* Ontario's Poverty Reduction Strategy Annual Report.

Ministry of Community and Social Services (11 April 1997). *Confidential cabinet office report: For special purpose welfare reform committee members only, meeting 3.* Ontario Works – Background/Reference Material 1996. (RG10–407); Social Assistance & Employment – Social Assistance Reform/Welfare Reform (RG-29–90).

Ministry of Community and Social Services. (2006). *McGuinty government helping people break free of substance and welfare dependencies.* Archived, Ontario News Room. https://news.ontario.ca/archive/en/2006/03/21 /mcguinty-government-helping-people-break free of-substance-and -welfare-dependenc.html

Ministry of Community and Social Services. (2009). *8.4 addiction services initiative (ASI).* Ontario Works Policy Directives. https://www.mcss.gov .on.ca/documents/en/mcss/social/directives/ow/0804.pdf

Ministry of Community and Social Services. (2011a). *Ontario works policy directives.* https://www.mcss.gov.on.ca/en/mcss/programs/social/directives /ow/8_1_OW_Directives.aspx

Ministry of Community and Social Services. (2011b). *Results-based plan briefing book 2010–2011.* Ministry of Community and Social Services.

Ministry of Community and Social Services. (2012). *Results-based plan briefing book 2011–2012.* Ministry of Community and Social Services.

Ministry of Community and Social Services. (2013). *Results-based plan briefing book 2012–2013.* Ministry of Community and Social Services.

Ministry of Community and Social Services. (2014). *Results-based plan briefing book 2013–2014.* Ministry of Community and Social Services.

Ministry of Community and Social Services. (2015). *Results-based plan briefing book 2014–2015.* Ministry of Community and Social Services.

Ministry of Community and Social Services. (2016a). *Estimates briefing book 2015–2016.* Ministry of Community and Social Services.

Ministry of Community and Social Services. (2016b). *Ontario establishing income security reform working group.* https://news.ontario.ca/en/bulletin/40965/ontario-establishing-income-security-reform-working-group.

Ministry of Community and Social Services. (2017). *Estimates briefing book 2016–2017.* Toronto, Ontario.

Ministry of Community and Social Services. (2018). *Estimates briefing book 2017–2018.* Toronto, Ontario.

Mishler, E.G. (1991). *Research interviewing: Context and narrative.* Harvard University Press.

Montoya, I.D., & Atkinson, J.S. (2002). A synthesis of welfare reform policy and its impact on substance users. *American Journal of Drug Alcohol Abuse, 28*(1), 133. https://doi.org/10.1081/ada-120001285

Moore, D. (2004). Beyond "subculture" in the ethnography of illicit drug use. *Contemporary Drug Problems, 31*(2), 181–212. https://doi.org/10.1177/009145090403100202

Moore, D. (2007). *Criminal artefacts: Governing and users.* UBC Press.

Morgan, D.H.J. (2011). *Rethinking family practices.* Palgrave Macmillan.

Morrison, I. (1998). Ontario Works: A preliminary assessment. *Journal of Law and Social Policy, 13,* 1–46. https://digitalcommons.osgoode.yorku.ca/jlsp/vol13/iss1/1

Munro, D. (2015). Inside the $35 billion addiction industry. *Forbes.* https://www.forbes.com/sites/danmunro/2015/04/27/inside-the-35-billion-addiction-treatment-industry/?sh=425049c17dc9

Naji, L., Dennis, B.B., Bawor, M., Plater, C., Pare, G., Worster, A., Varenbut, M., Daiter, J., Marsh, D.C., Desai, D., Thabane, L., & Samaan, Z. (2016). A prospective study to investigate predictors of relapse among patients with opioid use disorder treated with methadone. *Substance Abuse: Research and Treatment, 10*(10), 9–18. https://doi.org/10.4137/SART.S37030

Nettleton, S., Neale, J., & Pickering, L. (2011). 'I don't think there's much of a rational mind in a drug addict when they are in the thick of it': Towards an embodied analysis of recovering heroin users. *Sociology of Health & Illness, 33*(3), 341–55. https://doi.org/10.1111/j.1467-9566.2010.01278.x

Ngabo, G. (22 January 2019). Video from Toronto shelters show 'inhumane' conditions, indicates shelter system is broken, advocate says. *The Toronto Star.* https://www.thestar.com/news/gta/2019/01/21/we-are-housing-people-in-places-that-are-not-shelters.html

Nussbaum, M.C. (2003). Capabilities as fundamental entitlements: Sen and social justice. *Feminist Economics, 9*(2–3), 33–59. https://doi.org/10.1080/1354570022000077926

O'Connor, J.S., Orloff, A.S., & Shaver, S. (1999). *States, markets, families: Gender, liberalism and social policy in Australia, Canada, Great Britain and the United States.* Cambridge University Press.

Oetting, E.R., & Donnermeyer, J. F. (1998). Primary socialization theory: The etiology of drug use and deviance. *Substance Use & Misuse, 33*(4), 995–1026. https://doi.org/10.3109/10826089809056252

O'Malley, P. (2004). *Risk, uncertainty and government*. The Glasshouse Press.

O'Malley, P. (2009). Responsibilization. In A. Wakefield & J. Fleming (Eds.), *The SAGE dictionary of policing* (pp. 276–7). Sage.

O'Malley, P., & Valverde, M. (2004). Pleasure, freedom and drugs: The uses of 'pleasure' in liberal governance of drug and alcohol consumption. *Sociology, 38*, 1, 25–42. https://doi.org/10.1177/0038038504039359

Ontario 360. (2019). Resetting social assistance reform. https://on360.ca /policy-papers/resetting-social-assistance-reform/

O'Reilly, M., & Parker, N. (2013). 'Unsatisfactory saturation': A critical exploration of the notion of saturated sample sizes in qualitative research. *Qualitative Research, 13*(2), 190–7. https://doi.org/10.1177/146879411 2446106

Orloff, A.S. (1993). Gender and the social rights of citizenship: The comparative analysis of gender relations and welfare states. *American Sociological Review, 58*, 303–28. https://doi.org/10.2307/2095903

Oxford Poverty and Human Dimensional Initiative. (2020). *Multidimensional poverty*. https://ophi.org.uk/research/multidimensional-poverty/

Parker, H.J., Aldridge, J., & Measham, F. (1998). *Illegal leisure: The normalization of adolescent recreational drug use*. Routledge.

Parker, H.J., Williams, L., & Aldridge, J. (2002). The normalization of 'sensible' recreational drug use: Further evidence from the North West England longitudinal study. *Sociology, 36*(4), 941–64. https://doi.org/10.1177 /003803850203600408

Parolin, M., & Simonelli, A. (2016). Attachment theory and maternal drug addiction: The contribution to parenting interventions. *Frontiers in Psychiatry*. https://www.frontiersin.org/articles/10.3389/fpsyt.2016.00152/ full

Pearce, L. (2002). Integrating survey and ethnographic methods for systematic anomalous case analysis. *Sociological Methodology, 32*(1), 103–32. https:// doi.org/10.1111/1467-9531.00113

Pearson, C., Janz, T., & Ali, J. (2013). *Mental and substance use disorders in Canada*. Statistics Canada Catalogue No. 82–624-X. https://www150 .statcan.gc.ca/n1/pub/82-624-x/2013001/article/11855-eng.htm

Peck, J. (2001). *Workfare states*. Guilford Press.

Peck, J., & Tickell, A. (2002). Neoliberalizing space. *Antipode, 34*(3), 380–404. https://doi.org/10.1111/1467-8330.00247

Peled, E., Gavriel-Fried, B., & Katz, N. (2012). I've fixed things up: Paternal identity of substance-dependent fathers. *Family Relations, 61*(5), 893–908. https://doi.org/10.1111/j.1741-3729.2012.00729.x

Pennisi, S., & Baker Collins, S. (2016). Workfare under Ontario works: Making sense of jobless work. *Social Policy & Administration, 51*(7), 1311–29. https://doi.org/10.1111/spol.12271

Pentti, S., Fagerlund, A., & Nyström, P. (2019). Flourishing families: Effects of a positive psychology intervention on parental flow, engagement, meaning and hope. *International Journal of Wellbeing, 9*(4), 79–96. https://doi.org/10.5502/ijw.v9i4.1003

Peralta, R.L., & Jauk, D. (2011). A brief feminist review and critique of the sociology of alcohol-use and substance-abuse treatment approaches. *Sociology Compass, 5*(10), 882–97. https://doi.org/10.1111/j.1751-9020.2011.00414.x

Petersen, A., & Wilkinson, I. (2015). Editorial introduction: The sociology of hope in contexts of health, medicine, and Healthcare. *Health, 19*(2), 113–18. https://doi.org/10.1177/1363459314555378

Phillips, D., & Pon, G. (2018). Anti-Black racism, bio-power, and governmentality: Deconstructing the suffering of black families involved with child welfare. *Journal of Law and Social Policy, 28*(1), 81–100. https://digitalcommons.osgoode.yorku.ca/jlsp/vol28/iss1/5

Pienaar, K., Moore, D., Fraser, S., Kokanovic, R., Treloar, C., & Dilkes-Frayne, E. (2010). Diffracting addicting binaries: An analysis of personal accounts of alcohol and other drug 'addiction.' *Health, 25*(5), 519–37. https://doi.org/10.1177/1363459316674062

Pinedo, M., Zemore, S., Beltrán-Girón, J., Gilbert, P., & Castro, Y. (2020). Black-white differences in barriers to specialty alcohol and drug treatment: Findings from a qualitative study. *Journal of Ethnicity in Substance Abuse*, 1–15. https://doi.org/10.1080/15332640.2020.1713954

Plante, C. (2018). Policy or window dressing? Exploring the impact of poverty reduction strategies on poverty rates among the Canadian provinces. *Journal of International and Comparative Social Policy, 35*(1), 112–36. https://doi.org/10.1080/21699763.2018.1549090

Polkinghorne, D.E. (1995). Narrative configuration in qualitative analysis. *International Journal of Qualitative Studies in Education, 8*(1), 5–23. https://doi.org/10.1080/0951839950080103

Pollack, S., & Caragata, L. (2010). Contestation and accommodation: Constructions of lone mothers' subjectivity through workfare discourse and practice. *Affilia, 25*(3), 264–77. https://doi.org/10.1177/0886109910375208

Pollini, R.A., O'Toole, T.P., Ford, D., & Bigelow, G. (2006). Does this patient really want treatment? Factors associated with baseline and evolving readiness for change among hospitalized substance using adults interested in treatment. *Addictive Behaviors, 31*(10), 1904–18. https://doi.org/10.1016/j.addbeh.2006.01.003

Prochaska, J., & DiClemente, C.C. (1992). Stages of change in the modification of problem behaviors. In M. Hersen, R. Eisler, & P. M. Miller (Eds.), *Progress in behavior modification* (pp. 184–218). Academic Press.

Prinstein, M.J., Brechwald, W.A., & Cohen, G.L. (2011). Susceptibility to peer influence: Using a performance-based measure to identify adolescent males at heightened risk for deviant peer socialization. *Developmental Psychology, 47*(4), 1167–72. https://doi.org/10.1037/a0023274

Public Safety Canada. (2022). Toronto Drug Treatment Court project. https://www.publicsafety.gc.ca/cnt/rsrcs/pblctns/drgtrtmnt-trnt/index-en.aspx

Pulkingham, J. (2015). Social assistance in British Columbia. In D. Béland & P. Daigneault (Eds.), *Welfare reform in Canada: Provincial social Assistance in comparative perspective* (pp. 143–50). University of Toronto Press.

Pulkingham, J., Fuller, S., & Kershaw, P. (2010). Lone motherhood, welfare reform and active citizen subjectivity. *Critical Social Policy, 30*(2), 267–91. https://doi.org/10.1177/0261018309358292

Pulkingham, J., & Ternowetsky, G. (1999). Neo-liberalism and retrenchment: Employment, universality, safety-net provisions and a collapsing Canadian welfare state. In W. A. Antony & D. Broad (Eds.), *Citizens or consumers: Social policy in a market society* (pp. 84–98). Fernwood.

Rabinow, P., & Rose, N. (2006). Biopower today. *Biosocieties, 1*(2), 195–217. https://doi.org/10.1017/S1745855206040014

Rapley, T. (2001). The art(fulness) of open-ended interviewing: Some considerations on analyzing interviews. *Qualitative Research, 1*(3), 303–23. https://doi.org/10.1177/146879410100100303

Raskin, J. (2002). Constructivism in psychology: Personal construct, psychology, radical constructivism, and social constructionism. In J. D. Raskin & S. K. Bridges (Eds.), *Studies in meaning: Exploring constructivist psychology* (pp. 1–25). Pace University Press.

Raskin, P.M. (2006). Women, work, and family: Three studies of roles and identity among working mothers. *American Behavioral Scientist, 49*(10), 1354–81. https://doi.org/10.1177/0002764206286560

Reith, G. (2004). Consumption and its discontents: Addiction, identity and the problems of freedom. *The British Journal of Sociology, 55*(2), 283–300. https://doi.org/10.1111/j.1468-4446.2004.00019.x

Reuter, P. (2006). Drug use. *Gender Issues, 23*(3), 65–79. https://doi.org/10.1007/BF03186778

Ribeiro, L.A., Sanchez, Z.M., & Nappo, S.A. (2010). Surviving crack: A qualitative study of the strategies and tactics developed by Brazilian users to deal with the risks associated with the drug. *BMC Public Health, 10*, 1–10. https://doi.org/10.1186/1471-2458-10-671

Ricciardelli, R., & Peters, A. (Eds.). (2017). *After prison: Navigating employment and reintegration.* Wilfrid Laurier University Press.

Rice, J.J., & Prince, M.J. (2013). *Changing politics of Canadian social policy* (2nd ed.). University of Toronto Press.

Richardson, L., Small, W., & Kerr, T. (2016). Pathways linking drug use and labour market trajectories: The role of catastrophic events. *Sociology of Health & Illness, 38*(1), 137–52. https://doi.org/10.1111/1467-9566.12344

Roberts, G., & Boardman, J. (2013). Understanding recovery. *Advances in Psychiatric Treatment, 19*, 400–9. https://doi.org/10.1192/apt.bp.112.010355

Roberts, M.L. (2002). True womanhood revisited. *Journal of Women's History, 14*(1), 150–5. https://doi.org/10.1353/jowh.2002.0025

Room, R. (2011). Addiction and personal responsibility as solutions to the contradictions of neoliberal consumerism. *Critical Public Health, 21*(2), 141–51. https://doi.org/10.1080/09581596.2010.529424

Rose, N. (1999). *Governing the soul: The Shaping of the private self* (2nd ed.). Free Association Books.

Roy, E., Vaillancourt, E., Morissette, C., Leclerc, P., Boivin, J.-F., Arruda, N., Alary, M., . . . Bourgois, P. (2012). Drug use patterns in the presence of crack in downtown Montréal. *Drug and Alcohol Review, 31*(1), 72–80. https://doi.org/10.1111/j.1465-3362.2011.00299.x

Rudzinski, K., McDonough, P., Gartner, R., & Strike, C. (2017). Is there room for resilience? A scoping review and critique of substance use literature and its utilization of the concept of resilience. *Substance Abuse Treatment, Prevention, and Policy, 12*, 41–76. https://doi.org/10.1186/s13011-017-0125-2

Rutherford, H., & Mayes, L. (2019). Parenting stress: A novel mechanism of addiction vulnerability. *Neurobiology of Stress, 11*, 100172. https://doi.org/10.1016/j.ynstr.2019.100172

Sælør, K.T., Ness, O., & Semb, R. (2015). Taking the plunge: Service users' experiences of hope within the mental health and substance use services. *Scandinavian Psychologist, 2.* https://psykologisk.no/sp/2015/05/e9/

Sanders, B. (2005). In the club: Ecstasy use and supply in a London nightclub. *Journal of the British Sociological Association, 39*(2), 241–58. https://doi.org/10.1177/0038038505050537

Schmidt, L., Zabkiewicz, D., Jacobs, L., & Wiley, J. (2007). Substance abuse and employment among welfare mothers: From welfare to work and back again? *Substance Use & Misuse, 42*(7), 1069–87. https://doi.org/10.1080/10826080701409644

Schneider, A., & Ingram, H. (1993). Social Construction of target populations: Implications for politics and policy. *The American Political Science Review, 87*(2), 334–47. https://doi.org/10.2307/2939044

Schoppelrey, S.L., Martinez, M., & Jang, S.M. (2005). Addressing substance abuse among TANF recipients. *Journal of Human Behavior in the Social Environment, 12*, 111–26. https://doi.org/10.1300/J137v12n02_06

Schwabe, L., Dickinson, A., & Wolf, O.T. (2011). Stress, habits, and drug addiction: A psychoneuroendocrinological perspective. *Experimental and Clinical Psychopharmacology, 19*(1), 53–63. https://doi.org/10.1037/a0022212

Sderstrm, K. (2012). Mental preparation during pregnancy in women with substance addiction: A qualitative interview-study. *Child and Family Social Work, 17*(4), 458–67. https://doi.org/10.1111/j.1365-2206.2011.00803.x

Sen, A. (2000). *Social exclusion: Concept, application and scrutiny.* Social Development Papers No. 1. Asian Development Bank. https://www.adb.org/sites/default/files/publication/29778/social-exclusion.pdf

Sen, A. (2005). Human rights and capabilities. *Journal of Human Development, 6*(2), 151–66. https://doi.org/10.1080/14649880500120491

Silva, S.A., Pires, A.P., Guerreiro, C., & Cardoso, A. (2013). Balancing motherhood and drug addiction: The transition to parenthood of addicted mothers. *Journal of Health Psychology, 18*(3), 359–67. https://doi.org/10.1177/1359105312443399

Simeon, R. (1994). *In search of a social contract: Can we make hard decisions as if democracy matters?* C. D. Howe Institute.

Simon-Kumar, R. (2011). The analytics of "gendering" the post-neoliberal state. *Social Politics: International Studies in Gender, State and Society, 18*(3), 441–68. https://doi.org/10.1093/sp/jxr018

Smith, D. (2011). A sociological alternative to the psychiatric conceptualization of mental suffering. *Sociology Compass, 5*(5), 351–63. https://doi.org/10.1111/j.1751-9020.2011.00369.x

Smith, J.P., & Book, S.W. (2010). Comorbidity of generalized anxiety disorder and alcohol use disorders among individuals seeking outpatient substance abuse treatment. *Addictive Behaviors, 35*(1), 42–5. https://doi.org/10.1016/j.addbeh.2009.07.002

Smith-Carrier, T. (2017). Reproducing social conditions of poverty: A critical feminist analysis of social assistance participation in Ontario, Canada. *Journal of Women, Politics & Policy, 38*(4), 498–521. https://doi.org/10.1080/1554477X.2016.1268874

Smith-Carrier, T., & Lawlor, A. (2017). Realising our (neo-liberal) potential? A critical discourse analysis of the Poverty Reduction Strategy in Ontario, Canada. *Critical Social Policy, 37*(1), 105–27. https://doi.org/10.1177/0261018316666251

Smith-Carrier, T., & Mitchell, J. (2015). Immigrants on social assistance in Canada: Who are they and why are they there? In D. Béland & P-M. Daigneault (Eds.), *Welfare reform in Canada: Provincial social assistance in comparative perspective* (pp. 305–22). University of Toronto Press.

Smith-Carrier, T., Montgomery, P., Mossey, S., Shute, T., Forchuk, C., & Rudnick, A. (2020). Erosion of social support for disabled people in Ontario:

An appraisal of the Ontario Disability Support Program (ODSP) using a human rights framework. *Canadian Journal of Disability Studies, 9*(1). https://doi.org/10.15353/cjds.v9i1.594

Smith Cross, J. (2017). Ontario basic income pilot project starts in three cities. Residents of Hamilton, Lindsay and Thunder Bay will be first to receive guaranteed income as part of test. *Macleans*. https://www.macleans.ca/politics/ontario-basic-income-pilot-project-starts-in-three-cities/

Snyder, C. (1989). Reality negotiation – From excuses to hope and beyond. *Journal of Social and Clinical Psychology, 8*(2), 130–57. https://doi.org/10.1521/jscp.1989.8.2.130

Sobotka, T.C., & Stewart, S.A. (2020). Stereotyping and the opioid epidemic: A conjoint analysis. *Social Science & Medicine, 255*, 1–5. https://doi.org/10.1016/j.socscimed.2020.113018

The Social Assistance Review Advisory Council. (2010). *Recommendations for an Ontario income security review: Report of the Ontario Social Assistance Review Advisory Council*. Ministry of Community & Social Services.

Spronk, R. (2011). "Intimacy is the name of the game": Media and the praxis of sexual knowledge in Nairobi. *Anthropologica, 53*(1), 145–58.

Statistics Canada. (2022). Home alone: More persons living solo than everbefore, but roomies fastest growing household type. Statistics Canada The Daily. https://www150.statcan.gc.ca/n1/en/daily-quotidien/220713/dq220713a-eng.pdf?st=NnpfwCDU

Statistics Canada. (2019). Canadian income survey, 2017. *The Daily*. https://www150.statcan.gc.ca/n1/daily-quotidien/190226/dq190226b-eng.htm

Statistics Canada. (2020). *Low income statistics by sex, age, and family type*. https://www150.statcan.gc.ca/t1/tbl1/en/cv.action?pid=1110013501#timeframe

Stevens, E., Guerrero, M., Green, A., & Jason, L.A. (2018). Relationship of hope, sense of community, and quality of life. *Journal of Community Psychology, 46*(5), 567–74. https://doi.org/10.1002/jcop.21959

Strathearn, L., & Mayes, L.C. (2010). Cocaine addiction in mothers: Potential effects on maternal care and infant development. *Annals – New York Academy of Sciences, 1187*(1), 172–83. https://doi.org/10.1111/j.1749-6632.2009.05142.x

Strauss, A., & Corbin, J. (1998). *Basics of qualitative research: Techniques and procedures for developing grounded theory*. Sage.

Sumner, C. (1994). *Sociology of deviance: An obituary*. Open University Press.

Sutherland, E.H. (1947). *Principles of criminology* (4th ed.). J. B. Lippincott.

Szott, K. (2017). 'Heroin is the devil': Addiction, religion, and needle exchange in the rural United States. *Critical Public Health, 30*(3), 1–11. https://doi.org/10.1080/09581596.2018.1516031

Taekema, D. (2020). Hamilton-Niagara part of government pilot project to contract out employment services. CBC News. https://www.cbc.ca/news/canada/hamilton/contract-employment-services-ontario-1.5466860

Tang, J., Galbraith, N., & Truong, J. (2019). *Living alone in Canada*. Statistics Canada. https://www150.statcan.gc.ca/n1/pub/75-006-x/2019001/article/00003-eng.htm

Testa, M., Livingstone, J.A., & Leonard, K.E. (2003). Women's substance use and experiences of intimate partner violence: A longitudinal investigation among a community sample. *Addictive Behavior, 28*(9), 1649–64. https://doi.org/10.1016/j.addbeh.2003.08.040

Ti, L, Tzemis D, & Buxton, J.A. (2012). Engaging people who use drugs in policy and program development: a review of the literature. *Substance Abuse Treatment, Prevention, and Policy, 24*(7), 47–56. https://doi.org/10.1186/1747-597X-7-47

Tiessen, K. (2016). *Ontario's social assistance poverty gap*. Canadian Centre for Policy Alternatives Ontario. https://www.policyalternatives.ca/sites/default/files/uploads/publications/Ontario%20Office/2016/05/CCPA%20ON%20Ontario%27s%20social%20assistance%20poverty%20gap.pdf

Tonkens, E., Grootegoed, E., & Duyvendak, J.W. (2013). Introduction: Welfare state reform, recognition and emotional labour. *Social Policy and Society, 12*(3), 407–13. https://doi.org/10.1017/S147474641300016X

Trauma. (2014). In *Oxford world encyclopedia* (1st ed.). Online edition, np. Philips.

Tutty, L.M., Ogden, C., Giurgiu, B., & Weaver-Dunlop, G. (2013). I built my house of hope: Abused women and pathways into homelessness. *Violence Against Women, 19*(12), 1498–517. https://doi.org/10.1177/1077801213517514

Tweddle, A., & Aldridge, H. (2018). *Welfare in Canada, 2017*. Maytree. https://maytree.com/media-releases/new-report-welfare-in-canada-2017-looks-at-latest-welfare-rates-and-how-they-compare-to-poverty-measures/

Urbanoski, K., Inglis, D., & Veldhuizen, S. (2017). Service use and unmet needs for substance use and mental disorders in Canada. *Canadian Journal of Psychiatry, 62*(8), 551–9. https://doi.org/10.1177/0706743717714467

Van der Veen, R. (2012). Risk, risk perception, and solidarity. In R. Van der Veen, M. Yerkes, & P. Achterberg (Eds.), *Transformation of solidarity: Changing risks and the future of the welfare state* (pp. 13–30). Amsterdam University Press.

van Dijk, T.A. (1998). *Ideology: A multidisciplinary approach*. Sage.

van Dijk, T.A. (2013). CDA is NOT a method of critical discourse analysis. In *EDISO debate – Asociacion de Estudios Sobre Discuros y Sociedad*. Retrieved 12 January 2021, from http://www.edisoportal.org/debate/115-cda-not-method-critical-discourse-analysis.

Virokannas, E. (2011). Identity categorization of motherhood in the context of drug abuse and child welfare services. *Qualitative Social Work, 10*(3), 329–45. https://doi.org/10.1177/1473325011408480

Wachholtz, A., & Gonzalez, G. (2014). Co-morbid pain and opioid addiction: Long term effect of opioid maintenance on acute pain. *Drug and Alcohol Dependence, 145*, 143–9. https://doi.org/10.1016/j.drugalcdep.2014.10.010

Wagner, H.R. (2002). *Phenomenology of consciousness and sociology of the life-world: An introductory study*. University of Alberta Press.

Webb, J. (2021). Working for citizenship in the liminal space: Social reproduction in the emergency family shelter system. [Doctoral dissertation, York University]. https://library-archives.canada.ca/eng/services /services-libraries/theses/Pages/item.aspx?idNumber=1362902392

Webb, J., & Gazso, A. (2017). Being homeless and becoming housed: The interplay of fateful moments and social support in neo-liberal context. *Studies in Social Justice, 11*(1), 65–85. https://doi.org/10.26522/ssj .v11i1.1398

Weber, M. (1964). *The theory of social and economic organizations*. Free Press.

Weigers, W. A., & Chun, D. E. (2015). Stigma and resistance: The social experience of choosing sole motherhood in Canada 1965–2010. *Women's Studies International Forum, 51*, 42–55. https://doi.org/10.1016/j.wsif .2015.05.001

Weinberg, C. M. (2013). Hope, meaning, and purpose: Making recovery possible. *Psychiatric Rehabilitation Journal, 36*(2), 124–5. https://doi.org /10.1037/prj0000011

Weinberg, D. (2011). Sociological perspectives on addiction. *Sociology Compass, 5*(4), 298–310. https://doi.org/10.1111/j.1751-9020.2011.00363.x https:// doi.org/10.1080/1478601X.2018.1437036

West, R. (2001). Theories of addiction [Editorial]. *Addiction, 96*(1), 3–13. https://doi.org/10.1046/j.1360-0443.2001.96131.x

White, L.A. (2012). Must we all be paradigmatic? Social investment policies and liberal welfare states. *Canadian Journal of Political Science, 45*(3), 657–83. https://doi.org/10.1017/S0008423912000753

White, V. (2017). The addiction crisis means the rich get treatment, the poor go to jail or die. *Ottawa Citizen*. https://ottawacitizen.com/opinion /columnists/white-the-addiction-crisis-means-the-rich-get-treatment -the-poor-go-to-jail-or-die

Widdicombe, S. (1998). Identity as an analysts' and a participants' resource. In C. Antaki & S. Widdicombe (Eds.), *Identities in talk* (pp. 190–206). Sage.

Williams, M. (2000). Interpretivism and generalisation. *Sociology, 34*(2), 209–24. https://doi.org/10.1177/S0038038500000146

Wincup, E. (2011). Carrots and sticks: Problem drug users and welfare reform. *Criminal Justice Matters, 84*(1), 22–3. https://doi.org/10.1080/09627251.2011 .576025

Wincup, E., & Monaghan, M. (2016). Scrounger narratives and dependent drug users: Welfare, workfare and warfare. *Journal of Poverty and Social Justice, 24*(3), 261–75. https://doi.org/10.1332/175982716X14721954315084

Windsor, L.C., Dunlap, E., & Golub, A. (2011). Challenging controlling images, oppression, poverty, and other structural constraints: Survival strategies among African-American women in distressed households. *Journal of African American Studies, 15*(3), 290–306. https://doi.org/10.1007/s12111-010-9151-0

Wodak, R., & Meyer, M. (2016). *Methods of critical discourse analysis* (3rd ed.). Sage.

Wong, P.T. (2013). *A meaning-centered approach to addiction and recovery.* http://www.drpaulwong.com/meaning-centered-approach-addiction-recovery/

Working report # 2. Ontario Centre for Workforce Innovation. https://ocwi-coie.ca/wp-content/uploads/2018/06/Singles-Study-Report-2-Walk-A-Mile-In-Their-Shoes-FINAL.pdf

World Health Organization. (2004). *Neuroscience of psychoactive substance use and dependence.* World Health Organization. http://www.who.int/substance_abuse/publications/en/Neuroscience.pdf.

World Health Organization. (2020). *Lexicon of alcohol and drug terms.* World Health Organization. https://www.who.int/substance_abuse/terminology/who_lexicon/en/

Wu, N.S., Schairer, L.C., Dellor, E., & Grella, C. (2010). Childhood trauma and health outcomes in adults with comorbid substance abuse and mental health disorders. *Addictive Behaviors, 35*(1), 68–71. https://doi.org/10.1016/j.addbeh.2009.09.003

Yalnizyan, A. (1994). Securing society: Creating Canadian social policy. In A. Yalnizyan, T.R. Ide, & A. J. Cordell (Eds.), *Shifting time: Social policy and the future of work* (pp. 17–71). Between the Lines.

Yang, L.H., Kleinman, A., Link, B.G., Phelan, J.C., Lee, S., & Good, B. (2007). Culture and stigma: Adding moral experience to stigma theory. *Social Science & Medicine, 64*, 1524–35. https://doi.org/10.1016/j.socscimed.2006.11.013

Young, L. (2016, October 6). More fentanyl deaths in Ontario but where are the detox programs? *Global News.* https://globalnews.ca/news/2987731/more-fentanyl-deaths-in-ontario-but-where-are-the-detox-programs/

Younglai, R., & Yukselir, M. (2017). Who are Canada's 1% and highest paid workers? *The Globe and Mail.* https://www.theglobeandmail.com/news/canada-1-per-cent-highest-paid-workers-compare/article36383159/

Zafar, A. (2020). Canada's opioid crisis killed 13 people a day in 2018, prevention report shows. *CBC News.* https://www.cbc.ca/news/health/opioid-poisoning-parachute-1.5789654

Zedini, A. (2020). Profiling the fuzzy latent structure of multidimensional poverty: Toward valuable insights for poverty policymakers. *Journal of Economic Issues, 54*(2), 535–49. https://doi.org/10.1080/00213624.2020.1757978

Zilkowsky, D. (2001). Canada's national drug strategy. *Forum on Corrections Research, 13*(3), 3–4.

Zinn, J.O. (2013). Introduction: Risk, social inclusion and the life course. *Social Policy and Society, 12*(2), 253–64. https://doi.org/10.1017/S1474746412000681

Zizys, T. (2011). *Working better: Creating a high-performing labour market in Ontario.* Metcalf Foundation.

Zlotorzynska, M., Milloy, M.-J. S., Richardson, L., Nguyen, P., Montaner, J.S., Wood, E., & Kerr, T. (2014). Timing of income assistance payment and overdose patterns at a Canadian supervised injection facility. *International Journal of Drug Policy, 25*(4), 736–9. https://doi.org/10.1016/j.drugpo.2014.03.014

Index

www.ingramcontent.com/pod-product-compliance
Lightning Source LLC
Chambersburg PA
CBHW020454030426
42337CB00011B/111